Pandemia

Pandemia

How Coronavirus Hysteria Took Over Our Government, Rights, and Lives

Alex Berenson

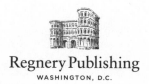

Regnery Publishing
WASHINGTON, D.C.

Regnery® is a registered trademark and its colophon is a trademark of Salem Communications Holding Corporation

Cataloging-in-Publication data on file with the Library of Congress

ISBN 978-1-68451-248-5
eISBN 978-1-68451-249-2
Library of Congress Control Number: 2021946362

Published in the United States by
Regnery Publishing
A Division of Salem Media Group
Washington, D.C.
www.Regnery.com

Manufactured in the United States of America

10 9 8 7 6 5 4 3 2 1

Books are available in quantity for promotional or premium use. For information on discounts and terms, please visit our website: www.Regnery.com.

For Harvey, who fought to the end

When you have eliminated the impossible, whatever remains, however improbable, must be the truth.
—Sherlock Holmes

Go and try, you'll never break me.
—"Welcome to the Black Parade," My Chemical Romance

CONTENTS

1

Welcome to Pandemia

At the beginning, the *very* beginning, the hide-in-the-basement, stock-up-on-bottled-water, shut-down-the-world-the-plague-is-here panic made sense.

Maybe.

But within a few weeks, even as the United States and Europe had just begun lockdowns, anyone paying attention could see the cure was worse than the disease. In our desperation to control Covid-19, we had done more damage to ourselves and the world than the virus ever could.

By then, though, it was already too late.

This is the true story of how media hysteria, political partisanship, overreliance on unproven technology, and scientific illiteracy brought the United States and the world to the brink of breakdown.

The true story of how we trashed civil liberties we had treasured for generations. How we denied school to our children and destroyed small businesses.

The true story of how we locked down and hid our faces from one another on the thinnest possible evidence. Of how a public health emergency became big business overnight, as governments spent trillions of dollars to fight the coronavirus—and unnecessary lockdowns destroyed small businesses, hugely enriched giant corporations, and forced people off paid employment onto government checks. How we spent a year hiding the risks and overestimating the benefits of vaccines based on a radical new biotechnology. And how we then tried to force the shots on tens of millions of unwilling Americans—while censoring those who raised questions about them.

All in response to a virus much less dangerous than the Spanish flu, much less Ebola. A virus that is less dangerous to healthy children and young adults than influenza. A virus that does most of its damage to people at or very near the end of their lives. A virus that killed slightly more people worldwide than diarrhea or Alzheimer's disease in 2020.

This is the true story many of you have never heard.

Not because I have a magic source at the Centers for Disease Control passing me thumb drives with hidden information. The facts that I and a handful of other journalists and "skeptics" have reported since March 2020 are readily available in government documents and hospital records and scientific papers.

No, the facts you're about to read aren't secrets.

The secret is in the perspective.

For the last two years, I have tried to approach Covid-19 and the vaccines for it as I do every story I write as a reporter—looking at evidence with an open mind and evaluating risks realistically. I have tried to compare lockdowns and other Covid policies to previous consensus views on the right way to manage epidemics.

Unfortunately, the media, especially the American media, committed early on to portraying the coronavirus as far riskier than it was and the vaccines as safer. Elite outlets like the *New York Times* went out of their way to foment panic and ignore positive news. Throughout 2020, many scientific studies offered reassuring data, especially the low risks Sars-Cov-2 posed to kids and young adults and their safety in schools. Practically everything pointed the same way.

Meanwhile, the models that had predicted apocalyptic outcomes proved wrong. Aside from a few bad days in New York City in March and April 2020, American hospitals were never close to being overrun. In fact, they were so empty in the spring of 2020 that many laid off workers. Even in New York, the field hospitals and medical ships went largely unused.

But no one seemed to notice, much less care.

Instead the *Times*, CNN, and the rest fixated on a single number, the count of Americans who had (reportedly) died from the coronavirus. Cable networks offered real-time tallies. The *Times* ran a special edition when the figure reached one hundred thousand.

They never put the figure in context. They never explained that our methods for recording Covid-linked deaths were likely producing over-counts. Or that even with our aggressive counting, the Covid death figure represented just over 10 percent of all American deaths in 2020.

Most important, they never explained honestly that Covid almost exclusively targeted the very old and sick.

Instead they went the other way, searching desperately for outlier cases—the handful of coronavirus deaths of people under fifty without preexisting conditions. Inevitably, they made mistakes, as when the *Times* called the murder of a twenty-seven-year-old Iowa man a Covid death.

Reporters are crucial watchdogs against government mistakes and overreach. *All* of government. But the media's hatred for Donald Trump blinded journalists to the power that state governors and unelected scientific and medical advisors wielded as the epidemic unfolded.

As Covid hit, governors in many states seized unprecedented control of their citizens. They refused to reopen schools. They imposed draconian rules on businesses. They forced people to wear masks, even outside.

Journalists didn't question these monumental intrusions. They cheered them, while ignoring scientists who challenged the conventional narrative.

Hugely powerful social media companies such as Facebook and tech giants such as Google and Amazon went even further. Those corporations blocked videos and books and groups that questioned the value of the lockdowns—from which these same corporations have profited enormously. The social media companies worked with organizations such as the World Health Organization to become quasi-governmental censors. In suppressing honest debate and dissent, they set a dangerous precedent—and fed the rise of wilder conspiracy theories.

Yet they couldn't silence everyone.

This is the true story of how—to my surprise—I became a leading voice calling for an end to lockdowns and a return to normality. How the strange intimacy of celebrity in the age of social media enveloped me. My Twitter follower count grew from 7,000 to 200,000 in months, and then to over 300,000 in 2021. Some people told me I had kept them sane. Others said I was a psychopath who didn't care how many people Covid killed.

People followed my feed to get information they couldn't find anywhere else. I tried to source my tweets, offering links to the material I quoted. I wanted my readers to judge for themselves whether I had fairly represented it. I knew I had.

I will do the same in this book. I want to be as transparent as possible.

But it wasn't the information I offered that made people love or hate my feed—and me. It was my tone: enraged at the lockdowns, prodding, often sarcastic. I didn't treat the epidemic with fear. Instead I insisted that "virus gonna virus." I wrote about "Team Reality" and "Team Apocalypse." I called masks "face diapers" and complained of "Neils and Karens" who wouldn't leave their houses. I created an Orwellian "Department of Pandemia" to announce rules about "the thing."

Even readers who supported me occasionally told me I was going too far, that I needed to remember that the coronavirus really did kill people.

But I believed I needed to speak out in a way that couldn't be ignored. I believed mainstream reporters were offering worst-case scenarios for reasons both economic and political. Panic was good for page views and terrible for Donald Trump. And most reporters at places like the *New York Times* hate Trump with a passion that can't be overstated. (As for me, I'm a registered independent whose politics are that it is impossible to be too cynical.)

On April 16, 2020, I tweeted:

> Against hysteria, satire. Against storytelling, data. Against groupthink, reporting. Against authoritarianism, bravery. Most of all: Against millennialism, realism. And hope.[1]

Against hysteria, satire. And if that satire sometimes cut too deep or went too far, I had to accept the consequences.

"I can't tell if you are super angry or if you are enjoying yourself," a journalist said to me in June 2020. My answer: "Why not both?"

Day by day and hour by hour, the cause of fighting for the truth—and against our overreaction to Sars-Cov-2—took over my life.

Vanity Fair published two hit pieces on me. I went to war with the *Times*, a newspaper where I had worked for a decade. Old friends stopped speaking to me. Sometimes they publicly attacked me. My marriage staggered under the weight of my Twitter obsession.

Most painful of all, my father, who was dying of cancer, grew angry with me for pressing against lockdowns. He accused me of not caring about him. My stance became a subject we couldn't discuss.

Until, in May 2020, he died. (Not of Covid. Of leukemia.)

I didn't mourn him properly.

My wife was right, my friends were right. I was obsessed. I couldn't stop fighting. Couldn't and wouldn't. Can't and won't. Because our response to the coronavirus is the worst public policy mistake worldwide in at least a century, since World War I, when Europe's leaders sent millions of young men to their graves for reasons they couldn't even explain. A generation after the fall of the Berlin Wall, we have run the other way, tearing up human liberty around the world.

The people who have caused the panic show no sign of letting up, no sign they plan to let us get back to normal anytime soon. If ever.

Yes, lockdowns in the United States have ended—but countries such as Australia and New Zealand show just how fragile our freedoms have become.

Meanwhile, we are still suffering from intrusive rules that vary state to state and country to country. Since the beginning of the pandemic, they have included "social distancing," mask requirements, school closings, bans on indoor dining, endless testing of college students, aggressive contact tracing, travel restrictions, quarantines for people without symptoms, and now vaccine mandates.

Yet despite the enormous cost of these measures, despite their intrusion on our civil liberties, *none* of them been shown to slow the spread of Covid. We engaged in a game of viral theater at incalculable cost, both real and psychic—particularly to children and teenagers, who were denied normal schooling and social interaction.

In August 2020, the Centers for Disease Control reported that 25 percent of adults ages eighteen to twenty-four said they had seriously considered suicide during the month of June. That figure was more than double the percentage who had reported doing so in a similar survey in 2018. These young adults are at essentially no risk from the coronavirus. But we made them terrified for their futures and locked them up to grapple adolescent angst, drug problems, or depression alone.

This is the true story of the pandemia: one part pandemic, five parts hysteria. Neither shaken nor stirred, but heated in a thermal cycler—also known as a PCR machine (another obscure and complex technology that played a crucial role in bringing us this crisis).

The coronavirus epidemic could not have happened a generation ago. Or a decade ago. *But not because of the virus.*

At the beginning, the *very* beginning, when the panic made sense, the novel coronavirus seemed special. Exceptional. It could lurk for weeks before suddenly cutting down its victims, we were told. It spread like the common cold but killed far more aggressively than influenza, we were told. It colonized the nose and mouth for maximum infectivity before suddenly moving into the lungs for maximum lethality, we were told.

But a lot of what we were told wasn't true. We've learned now that Sars-Cov-2 isn't particularly lethal and that its contagiousness varies widely in different settings. Most people without symptoms don't spread it much. Really, the novel coronavirus is just…a virus. It has one truly unusual symptom—many infected people temporarily lose their senses of smell and taste.

Not exactly Ebola, which has a 50 percent fatality rate.

So why was our response to this rather ordinary virus so different from our reaction to any other disease in human history? *Because it could be.* Because in our foolish brilliance we have created information technology indistinguishable from magic.

We closed offices and schools *because we could.* We now have the internet bandwidth for white collar workers to stay home—and for students to "learn" remotely, on their computers.

We counted and publicized deaths obsessively—and still do—*because we can.* We have database software that enables hospitals and health departments to aggregate information in real time.

We distribute that information to everyone instantaneously, through social and conventional media, *because we can.* We are not just choking on data, we are stuffing it down our throats. Yet we are desperate for more each moment. Many of us seem almost addicted to tracking the toll of the coronavirus. We know we should stop, but we can't.

We test endlessly for the virus *because we can.* Polymerase chain reaction (PCR) machines make the virus's RNA into DNA and that DNA into more DNA. They let us find a single fragment of the virus and multiply it a trillion times. A trillion is a million million, a thousand thousand thousand thousand. It is a number no one can really grasp.

And the mRNA Covid vaccines—created, developed, and put into use worldwide in under a year, faster than almost any other drug or vaccine in history—are only the latest example of our scientific brilliance.

But we are playing magic tricks *on ourselves*. We have forgotten a crucial fact: These medical wonders come at the highest possible price. When we multiply a viral fragment a trillion times, we get a positive test result in many people who never will be sick.

Then we tell those healthy people that they're ill, and we make them—and the people around them—stay home.

Our magic has made us insane.

Long before the coronavirus, physicians had a phrase for the havoc that over-testing healthy people can wreak: the medical cascade. A single unusual result on a medical test causes doctors to recommend more tests. Those tests can lead to drugs or surgeries, even for patients with no symptoms. Men have their prostates removed. Women are given chemotherapy for breast cancer. The temptation to *do something* is overwhelming. The financial incentives don't hurt either.

When it comes to Covid, all of us everywhere have been riding that cascade—even if we haven't had a single test.

Nowhere are the incentives stronger and the cascade more powerful than in the United States, with its incredibly expensive health care system. In 1960, Americans spent $27 billion on health care, or about $235 billion adjusted for inflation. That figure represented 5 percent of our overall economy.

In 2019, Americans spent $3.6 trillion—$3,600 billion—on health care. That represents a more than fifteen-fold increase in fewer than sixty years, *after* accounting for inflation. Medical spending is now almost 20 percent of the overall economy, more than energy and real estate combined.

Other rich countries don't spend as much, but the trend is the same. We have medicalized our societies. Worse, hospitals themselves have proven remarkably effective vectors for spreading the coronavirus.

This dynamic was obvious almost immediately. As Italian physicians wrote in March 2020, "Coronavirus is the Ebola of the rich. . . . It is not particularly lethal, but is very contagious. The more medicalized and centralized the society, the more widespread the virus."[2]

Yet weirdly, even as our societies have become more medicalized, our experience of death has turned more remote. Death itself is more horrifying and unthinkable than ever. Serious technologists now truly believe they will be able to cheat the reaper for all eternity by uploading their consciousnesses into the ether.

More than three million Americans died in 2020, but we hide many of those deaths in nursing homes and hospices. My father could not imagine his passing even as it was on him, but the denial that is understandable and perhaps even merciful for the individual pilgrim on his final journey will not work for society as a whole. Not if our denial about the mortality of the aged and sick comes at the cost of denying children a chance at full lives of their own.

Please understand: *I am not saying Sars-Cov-2 is not real. I am not saying it does not kill people.*

What I am saying is that our response to the coronavirus has been vastly disproportionate. The coronavirus has not disrupted the food chain (though the lockdowns threatened to do so). It has not overrun hospitals (though vaccine requirements for reluctant nurses are putting the system under enormous stress). It kills fewer American children than drowning, cancer, abuse, or a dozen other conditions.

We panicked anyway.

Sars-Cov-2 did a fraction of the damage we feared it would when it first escaped China. But the dangers it has revealed are here to stay. The medicalization of society is not going away. Neither is our reliance on advanced technology and the power of the companies that provide it.

Fed by anger at Trump, conventional media outlets stoked the coronavirus panic. The panic was the pull. But the push came from two incredibly powerful industries, technology and health care.

Now Trump is gone. But we've set a precedent. A terrible precedent. The temptation to panic—over another coronavirus, a bad flu strain, a drug-resistant tuberculosis—will only keep growing harder to resist, unless we stop it.

We need to fight the pandemia—the hysteria about the pandemic—and stand up for the old normal.

Or before we know it, the old normal will be gone.

2

Happy New Year

The first reports came hours before the end of 2019, as the world celebrated New Year's Eve.

On December 31, authorities in Wuhan, a city of ten million in central China, announced several cases of atypical pneumonia. The origins of the disease were unknown, but it did not appear to spread from person to person, the authorities said.

Doctors in Wuhan weren't so sure.

A day earlier, Dr. Li Wenliang, an ophthalmologist, had warned other physicians on a message board that Wuhan Central Hospital had pneumonia patients who were not responding to typical treatments. The doctors and their families should "take precautions," Li wrote. He worried the disease was related to SARS, which had emerged from China almost two decades earlier. SARS—the letters stood for severe acute respiratory syndrome—killed almost 10 percent of the eight thousand people it infected before being contained in July 2003.

Li wanted his warning to stay private.

"Don't circulate this information outside of this group," he wrote. But by New Year's Day, it had leaked to Chinese chat rooms. On January 3, police in Wuhan forced Li to sign a letter that said he had "severely disturbed the social order."[1]

But like the pneumonia cases, the rumors kept spreading. On January 6, the *New York Times* took note. "China Grapples with Mystery Pneumonia-Like Illness," its headline ran. The story reported, "Beijing is racing to identify a new illness that has sickened 59 people as it tries to calm a nervous public."[2]

Two days later, the *Times* followed up, reporting that Chinese scientists had identified the virus behind the illness. Like the first SARS, it was a coronavirus, so named for its distinctive shape. Coronaviruses consist of globes that have a "corona" of proteins spiking out in all directions, ready to attach to receptors on cells and invade them. They are ugly little beasts.

Still, scientists have generally not viewed coronaviruses as particularly dangerous, aside from SARS and another recent arrival called MERS. Most cause only cold-like symptoms in people. "The new coronavirus doesn't appear to be readily spread by humans, but researchers caution that more study is needed," the *Times* reported.[3]

By then, Chinese government officials had good reason to believe otherwise. Physicians were seeing clusters of cases that infected entire families, a strong signal that the disease could spread person to person.[4]

For the next ten days, the Chinese government and the World Health Organization (WHO) played down the seriousness of the new illness and the risk it could spread among people. On January 14, the WHO famously tweeted, "Preliminary investigations conducted by the Chinese authorities have found no clear evidence of human-to-human transmission of the novel coronavirus."[5]

As part of the United Nations, the World Health Organization is inherently political, trying to balance pressures from member states. The coronavirus pandemic turned into a political crisis almost as soon as it started.

Throughout January, China stonewalled attempts by American and other foreign physicians, scientists, and journalists to understand what was happening in Wuhan. As early as January 6, the White House offered to send experts from the Centers for Disease Control to Wuhan. The Chinese rejected the offer, along with others later in January.[6]

Only on January 28 did Beijing finally agree to accept a World Health Organization team. It took almost two weeks more before China actually allowed the team onto its soil.

Even if the WHO and China had sounded the alarm in early January, it might already have been too late. Studies of stored blood and wastewater samples would later show that the coronavirus had already jumped to the United States and Europe by December. Also, given the fact that both SARS and the swine flu of 2009 had turned out to be far less serious than initially feared, other countries might have resisted aggressive action without first-hand evidence the virus might be dangerous.

But a few extra weeks of warning could only have helped. And no one can doubt that as the virus exploded in Wuhan in mid-January, the Chinese government hid crucial information about it. The most brazen example came on January 12. Just one day after a laboratory in Shanghai sequenced the coronavirus genome and published it online, China closed the lab for "rectification."[7]

Why was China so desperate to hide information about the virus? I will return to that question near the end of this book, when I discuss the potential origins of Sars-Cov-2.

But China's censorship efforts could not hide the fact that coronavirus patients were filling hospitals in Wuhan and infecting nurses and doctors. On January 20, China acknowledged the obvious truth that human beings could pass the virus to one another.[8] Meanwhile, Chinese officials quietly told groups of Chinese expatriates to buy all the gloves, masks, and respirators they could find anywhere in the world.

"In Nagoya, Japan, volunteers drove to pharmacies and bought 520,000 masks in three days," *Bloomberg BusinessWeek* reported in September 2020.[9] By the end of February, the volunteers had shipped 2 billion masks and 500 million other pieces of protective equipment to China, worsening shortages in the United States and elsewhere.

The next shock came on January 23, when China locked down Wuhan and other cities in Hubei province, preventing at least thirty-five million people from traveling. Airports and train and bus stations were closed. Police officers and soldiers blocked roads. At the time, China had reported only five hundred cases and eighteen deaths from the coronavirus, though journalists and scientists agreed that the figures did not match the reality on the ground.

By then the world's attention was focused on the crisis in China and whether it might be contained. In Wuhan, "anxiety and anger prevailed as worried residents crowded into hospitals,"[10] the *Times* reported.

Social media fanned the panic. Videos posted to Chinese sites and shared to Reddit and Twitter showed men welding apartment doors shut and people collapsed in the streets. One disturbing video revealed body-bagged corpses filling hospitals.[11] In a YouTube video posted on January 28, a Wuhan resident warned, "It's like living in hell, waiting for death."[12]

Sars-Cov-2 was not the first viral outbreak in the age of social media. An Ebola outbreak had received attention in 2014. But in that first month of 2020, with the new coronavirus mostly confined to China, Twitter and Facebook amplified the worldwide panic while simultaneously turning the epidemic into what felt at times like a video game: "Beat the Virus." *How many cases today? How many dead today? How quickly can the Chinese build field hospitals?* The coronavirus lacked the visceral melting-corpse horror of Ebola, but it offered the real risk of mass death—terror close enough to be thrilling, yet still safely an ocean away.

Until it wasn't. By late January, the epidemic had clearly broken out of Wuhan and Hubei province. China reported cases in megacities including Beijing and Shanghai. The Chinese government ramped up its response, quickly building field hospitals that could take patients from Wuhan's overcrowded medical centers. Police and soldiers tightened the already draconian lockdown. Almost no one was allowed outside. Even food shopping was strictly limited.[13]

Yet on January 31, when President Donald Trump announced he was banning almost all foreign nationals from traveling to the United States if they had visited China in the previous two weeks, he faced condemnation.

"WHO chief says widespread travel bans not needed to beat China virus," Reuters reported on February 3.[14] The Chinese government complained even more loudly. "Beijing is growing increasingly angry at countries imposing harsh travel restrictions," Bloomberg reported.[15]

In an early sign of the political and media wars to come, Democrats and journalists quickly criticized the Trump ban as useless or even counterproductive. "Health experts warn China travel ban will hinder coronavirus response," claimed Stat News, which covers drug and biotechnology companies.[16] A Democratic member of Congress warned that a travel ban might inflame anti-Asian sentiment.[17]

These criticisms would seem quaint by mid-March, as country after country closed its borders in efforts to control the coronavirus. In fact, travel bans appear to have little chance of working unless they are applied rigorously and early in an epidemic, ideally by island nations such as New Zealand, which can more easily close their borders, or by repressive nations such as China, which can also restrict internal movement. Still, like other aggressive public health measures that were rejected until last year, the bans have become standard practice. More than a year after the epidemic began, international travel is still restricted.

The days after the travel ban marked a kind of phony war. The number of cases in China leveled off by mid-February. The expected mass breakouts in Shanghai and other megacities never happened. Cases spiked in Iran and South Korea. An outbreak aboard the *Diamond Princess* cruise ship grabbed attention. But it began to seem as though the world had somehow escaped the worst of the novel coronavirus, which on February 11 was officially titled Sars-Cov-2, a name that carefully omitted any reference to where it had first appeared.[18]

In mid-February 2020, I flew to New Zealand. A group fighting cannabis legalization there had invited me to talk about my non-fiction book *Tell Your Children*, which discusses the mental health effects of cannabis. I was somewhat worried about the trip, but not enough to cancel it (lucky me, New Zealand is a beautiful place, and if I hadn't gone then I wouldn't have had the chance for years). No one I met there seemed overly concerned about the coronavirus. Even when I flew back through San Francisco on February 22, the airport seemed almost normal. Only a few people wore masks.

    We were all wrong, though. Sars-Cov-2 had already hitched rides all over the world. The real action was just about to start.

3

In the Beginning

The Spanish flu was the first modern pandemic.

Its horrors began in the last year of World War I. It spread by railroad, automobile, and even airplane across the United States and Europe as soldiers returned home. It was unpredictable and vicious. Doctors had considered respiratory infections a disease of the elderly. The Canadian physician William Osler famously called pneumonia "the friend of the aged" because it killed quickly and relatively painlessly.[1] (Ironically, Osler himself died of pneumonia in 1919.)

But the Spanish flu mowed down not just older people but healthy children and young adults, too. They coughed so hard they broke ribs and tore muscles in a desperate effort to breathe. Their faces and bodies turned blue as they struggled for oxygen.[2]

The epidemic came in three waves, in the spring and fall of 1918 and the spring of 1919. The fall crisis was the most severe. Undertakers and coffin makers were overwhelmed. Bodies were left covered in ice as they festered, awaiting burial.[3]

"It is simply a struggle for air until they suffocate," a doctor at an army base near Boston wrote in September 1918. "It is horrible. One can stand to see one, two, or twenty men die, but to see these poor devils dropping like flies gets on your nerves."[4]

We will never know exactly how many people the Spanish flu killed. But the best estimates are that about 50 million people died worldwide, almost 3 percent of the global population at the time. The equivalent figure today would be 220 million people. The United States escaped relatively lightly, with about 675,000 dead, less than 0.7 percent of the American population at the time. Still, that figure would be equal to about 2.2 million today.[5]

The horrors of the pandemic provoked a worldwide scientific and medical response. Doctors and researchers raced to understand why this flu was so deadly—and how to prevent it.

They even ran experiments to see if they could use phlegm from infected people to sicken healthy volunteers. In one case, the "volunteers" were actually inmates at a navy prison who had been promised pardons if they participated. Today, such an experiment would rightly be banned as unethical.[6]

Meanwhile, public health experts measured the spread of the flu, tracking cases and deaths daily. A relatively young branch of medicine, public health had emerged in the nineteenth century in response to epidemics of cholera and other diseases that ran rampant in overcrowded cities.

Two mid-nineteenth-century British scientists, John Snow and William Farr, led the way, helping create a discipline that would become known as epidemiology. Snow and Farr used statistical and mapping tools to analyze how diseases spread. In 1854, Snow famously mapped a cholera epidemic in central London and proved it was centered on a water pump on Broad Street. He convinced the city to remove the pump's handle, and the outbreak quickly ended.[7]

Around the same time, Farr showed that epidemics often rose and fell in remarkably similar patterns, no matter the underlying disease.

Illnesses that spread quickly and caused exponential growth in cases and deaths tended to burn out equally fast. Later epidemiologists would call this finding Farr's Law and use it to predict the course of epidemics. Farr's Law would provide crucial clues to the path of the coronavirus epidemic—for anyone who cared to look at it.

Farr also theorized that outbreaks would seem deadlier at first then they really were. Vulnerable people would die quickly, while healthier people might struggle and be hospitalized but would ultimately recover. Thus the number of deaths relative to the number of cases would be higher at the beginning of the epidemic than later.

Along the way, Farr offered commonsense suggestions to reduce outbreaks: "The dead should no longer be buried where they are surrounded by crowded dwellings.... And there is assuredly no reason why thousands of cattle, sheep, horses, animals of every kind—sometimes affected with epizootic diseases—should be gathered together."[8]

Almost two centuries later, China would *still* be ignoring this advice. It allowed "wet markets" in its crowded cities where live animals, both wild and farm-raised, were sold as food.

In the late nineteenth and early twentieth centuries, reformers known as Progressives in the United States mandated basic public health standards, such as requiring apartment buildings to have indoor plumbing. Cities became cleaner and healthier. People began to live much longer. Between 1885 and 1915, life expectancy soared from forty-one to fifty-four years, an astonishing gain in just one generation. (Had life expectancy kept increasing at the same pace since then, the average American child born now could expect to live to one hundred. Unfortunately, the gains have slowed.)

But the Spanish flu temporarily turned back the clock, killing as no plague had for many years. It tore across the East Coast and Midwest before spreading to California and even Alaska. With little federal guidance, cities and states were left to their own devices.

Local public health departments temporarily shut schools, churches, and taverns, and even restricted funeral attendance. A few cities, especially in California, recommended or required gauze masks. San Francisco enforced its rules particularly strictly. Police there arrested almost three hundred people for refusing to wear masks.[9]

Still, the epidemic seemed to wax and wane on its own. In city after city, both where public health measures were strict and where they were not, cases peaked within a few weeks after the first infection was seen, then plunged again.

Shortly after the epidemic ended in 1919, Dr. W. H. Kellogg, the executive officer of the California State Board of Health, published a "Summary of Conclusions Reached as a Result of the Study of the Control Measures Adopted."[10]

In other words, what, if any, public health rules had been most helpful?

When he compared the course of the epidemic in different cities, Kellogg found that most regulations had made little difference. He was particularly dismissive of masks.

"The very complete records at the disposal of the California State Board of Health indicate conclusively that the compulsory wearing of masks does not affect the progress of the epidemic," he wrote. Three eastern cities that had no mask rules had seen the same course of the epidemic as San Francisco.

Worse, nearly all the nurses at San Francisco Hospital had been infected, even though they wore masks while treating patients. Kellogg speculated one reason mask rules might fail was that people took off their masks when they most needed them, when they were in close contact with friends.

Nor did mass closings seem to matter, Kellogg wrote. Instead, he argued that self-isolation of sick people appeared to be the most effective tactic against the flu. But governments didn't have the resources to track mildly ill people, much less make them stay home. Instead the infected had to be convinced to do so themselves. "This measure depends more on the individual citizen than the health officer."

Scientific efforts to isolate the pathogen that caused the Spanish flu were equally halting. And despite their best efforts, the scientists of the time lacked the tools to figure out how the influenza virus spread on either the cellular or environmental level. They also had no way to know why this particular strain of flu was so dangerous.

In the seventeenth century, scientists had used primitive microscopes to see bacteria—tiny living microorganisms—for the first time.[11] In the late nineteenth century, the German physician Robert Koch showed how cholera and other bacteria could spread infectious diseases from person to person.

Then physicians discovered that some diseases could spread through fluids that had been strained through material with pores fine enough to catch all bacteria. They realized that the pathogens causing those infections must be even smaller than bacteria, too tiny to be filtered out. They used the word virus to describe these invisible scourges.

Slowly, scientists linked more diseases to viruses. But it was only in 1926—seven years after the Spanish flu epidemic ended—that an American doctor named Thomas Rivers made the crucial observation that, unlike bacteria, viruses could not reproduce on their own. Instead, they needed a living host.

"Viruses appear to be **obligate parasites** [emphasis added] in the sense that their reproduction is dependent on living cells," Rivers wrote. A monograph on Rivers would call his realization "probably one of the most important single statements ever made in the history of virology."[12]

Five years later, the advent of the electron microscope enabled virologists to see their tiny quarry for the first time. Viruses came in many different shapes and sizes. Some were nearly as large as small bacteria. Others were barely larger than a few clusters of atoms.

But in 1918 and 1919, scientists couldn't even see viruses, much less understand how they replicated. The seminal breakthrough from James Watson and Francis Crick, who figured out that all life depended on genetic material stored as long strands of amino acids, was a generation away.

Thus the physicians of the era had little chance to understand how the Spanish flu wreaked its havoc. About all they could do was treat symptoms such as fever and hope the infected would recover on their own.

The irony here is rich. A century later, scientists and physicians have made incredible progress in understanding how viruses survive and replicate. We have fully unlocked the genome of viruses such as influenza and the coronavirus. We know what these viruses look like, how they hide from our immune systems, how they attack our cells.

Yet we have made far less progress in understanding how viruses spread. We still don't know exactly how long an infected person is contagious, or why some people seem to be "superspreaders" while others don't spread illness at all. Further, so-called "supportive care" is still the core of our treatment for people stricken with the flu. Antivirals such as Tamiflu, developed at great expense, are only marginally effective.

Doctors sometimes joke that if patients get good medical care, they will recover from the flu in a week. Without help, they'll need seven days.

Fortunately, even without lockdowns or vaccines or year-long school closures, the Spanish flu did pass. It was forgotten surprisingly quickly. Perhaps we shouldn't be surprised. Though fifty million dead may shock us, people a century ago were more accustomed to facing their mortality. Medicine was advancing, but women still routinely died in childbirth. Without effective antibiotics, infections could prove deadly even to the young and healthy. Political leaders were much more ruthless too, even in democracies. European governments had just sacrificed millions of their citizens for a pointless war—without much protest even from the men being sent to the slaughter.

The decades that followed the Spanish flu saw a worldwide depression, another world war, and then the rise of nuclear arsenals with the power to destroy all human life. The twentieth century's worst epidemic became a historical footnote. Infectious diseases became less fearsome. Even before scientists learned the secrets of DNA and RNA, they had begun to craft effective vaccines against feared viral killers. The discovery of penicillin made bacterial infections far more treatable.

Still, the flu did not disappear.

In 1957, an outbreak that began in China killed about 116,000 Americans, the equivalent of 230,000 today. In 1968, what became known as the Hong Kong flu killed another 100,000 Americans. Both outbreaks received little attention. They led to no calls for masks, much less school closings, quarantines, or lockdowns.

In fact, Woodstock—the concert where hundreds of thousands of people gathered for days at a farm in Upstate New York—is just one of the many mass gatherings that took place during the Hong Kong epidemic. The contrast with our panic over the coronavirus is stunning, and proof of how much our attitude towards infectious diseases has changed in the last few years.

4

All the Wrong Lessons

After the Hong Kong flu faded away in 1969, the United States faced no major respiratory virus epidemics for more than a generation. Scientists and governments focused on chronic diseases that burdened aging societies and were often worsened by smoking and obesity. The United States declared a mostly unsuccessful war on cancer, even as heart disease remained the nation's leading killer.

Meanwhile, a public health panic in 1976 about a possible influenza crisis backfired. Expert predictions that a "swine flu" outbreak might become another Spanish flu proved wildly wrong. A hastily made vaccine was blamed for hundreds of cases of Guillain-Barre syndrome, a neurological ailment that can lead to muscle weakness, paralysis, and even death.[1]

The next infectious disease emergency had nothing to do with influenza or any respiratory virus. In 1981, physicians in New York and Los Angeles began seeing an unusual pattern of diseases. Healthy young gay men fell ill with pneumonia and a rare cancer called Kaposi's sarcoma and died quickly. Their immune systems appeared ravaged, unable to cope with even simple infections. Doctors named the disease acquired immunodeficiency syndrome, or AIDS. A hunt for the virus that might cause AIDS began.

By 1983, scientists had found the culprit, which was ultimately named HIV, the human immunodeficiency virus.[2] HIV was so dangerous because it aimed directly at the immune system. It infected and destroyed T-cells, the core of our immune response, leaving the body open to attack from other pathogens.

Before effective medicines were invented, HIV killed more than 95 percent of people it infected, making it the most lethal virus the world had ever seen.[3] But HIV took years to wreak havoc, so infected people could pass it on without knowing they were sick.

Even before the virus was discovered, researchers had begun the search for treatments. By 2000, they had largely succeeded. The defeat of HIV is one of the great scientific, medical, and pharmaceutical industry triumphs of the twentieth century.

Politically, however, the story is more complicated.

Physicians quickly realized that most people infected with HIV were either gay men or intravenous drug users—both marginalized groups. Even as deaths topped two thousand by the end of 1984, the Reagan administration was slow to acknowledge the threat. Ronald Reagan himself did not mention AIDS in public until September 1985.[4]

In response, gay rights groups began aggressive protests, proclaiming "Silence = Death." Even as research spending increased, the groups turned their ire on the National Institutes of Health (NIH) and the Food and Drug Administration (FDA). They said the NIH and FDA were moving too slowly to find treatments. Among their top targets was a forty-something physician from Brooklyn, Dr. Anthony Fauci.

Fauci was an energetic bantam with oversized glasses and a helmet of dark brown hair. He had captained his high school basketball team at Regis High School in Manhattan despite being only five foot seven. "He was ready to drive through whoever was in his way," one team-mate would recall to the *Wall Street Journal* more than sixty years later.[5] Another called him a "ball of fire." (Despite his relentless drive, the Regis team lost the first sixteen of seventeen games it played with Fauci as captain.)

After graduating medical school and completing his residency in internal medicine in 1968, Fauci joined the National Institute of Allergy and Infectious Diseases (NIAID), part of the National Institutes of Health. In doing so, he avoided military conscription and potential service in Vietnam.

He recalled in a 2014 interview, "At the time, the Vietnam War was on and all doctors were drafted, and you could either go into the Army, the Air Force, the Navy, or the Public Health Service (the NIH or the CDC). As it turns out, I got into the NIH."[6] Fauci moved up the ranks of the NIAID, and in 1984 he was named its director. He found himself in the crucible of the AIDS crisis.

In 1988, Larry Kramer, a leading AIDS activist, blasted Fauci in a San Francisco newspaper for "inaction [that] is causing today's increase in HIV infection."[7] In May 1990, a thousand AIDS activists occupied NIH headquarters in Maryland. Eighty-two were arrested.[8]

Media outlets were sympathetic to the activists, many of whom were young and sick with AIDS. Fauci also had a mostly positive attitude towards them, brushing off their complaints about him as political theater. After the Bethesda protest, he said he had "great empathy" for them, while he also defended the pace of federal research. In fact, the Food and Drug Administration had approved the first drug for HIV in 1987, only six years after physicians first recognized AIDS as a disease.

But Fauci went further than simply sounding empathetic. Recognizing HIV's lethality, he worked with activists to speed the process of drug development. Kramer recalled in a 2006 interview, "We had relationships with drug companies; we had a few treatments that needed to be tested and a lot of dying patients who were desperate to test them. What it needed was a government official to make the first move, and that's what Tony Fauci did."

Of course, none of that might have mattered if the scientists actually *doing* the research hadn't found effective HIV treatments. But they did. By 1996, the first effective multi-drug treatments for AIDS became available. The same activists who had previously attacked Fauci now lionized him. "Dr. Fauci has become the only true and great hero in all of this," Kramer said.[9]

Having the activists on his side helped Fauci in another, more tangible way—the harder they pushed for funding, the bigger his research budgets became. In 1984, when he took over the National Institute for Allergy and Infectious Diseases, it was the fifth-largest of the NIH's departments, with a budget of $320 million.

By 2005, its budget had increased almost 15-fold, to $4.5 billion. That figure was 50 percent more than the government spent on basic research into heart and lung diseases that killed far more people than HIV. Only the National Cancer Institute had a bigger budget.[10] Those billions made Fauci among the most powerful scientists in government.

Along the way, Fauci learned several lessons that he would return to when Sars-Cov-2 arrived in 2020: large-scale epidemics are political as well as medical crises; the media often fixates on death counts; and developing treatments fast is more important than dotting every *I* or crossing every *T*.

Only the fact that HIV killed nearly everyone it infected, while the opposite was true for the coronavirus, escaped him.

HIV grabbed the world's attention, but other infectious diseases were mostly forgotten, aside from the occasional Ebola outbreak. That amnesia began to change in 2001, though. In the deadliest biological weapons attack in United States history, a series of anthrax attacks killed five people and injured seventeen more. Media outlets and policymakers seized on the risk that al-Qaeda might use bioweapons in terror attacks, although the practical obstacles were enormous. Then the 2003 SARS outbreak, with its 10 percent infection fatality rate, generated headlines.

In 2005, President George Bush ordered the federal government to update its plans for an epidemic, whether natural or a bioterror attack. Centers for Disease Control (CDC) scientists began working on a report that would guide the federal response.

The process centered on questions over what epidemiologists and infectious disease experts call "non-pharmaceutical interventions," or NPIs—a catch-all public health term for ways of slowing the spread of a disease besides medical treatments. NPIs can be as basic as encouraging sick people to wash their hands, or as aggressive as shutting down whole countries.

As the work progressed, computer models that simulated how an epidemic might spread became increasingly important. The models showed that closing schools and encouraging telecommuting could slow the spread of a virus.

In April 2020, the *New York Times* explained how the plan for lockdowns had gained momentum:

> Fourteen years ago, two federal government doctors, Richard Hatchett and Carter Mecher, met with a colleague at a burger joint in suburban Washington for a final review of a proposal they knew would be treated like a piñata: telling Americans to stay home from work and school the next time the country was hit by a deadly pandemic.
>
> When they presented their plan not long after, it was met with skepticism and a degree of ridicule by senior officials....[11]

Dr. Mecher, an internist at the Department of Veterans Affairs, had connected with Robert Glass, a computer scientist at Sandia National Laboratories. For a science project, Glass's fourteen-year-old daughter Laura had made a simple model of the way school and business closures might slow the flu. Glass built on his daughter's work to create a simulation "proving" lockdowns could reduce an influenza epidemic in a hypothetical town of ten thousand people by 90 percent. "Dr. Mecher received the results at his office in Washington and was amazed," the *Times* reported.

Robert and Laura Glass ultimately became the first two authors of a paper published in *Emerging Infectious Diseases*, a Centers for Disease Control journal, about the simulation. Sure enough, it showed the "mitigation strategies" worked.

It is crucial to remember *these models were essentially not based on real-world data*. Almost no real-world data about efforts to reduce flu epidemics existed in 2005. The modelers depended on small studies on hand-washing and other simple interventions. They also used reports about masks and quarantines during the 1918 epidemic. But mainly they were guessing, as they admitted. A 2007 paper in the *Proceedings of the National Academy of Sciences* acknowledged, "A recent review, however, concluded that the evidence base for recommending such interventions is limited, consisting primarily of historical and contemporary observations, rather than controlled studies."[12]

Still, the modelers gained ground as the debate progressed. After more than a year of back and forth, the CDC released its report in February 2007. The report divided epidemics into five categories, ranging from typical seasonal flu that killed fewer than 90,000 Americans to a Spanish-flu type epidemic killing more than 1.8 million.[13]

Steps such as school closures of up to twelve weeks were recommended only for the most serious outbreaks, those expected to kill more than 900,000 people. The report did not even mention the possibility of complete societal lockdowns.

Still, an official government document had now recommended restricting public gatherings. And when the CDC revised its planning forecast a decade later, *it removed the different categories of epidemics*. The change gave lawmakers more flexibility to impose strict measures. Suddenly a virus that might kill 200,000 people was officially viewed no differently from one that could kill 2 million.[14]

But even after the 2017 revisions, the CDC never publicly contemplated broad lockdowns. In 2019, the World Health Organization issued an even more detailed report on the ways governments should handle epidemics. It, too, did not discuss broad lockdowns.[15]

And even before the CDC put its first report together in 2007, scientists with expertise fighting infectious diseases worried that aggressive interventions wouldn't work and might backfire.

Among the most vocal critics of the recommendations for lockdowns was Dr. Donald Henderson. Henderson, a recipient of the Presidential Medal of Freedom, had led the successful effort to eradicate smallpox, once among the world's most feared diseases.

In December 2006, Henderson and three other scientists authored an eleven-page paper called "Disease Mitigation Measures in the Control of Pandemic Influenza." After outlining lockdown measures, they posed the question, "We must ask whether any or all of the proposed measures are epidemiologically sound...[and] consider possible secondary social and economic impacts."[16]

The authors argued that efforts to slow the spread of the flu in past epidemics had largely failed. They attacked quarantines, travel bans, and school closings of more than two weeks as likely counterproductive. They did not even mention full lockdowns, presumably because they viewed those as so unlikely.

Near the end of the paper they made a heartfelt plea for governments to focus on supporting medical systems and otherwise allow life to go on: "Experience has shown that communities faced with epidemics or other adverse events respond best and with the least anxiety **when the normal social functioning of the community is least disrupted.** Strong political and public health leadership to provide reassurance and to ensure that needed medical care services are provided are critical elements" [emphasis added].

Similarly, a 2006 report from the Institute of Medicine, a federally chartered non-partisan group that offers advice on tough health questions, warned against over-relying on models.[17] "Models should be viewed as aids to decision-making, rather than substitutes for decision-making," the report warned. Unfortunately, "in the midst of a crisis, there will be pressure for government to employ public health interventions, even in the absence of proven benefits."

Fourteen years later, we would learn how prescient that warning had been.

5

Globetrotting

The second phase of the coronavirus epidemic began on Friday, February 21, 2020, when Italian authorities cut off ten northern towns where the virus had spread.[1]

Italy's announcement marked the first lockdowns outside China. Yet after those massive Chinese quarantines, the plan had an odd precision. *We don't need to shut down the country, or even a province. If we keep away from these fifty thousand people, we'll be fine. This respiratory virus definitely hasn't spread to the rest of the country.*

The world, including the financial world, seemed to share Italy's calm. After all, the United States hadn't reported any deaths from the coronavirus. On Wall Street, the Standard & Poor's (S&P) 500 Index fell less than 1 percent the day of the Italian announcement. It had reached an all-time high only two days before.

Then the bottom dropped out. In the four days after the quarantine, the number of Italian coronavirus cases rose from 3 to 280.[2] South Korea and Iran also reported fast-growing caseloads.

Meanwhile, President Trump repeatedly minimized the crisis. On February 25, Trump told reporters that the Chinese appeared to have the virus "under control, so I think that's a problem that's going to go away." The next day, in response to reports that fifteen Americans had tested positive, Trump said, "You have 15 people, and the 15 within a couple of days is going to be down to close to zero, that's a pretty good job we've done."[3]

The comment would be the first of many that would haunt Trump through Election Day.

Even at the time, it appeared tin-eared. Sars-Cov-2 was moving unchecked across Europe and Asia. How could the United States possibly escape? But aside from his January 31 China travel ban, Trump had taken little action. He had done even less to prepare Americans mentally for the possibility the coronavirus might hit the United States in force.

In those crucial weeks in February and early March, Trump seemed to view the virus mostly as a political and public relations problem. On March 6, he complained that allowing Covid-infected passengers to leave a cruise ship near San Francisco was a mistake because it would cause the reported number of American infections to rise.

"I don't need to have the numbers double because of one ship that wasn't our fault. . . . I'd rather have them stay on, personally," the president said.[4]

Trump's fumbling comments led to a ripple of bad publicity that presaged the tidal wave to come. And they did little to calm anyone. During the last week of February, the S&P fell about 10 percent.

On Saturday, February 29, the coronavirus officially took its first life on American soil. A fifty-something resident of a nursing home outside Seattle died shortly after being infected.[5] Authorities warned that more than fifty other residents and staff members at the facility were showing signs of pneumonia. Worse, they could not find a connection between the nursing home and anyone who had traveled to China—proof that community transmission inside the United States was occurring.

In a sign of the seriousness of the news, Trump announced the death at a news conference. By then, Sars-Cov-2 had become the most important story not just online but off, not just in the United States but around the world. Stores ran short on cleaning products and masks. CNN reported on February 29 that the cost of a box of 100 dust masks on Amazon had risen from $8 to $200 in days.[6]

The run on masks came even as public health experts discouraged civilians from buying either standard surgical masks or higher-end protective respirators called N95s. "There is no role for these masks in the community," Dr. Robert Redfield, the director of the CDC, said at a congressional hearing on February 27.

Three days later, Dr. Jerome Adams, the surgeon general, went further.

"You can increase your risk of getting it by wearing a mask if you are not a health care provider," Adams said in an interview on Fox News. "There are things people can do to stay safe. There are things they shouldn't be doing and one of the things they shouldn't be doing in the general public is going out and buying masks."[7]

Yet the shortages worsened by the day—made worse by China's efforts to hoover up every mask it could find. (Amazingly, in its February 29 article, CNN simultaneously called Americans "scared" for buying masks and wrote glowingly of efforts by Chinese Americans to send thousands of masks to their relatives and friends in China.)

On March 3, the World Health Organization issued a press release warning that hospitals, doctors, and nurses around the world faced shortages of personal protective equipment (PPE)—masks, gloves, respirators, and face shields. "Supplies can take months to deliver and market manipulation is widespread, with stocks frequently sold to the highest bidder," the WHO said. It called for an immediate 40 percent increase in production worldwide.

The run on masks both reflected and amplified the panic spreading worldwide. Over the next several days, more infections and deaths were reported in Washington State, and other states began to report their own cases. Yet outside of China, and to a lesser extent Iran, the horrors were mostly theoretical. The world appeared to be functioning normally.

Then, on March 6, a doctor in Bergamo, a city at the center of northern Italy's outbreak, published a desperate Facebook post warning that conditions were far worse than anyone understood.

"I want to fight this sense of security that I see," Dr. Daniele Macchini wrote. Pneumonia patients filled his hospital, the emergency room was "collapsing," and "every ventilator becomes like gold." Sars-Cov-2 was far more dangerous than influenza, he wrote: "One after the other the poor unfortunates present themselves in the emergency room. They have anything but the complications of a flu. Let's stop saying it's a bad flu."

Macchini finished with a plea: "Please share this message. We must spread the word to prevent what is happening here from happening all over Italy."[8]

He was more successful than he could have imagined. His original post in Italian was shared forty thousand times on Facebook. Then a Swiss epidemiologist translated much of it into English and tweeted it, leading to thirty-six thousand retweets and articles everywhere from the *Financial Times* to the *New York Post*.[9] Tens of millions of people saw Macchini's warning.

The videos and social media posts from China had been frightening. But with so few independent reporters in Wuhan, no one could be sure how much China's state-run propaganda machine might be distorting the epidemic. None of those caveats applied to Macchini's frantic warning.

His post, as much as anything else, helped set the stage for what came next.

On March 9, Italian prime minister Giuseppe Conte announced a lockdown covering all sixty million people in Italy. Even China had not tried to quarantine its entire population. Conte said Italy had no choice. "We all have to renounce something," he said, calling for shared sacrifice.

All outdoor gatherings were forbidden. Schools and universities would be closed. The restrictions would last through April 3.[10]

Two days later, Italy further tightened its rules, closing bars, restaurants, and retailers aside from essential services such as grocery stores. For the first time since World War II, an advanced democracy had asserted the right to interfere in the most basic aspects of its citizens' lives. The Italian government made the extraordinary move in a matter of days, with almost no public discussion or debate.

Yet, by March 9, when Italy imposed its first lockdown, the country had suffered only about nine thousand coronavirus cases and five hundred deaths. With one of the world's oldest populations and harsh northern winters, Italy regularly suffered severe winter flu epidemics. In the winter of 2014–2015 and again in 2016–2017, influenza and other flu-like illnesses had killed more than forty thousand Italians—*eighty times* as many as had died from the coronavirus at the time of the lockdown.

Yet almost no one anywhere in the world questioned whether Italy had overreacted. The only question for the rest of Europe and the United States seemed to be when they too would follow Italy into lockdown. With the virus spreading uncontained, no one had real reason to believe that Italy was different than anywhere else.

"Bottom line, it's going to get worse," Dr. Anthony Fauci said at a congressional hearing on March 11.

By then Fauci had become the face of the coronavirus response in the United States—and worldwide.

Anthony Fauci was a member of the federal coronavirus task force, but he didn't head it. He was not the most senior physician or scientist in the American government. He was not the head of the National Institutes of Health or the Centers for Disease Control. He was not the surgeon general or the secretary of Health and Human Services.

But the White House's toxic relationship with the media was spiraling to new depths, and reporters saw anyone close to Trump as tainted and untrustworthy. In addition, Redfield, who as CDC director should naturally have been the face of the federal response, lacked Fauci's gravitas.

Worse, Redfield's reputation never recovered from a crucial misstep in early February. The CDC sent Covid test kits that didn't work to state health laboratories and refused to let other labs create their own tests.[11]

As a result, Covid surveillance was badly hamstrung during February. With test kits nearly nonexistent, authorities made them available only to people who had traveled from China or could prove direct contact with an infected person.

Though the epidemic would almost certainly have exploded anyway, more early tests would have given the public a better sense of how quickly Sars-Cov-2 was spreading.

Instead, the virus spread silently across the country, especially the Northeast, setting the stage for a massive wave of cases in late March. The testing fiasco did not cost Redfield his job, but it tainted him. Fauci emerged unscathed.

Long before the testing mess, Fauci had become more powerful than his relatively modest title suggested. In 1989, he turned down an overture from President George H. W. Bush to run the entire National Institutes of Health, preferring to stay at NIAID and keep control over AIDS research—and his fast-growing budget.[12] ("This is not the time for the general to leave the battlefield to go back to the Pentagon," he had told *Science* magazine in September 1989. The comment, like others he would make over the next twenty-five years, revealed more about Fauci's opinion of himself than he may have intended.[13])

Fauci cultivated both Congress and the White House. "One of the first things is to understand the relationships between people in power," he said in a 2014 interview.[14] "I never in my wildest dreams would have thought that I would become adviser to five separate Presidents."

George W. Bush, who had met Fauci when his father was vice president, respected Fauci so much that in 2008 he awarded Fauci the

Presidential Medal of Freedom. The award is one of the two highest given to civilians in the United States.

Fauci did have one flaw, Bush said. "Sometimes he forgets to stop working. He regularly puts in 80-hour weeks....He's even found notes on his windshield left by coworkers that say things like, 'Go home. You're making me feel guilty.'"[15]

Fauci proved equally willing to work with Democrats. After Bill Clinton defeated Bush in 1992, Fauci regularly briefed Clinton in the Oval Office.[16]

But if Fauci was a consummate inside player, he also recognized the importance of the media. He spent decades cultivating relationships with the reporters who covered science and infectious diseases for elite media organizations such as the *New York Times* and the *New Yorker.*

Those veteran reporters would lead coverage of the coronavirus for their outlets—which shaped the attitudes of the rest of the media. Fauci directly cultivated younger reporters too, in the simplest possible way. He made himself available.

"When reporters call Dr. Fauci, he calls them back," the *Times* reported on March 8.[17] The article was a perfect illustration of *why* he called them back. It began, "Dr. Anthony Fauci, the nation's leading expert on infectious diseases, is widely respected for his ability to explain science without talking down to his audience—and lately, for managing to correct the president's pronouncements without saying he is wrong."

So even after Trump put Vice President Mike Pence in charge of the coronavirus task force on February 25, Fauci was still the go-to guy: the task force's most important member, the one the media respected more than any other—and far more than Trump or Pence.

In the months to come, he would use that power to make sure the United States responded to the coronavirus as aggressively as possible, whatever the cost.

6

Fifteen Days

On Monday, March 9, 2020, Rudy Gobert—a seven-foot-one center for the Utah Jazz known for his tough defense—talked to reporters at a press conference after a Jazz practice. With the coronavirus spreading, the National Basketball Association had banned journalists from locker rooms. It mandated press conferences instead. Gobert mocked the new rule by wiping his hands on every microphone at the podium where he spoke.[1]

Two days later, Gobert became the first professional athlete to test positive for Sars-Cov-2.

In the year-plus since, Gobert's story has largely been forgotten. He recovered quickly, though his sense of smell did not return for months.[2]

At the time, though, Gobert faced swift condemnation. *How could this overpaid oaf have been so cavalier? How could he have put his teammates and the reporters who cover him at risk? Doesn't he understand how serious this virus is? Or how contagious? Bet he does now!*

Within twenty-four hours, Gobert abjectly apologized on Instagram. "I was careless and make no excuse," he wrote. "I hope my story serves as a warning."

Still the brickbats kept coming. "Gobert was a goob," a columnist in Oklahoma wrote on March 15. "A moron. An idiot."[3] The response was an early example of what became a major theme in coronavirus coverage: the media's open efforts to shame anyone who appeared not to be taking the epidemic seriously enough—especially anyone young.

But Gobert's positive test hurt more than just his reputation.

Hours after the news broke, the NBA suspended its season "until further notice," even as games were still being played. The decision created palpable shock. In a live interview on ESPN from the American Airlines Center in Dallas, with players feet away on the court, Dallas Mavericks owner Mark Cuban said he didn't even know if his children would go to school in the morning.

"It's like something out of a movie," Cuban said.[4]

The National Hockey League and college basketball leagues followed the NBA's lead the next day, leading to a bizarre spectacle just past noon at Manhattan's Madison Square Garden. Creighton and St. John's Universities played the first half of a game—and then didn't come back after halftime. The game was called, its first twenty minutes erased from history.

The suspension of college and professional sports fanned the panic. Even after the September 11 terrorist attacks, sports had paused only momentarily; by September 21, 2001, baseball was being played again even in New York City.[5] But in March 2020, neither the NBA nor any other league offered any potential timetable for resuming games.

March 11 was also the day Tom Hanks and Rita Wilson, Hanks's wife, announced from Australia they had been infected. Hanks, one of the world's most recognizable movie stars, was the first A-list celebrity known to have contracted the coronavirus. In a statement to the media, Hanks did not overplay the severity of the symptoms he or Wilson had suffered: "We felt a bit tired, like we had colds, and some body aches. Rita had some chills that came and went. Slight fevers too."[6]

No matter. The announcement added to the grim sense that Sars-Cov-2 was everywhere and that no one, no matter how wealthy or careful, would escape it.

Along with the Gobert and Hanks announcements, the World Health Organization made its own news on March 11, declaring the coronavirus a "pandemic" for the first time. To public health experts, epidemics and pandemics are not the same. An epidemic is a disease outbreak in one country or region. A pandemic is an epidemic that has spread uncontrolled across multiple regions—an epidemic of epidemics.

On a conference call with reporters, Tedros Adhanom Ghebreyesus, the Ethiopian biologist who was the WHO's director-general, did not mince words:

> WHO has been assessing this outbreak around the clock and we are deeply concerned both by the alarming levels of spread and severity, and by the alarming levels of inaction....
>
> Pandemic is not a word to use lightly or carelessly. It is a word that, if misused, can cause unreasonable fear, or unjustified acceptance that the fight is over, leading to unnecessary suffering and death.[7]

Since late February, coronavirus infections outside China had risen 13-fold, Ghebreyesus said. The number of countries reporting infections had tripled. The world now had more than 118,000 cases in 114 countries, with almost 4,300 deaths. Ghebreyesus called on countries to step up their efforts to test for infected people and trace their contacts.

Ghebreyesus didn't say so explicitly, but anyone with a calculator could do the math. Based on his figures, the coronavirus was killing 3.6 percent of the people it infected. That percentage translated into thirty-six out of every one thousand people, a horrifically high death rate considering how quickly the virus seemed to spread.

By way of comparison, standard influenza strains were believed to have a death rate of 0.05 percent to 0.1 percent. At the high end, that translated into one death out of every one thousand infections—1/36 of the coronavirus's rate.

Later in the call, Dr. Mike Ryan, the head of the WHO team responsible for containing and treating Covid, said hospitals and entire health systems might collapse if countries did not move quickly to stop the virus: "The difficulty is that if you do not try and suppress this virus it can overwhelm your health system, so there have to be very strong efforts made to suppress infection, to push the infection back because at the very least it will take the pressure—it will **flatten the curve** and allow your health system to remain in control and achieve some success in reducing case fatality" [emphasis added].

Ryan's promise to "flatten the curve" was a neat bit of epidemiologic jargon. The phrase meant slowing the spread of the virus to reduce the peak number of infections. Instead of a mountain, the graph of infections would look more like a ridge, longer but lower and less steep. That way Covid would be less likely to swamp hospitals, doctors, and nurses.

To take a simple example: If medical centers in a city with 1,000 hospital beds faced 50 new coronavirus cases every week for a year, they could handle the cases easily (assuming each patient needed exactly one week of care). But if all 2,600 cases arrived the same week, the hospitals would face dire shortages. Coronavirus patients, and other patients, might die untreated.

In the days to come, "flatten the curve" would become the pandemic's first mantra. Politicians and public health experts would repeat the magic words over and over. *Flatten the curve to slow the spread. Flatten the curve, save lives.* And most important: *Fifteen days to flatten the curve.* Flattening the curve became a goal we could all agree on, a positive reason to lock down—temporarily.

But on March 11, 2020, most people hadn't yet heard the phrase. And the panic rose even further when President Trump, in a primetime speech from the Oval Office, declared that he was banning all travel from Europe for thirty days. One year later, NPR would rightly declare March 11 "The Day Everything Changed."[8]

As March 2020 fades into memory, it is easy to forget how panicked the United States and world became that month. Stock markets worldwide plunged. On March 11 and 12, the Standard & Poor's 500 fell 13.5 percent. In barely three weeks, the index had lost nearly one-quarter of its value, in one of the sharpest and fastest declines in its history.

It wasn't just investors. Shoppers were no longer merely emptying grocery stores. They were stocking up on guns, too.

About two million firearms were sold in the United States in March, the second-highest monthly figure ever. "People are nervous that there's a certain amount of civil disorder that might come if huge numbers of people are sick and a huge number of institutions are not operating normally," a law professor and expert on the gun industry told the *New York Times*.[9] "They may have an anxiety about protecting themselves."

City downtowns and suburban malls emptied as people stayed home. Mobile phone location tracking data showed a sharp decline in travel beginning March 8, with another drop the next week.

By Monday, March 16, school districts had begun to close, including New York City's, which gave only a day's warning before beginning its shutdown.[10] Bill de Blasio, the city's mayor, said he had not expected "in a million years" he would need to shut schools.

Across the Atlantic, European countries followed Italy's lead and shut their borders. Spain imposed a quarantine on March 14, France on March 16.

What the public learned only in pieces over the next few days was that researchers at Imperial College London had spent the week of March 9 making terrifying predictions to British, European, and American leaders.[11]

On March 15, *Le Monde* explained how the Imperial College team, led by a physicist-turned-epidemiologist named Neil Ferguson, had influenced French president Emmanuel Macron:

> This modeling was carried out by epidemiologist Neil Ferguson of Imperial College in London. His team has been approached by several European governments to establish different scenarios for the progression of the epidemic....

> The results for France were presented Thursday, March
> 12 at the Elysee [the French presidential palace]. A few hours
> before the president solemnly addresses the French to explain
> the *"urgency"* of the situation.[12]

A lean, intense man who favored horn-rimmed glasses and swept his hair forward to hide a receding hairline, Ferguson was neither a medical doctor nor a virologist. He had earned a Ph.D. in theoretical physics from Oxford in 1994.

But after hearing a talk by another physicist-turned-epidemiologist about modeling the AIDS epidemic, Ferguson realized he could put his mathematical skills to real-world use. He left physics and turned to predicting epidemics.[13]

Of course, as skeptics had warned when the CDC put together its influenza response plan, the science of forecasting diseases can be *more* complex than physics. Models depend on many variables that can't be measured exactly, including the hardest to forecast of all—human behavior. Epidemiologists must estimate not only the deadliness and transmissibility of a pathogen, but also the ways people will respond as an epidemic goes on.

To highlight just a few of the questions a model must try to answer:

Not everyone spreads diseases equally well. Some infected people become "superspreaders," uniquely able to infect others. Who are they? Can they be found and quarantined quickly?

What about transmission by infected people who aren't yet showing symptoms? For how long will they be infectious? What about people who *never* show symptoms?

On the other hand, what percentage of the infected will need to be hospitalized? How many will require intensive care or ventilators?

Environments are also crucial. Does the virus spread quickly among children and in schools? What about apartment buildings or offices? Are surfaces a major channel for transmission, or is the pathogen primarily airborne? Do heat and humidity affect its viability?

We do not have complete answers for these questions even for influenza, which scientists have studied for more than a century. Trying to solve them in the case of the new coronavirus under the immense pressure of a pandemic was nearly impossible, even with scientists all over the world contributing to the effort.

If predicting an epidemic's course is hard, offering useful solutions to lessen its severity can be even harder, as Donald Henderson had warned in 2006. But despite—or perhaps because of—his lack of frontline experience, Neil Ferguson felt duty bound to try.

Over and over again.

In 2002, Ferguson made his first highly publicized prediction. He suggested that mad cow disease—a degenerative brain disorder—might kill as many as 100,000 people in Britain, or 150,000 if it also proved to be transmissible from sheep to humans.[14] Fewer than 180 Britons died.[15]

In 2005, Ferguson again grabbed attention when he warned that a strain of influenza called H5N1 could kill hundreds of millions of people. "Around 40 million people died in the 1918 Spanish flu outbreak," he told the British newspaper *The Guardian*. "There are six times more people on the planet now so you could scale it up to around 200 million people probably."[16]

It was perhaps a bad sign for Ferguson's skills as a mathematician that he couldn't figure out that the world's population in 2005 (6.5 billion) was not six times its 1918 population (1.8 billion), but about 3.5 times. Or that 40 million times six equaled 240 million, not 200 million.

In any case, Ferguson's prediction for the flu proved even more incorrect than his mad cow estimate. A total of forty-three people died from the H5N1 flu in 2005, according to the WHO, meaning Ferguson was off by a factor of millions.[17]

Yet Ferguson only became more important in the years that followed. By 2020, he headed the WHO Collaborating Centre for Infectious Disease Modelling. The center was based at Imperial College and offered the World Health Organization "rapid analysis of urgent infectious disease problems, notably outbreaks."[18]

In a front-page article on March 17, 2020, the *New York Times* explained how important Ferguson had become as world leaders struggled to respond to the coronavirus: "With ties to the World Health Organization and a team of 50 scientists, led by a prominent epidemiologist, Neil Ferguson, Imperial is treated as a sort of gold standard, its mathematical models feeding directly into government policies."[19]

Ferguson was also part of a semi-secret British government committee called the Scientific Advisory Group for Emergencies, or SAGE. SAGE first came together in 2009 amid fears of a potential swine flu epidemic. It quickly faced criticism for a lack of transparency and inaccurate projections. In July 2009, it estimated the swine flu might kill up to sixty-five thousand Britons—more than a hundred times the number who actually died.[20]

In 2011, a report from the British Parliament sharply criticized SAGE committees, whose membership changed with each emergency, for "an unnecessarily secretive way of working" and for failing "to adhere to any published guidance or code of conduct." Further, the report said, SAGE committees should focus on the "most probable scenarios" for emergencies, rather than worst-case projections.[21]

Nine years later, as the coronavirus emerged from China, SAGE largely ignored those suggestions. It operated without much, if any, oversight. It initially refused to disclose its members, supposedly to protect them from harassment. It kept both its meetings and recommendations secret.[22] It functioned essentially to give private advice to senior officials of the British government.

Not everyone in SAGE liked Ferguson. Some other scientists "bridled at his appetite for media coverage, which they said interfered with [SAGE's] work," as the *New York Times* would report. Still, he was the group's "undisputed star."[23]

Thus Ferguson enjoyed both a private channel to senior government officials and public influence as the voice making predictions through his Imperial College reports. By March 2020, he was in a uniquely influential position in Britain, and he was driving policies in the United States and continental Europe as well.

By mid-February, Ferguson had grown deeply frightened about the havoc the coronavirus might wreak. "This virus is probably the one that concerns me the most of everything I've worked on," he said on February 14.[24]

At a SAGE committee hearing on February 27, Ferguson first floated the idea that the virus might kill 500,000 people in Britain—the equivalent of more than 2 million in the United States.[25]

Despite the supposed precision of Ferguson's models, he based his estimate on the most basic math possible. He assumed the virus would infect four out of five people in the United Kingdom—about fifty million people—and that 1 percent of those would die.

The apparent catastrophe in Italy only worsened the fears of Ferguson and other SAGE members. British doctors who had spoken to colleagues in Italy warned that many more patients needed ventilators than they had expected. Medical staff were struggling to keep up. Ferguson said in an article published April 2 that the Italian problems "led to a 'sudden focusing of minds'" for him and other members of the SAGE committee.[26]

Meanwhile, China's experience breaking the epidemic in Wuhan appeared to offer a way out.

An influential paper from Xihong Lin, a biostatistician at Harvard University's School of Public Health, showed that the lockdown in Wuhan had essentially ended the spread of the virus immediately. Before January 22, the replication rate of the virus was 3.88, meaning that each infected person infected almost four more people.[27]

But the *very next day*, as China walled off Wuhan and Hubei province and forced its residents into lockdown, the replication rate fell dramatically to 1.25. The epidemic was still growing, but much more slowly. Then, beginning on February 2, China further tightened its rules, forcing people suspected of having the virus from their homes and into hotels. That way, they could no longer infect close family members.

That step broke the back of the virus, Lin found. The replication rate fell to 0.33, meaning that most infected people didn't pass the virus to *anyone* else. Since many people recovered from Covid in a week or less, cases dropped stunningly fast. In just weeks, the virus had nearly burned out in Wuhan.

Thus by March, China had controlled an outbreak that had appeared unmanageable in January.

The West had to follow suit, Ferguson believed. It faced a simple and stark choice: allow the virus to overrun its hospitals, or lock down and break the epidemic.

"Based on our estimates and other teams', there's really no option but follow in China's footsteps and suppress," he told the *New York Times* on March 16.[28]

But Western societies wouldn't accept such draconian steps.

Or would they? Again, the Italian experience proved crucial. The Italian government was notoriously weak. Yet Italians had accepted their lockdown almost overnight, despite the relatively low number of cases.

"People's sense of what is possible in terms of control changed quite dramatically between January and March," Ferguson would say later. Even after the Chinese lockdown, SAGE hadn't thought Western countries would tolerate lockdowns. "Then Italy did it. And we realized we could."[29]

But only if people were sufficiently terrified.

Fortunately, Ferguson had a model for that.

On Monday, March 16, Imperial College publicly released the forecast that it had previously shown only to policymakers. Under the anodyne title "Impact of Non-Pharmaceutical Interventions (NPIs) to Reduce Covid-19 Mortality and Healthcare Demand," it contained a terrifying forecast.

Over 2 million Americans and 500,000 Britons would die in a matter of months if governments did not shut their countries immediately. The epidemic would peak quickly and sharply. By the beginning of June, about 50,000 Americans would die of Covid each day.

Equally terrifying, an uncontrolled pandemic would cause coronavirus patients to destroy the hospital system. Within a month, hospitals would be out of intensive care beds. By mid-May, more than two million Americans would need intensive care, more than thirty times the number of beds available.

But the forecast was even *worse* than the topline figures suggested. Ferguson's model indicated that even strict "mitigation" efforts to slow the epidemic by isolating the infected, closing schools, and encouraging people over seventy to stay home might reduce the number of deaths only by half, to about one million in the United States.

Instead of mitigation, the report called for "suppression," which it defined as "social distancing of the entire population" and household quarantines or school closures. In other words, a strict and government-enforced lockdown, like Italy's.

Finally, it warned that those suppression efforts would "need to be maintained until a vaccine becomes available," a goal it estimated was at least eighteen months away. Temporary mitigation efforts would lead to a frustrating cycle of off-and-on restrictions. Only indefinite closures would work. It called suppression "the preferred policy option."

The report's impact was immediate and huge.

"A chilling scientific paper helped upend U.S. and U.K. coronavirus strategies,"[30] the *Washington Post* reported. "UK changes course amid death toll fears," the BBC said.[31]

Faced with the prospect of a worldwide economic meltdown, investors shed stocks en masse. The Dow Jones Industrial Average fell three thousand points, or almost 13 percent, on March 16. That same day the price of oil, a crucial economic indicator, fell three dollars a barrel, to twenty-eight dollars. Twelve days before, it had been over fifty dollars.

Social media accelerated the panic. Ferguson's report was perfect for Twitter. It had academic authority. It had dozens of authors. It was full of impressive-looking charts and graphs and written in punchy language one didn't need to be a scientist to understand.

No matter that it drew its world-changing conclusions on the thinnest possible evidence. It quickly went viral. "We can now read the Imperial College report on COVID-19 that led to the extreme measures we've seen in the US this week. Read it; it's terrifying," began a tweet that was liked 173,000 times.[32]

The Imperial College report turned lockdowns into a fait accompli— a step that couldn't be delayed, much less debated. Each day without "suppression" brought countries closer to the moment when the curves would go parabolic and the hospitals would crash.

Stay at home to flatten the curve. Public health organizations and cable news channels repeated the line over and over. Coronavirus messaging was proving like no other, coordinated to leave no room for doubt, no possibility for debate.

Yet even as the report was released, we had hints the virus might not be as catastrophic as it had seemed during those first days in Wuhan. The most notable evidence came from the *Diamond Princess* cruise ship. The ship had turned into a floating laboratory after Japan forced its passengers and crew to remain on board almost two weeks and the virus spread unchecked.

The ship had about 2,650 passengers and another 1,000-plus crew members. Despite the confined quarters and shared ventilation system, only 712 people contracted Covid. That figure was less than 20 percent of the total people on the ship. All by itself, that fact suggested that the coronavirus might not be as transmissible as early modeling had suggested.

The pattern of deaths was also striking. Of the 712 infected people, 14 eventually died, all passengers. That represented a death rate of 2 percent. But the 2 percent figure deeply overestimated Covid's risks on a national or worldwide basis. Why? Because the people aboard the *Diamond Princess* were mostly over 60, and thus far more susceptible to the virus than the general population.

Even among those people, Covid presented deeply uneven risks. The virus's dangers skyrocketed in people over 80. Four of the 14 deaths were people over 80, even though only 227 of the 3,700 people on board *Diamond Princess* were over 80.[33] Another 8 of the deaths were people between 70 and 80, the age of about 1,000 passengers. (The last two deaths included one woman in her sixties and one person whose age was not revealed.)

Early Italian data painted the same picture. By March 16, it showed that Covid almost exclusively killed people over 70. Of the first 1,700 Italians to die, not one was under 30. Only 13 were under 50. Nearly 9 in 10 of the deaths had occurred in people over 70. In fact, nearly as many Italians over 90 (yes, 90) died as under 70.[34]

Ferguson knew about the differences in the risks of coronavirus by age. He had to know, in order to make accurate death and hospitalization estimates. And his report didn't *entirely* ignore them. In a table on page 5, the report suggested the "case fatality ratio" would be 9.3 percent for people over 80, but only 0.15 percent for people in their forties. In other words, out of 11 people in their eighties who would develop symptoms of Covid, 1 would die. But only 1 in 670 people in their forties would die.

(An important note: The "case fatality ratio" is different from the "infection fatality ratio," or IFR. Many people who are infected with Covid never have symptoms. They may never be tested and not even know they are infected. So the case fatality ratio overstates Covid's real dangers. The best and truest measure is the IFR, which compares the *total* number of people who die to the *total* number infected, symptoms or no.)

Ferguson mentioned the age differences. But he didn't emphasize them. Despite all his charts and graphs, his report never provided the actual number of deaths he expected for people of different ages. Those figures would have shown that the epidemic was hugely concentrated in older people.

One person who understood where the real dangers lay was Dr. Fauci. On March 9—a full week before the Imperial College report—he told the editor of the *Journal of the American Medical Association*, "It's so clear that the overwhelming weight of serious disease and mortality is on those who are elderly and those with a serious comorbidity: heart disease, chronic lung disease, diabetes, obesity, respiratory difficulties."[35]

Fauci went on to say that anyone young and healthy who died of Covid-19 would be an "outlier."

He was right.

But Fauci and other public health experts rapidly changed course. They intentionally obscured the fact that the coronavirus posed only a tiny risk to healthy people under fifty. On March 18, Dr. Deborah Birx, a member of the federal coronavirus task force, cited "concerning reports coming out of France and Italy about some young people getting seriously ill."[36] Fauci made a similar comment a week later.[37]

Why? A March 22 paper from a SAGE subcommittee—kept hidden from the public at the time, but released months later—offered an answer. Only by pretending the virus posed a significant risk to everyone could governments ensure the public would accept lockdowns.

In the paper, entitled "Options for Increasing Adherence to Social Distancing Measures," unnamed members of the SAGE "behavioral science subcommittee" laid out the issue clearly:

> Perceived threat: A substantial number of people still do not feel sufficiently personally threatened; it could be that they are reassured by the low death rate in their demographic group....
>
> **The perceived level of personal threat needs to be increased among those who are complacent, using hard-hitting emotional messaging.** [emphasis in the original]

The authors also discussed the need for positive and negative reinforcement:

**Communication strategies should provide social approval for
desired behaviours....**

Social disapproval from one's community can play an
important role in preventing anti-social behaviour....**Consid-
eration should be given to use of social disapproval but with
a strong caveat around unwanted negative consequences.**[38]
[emphasis in the original]

To be sure, governments and public health agencies had long promoted some behaviors while discouraging others—drunk driving and
cigarette use, for example. But this campaign quickly became the most
aggressive propaganda campaign that democracies anywhere had conducted since World War I, if not ever.

A few skeptical scientists tried to push back as the frenzy—and the
lockdowns—spread. They were ignored.

■ ■ ■

And on March 19, lockdowns crossed the Atlantic, as California's
Gavin Newsom became the first governor to announce a "stay-at-home"
order for his state. California, with a population of forty million, had
fewer than two thousand cases at the time, and fewer than twenty deaths.

Of course, reporters didn't *have* to follow along.

During the HIV epidemic, newspapers had questioned public health
pronouncements and warned against government overreach. As early as June
1983, the *New York Times* had published an opinion piece titled "AIDS and
Civil Liberties," citing the "danger that the judicial and political systems will
fall prey to the irrational demands of a frightened public and impose groundless and onerous regulations that result in the widespread loss of freedom."[39]

The response to Covid was different.

Whether out of ignorance of Covid's minuscule risks to the young,
a cynical realization that fear would drive ratings and clicks, anger at

Donald Trump, or the genuine desire to beat the virus at any cost, reporters happily followed the government's diktats.

Following the Imperial College report, teenagers and young adults on spring break became a particular subject of the media's ire. On March 19, a twenty-five-year-old offered "an open letter to my peers partying on the beach" on CNN.com, begging them to go home. "We'll get back to brunches and concerts once we've taken action, flattened the curve and shared social media posts about the importance of young people laying low," she wrote.[40]

Four days later, Global News, a Canadian website, reported:

> The internet has a new word for all the spring breakers, partygoers and hoarders behaving selfishly during the new coronavirus threat.
>
> They're calling those people "COVIDIOTS," a nickname inspired by the COVID-19 disease, which appears to be bringing out the worst in a minority of people, even while others practice generosity and social distancing.[41]

Generosity *and* social distancing. Was there even a difference?

By then, though, spring break had become a sideshow. Reporters were focused on New York City, where a disaster that dwarfed the crises in Wuhan and northern Italy appeared to be unfolding.

7

Following the Science

While the world hunkered down, scientists and physicians raced to understand the biological underpinnings of Sars-Cov-2. They hoped to find the virus's Achilles' heel—or at the least reduce the suffering of Covid patients and increase their odds for survival.

The effort began in earnest on January 11, with the publication of the complete genome for Sars-Cov-2—the basic building blocks of the virus. The release of the genome ended any doubts that the cause of the illness sweeping Wuhan was in fact a coronavirus similar to the original SARS.

The Sars-Cov-2 genome consisted of a single strand of RNA containing almost thirty thousand nucleotides, each of which was one of four tiny molecules—adenine, cytosine, guanine, or uracil, known by the letters A, C, G, and U. The tens of thousands of nucleotides were linked together one by one to form the entire strand.

The virus's genome could be written down, one letter after the next, each letter representing one nucleotide. To our eyes, the resulting text looked like nonsense:...GUCAACAAC....[1]

Yet the letters weren't nonsense. They were a code our bodies had the natural ability to decrypt. Just as the nucleotides in human DNA determine the color of a person's eyes, the nucleotides in the virus's RNA strand determined the exact structure of Sars-Cov-2.

The publication of the genome was a major step forward in the fight against the virus. Scientists everywhere could design diagnostic tests to detect it. On January 21, European researchers published the results of a test that they said could accurately find the new coronavirus.[2]

The test was called a PCR test, the letters standing for polymerase chain reaction. It looked for specific chains of nucleotides unique to Sars-Cov-2 and then used a complex chemical process to multiply those chains until they could be easily detected. In theory, the test was both specific and sensitive. In other words, it could find almost all Sars-Cov-2 infections but not be fooled by similar viruses.

Since its invention in 1984, PCR testing had become crucial to biotechnology research. Kary Mullis, its inventor, shared a Nobel Prize in Chemistry in 1993 for his work.[3] Scientists all over the world had experience with it. It immediately became the core test to find Covid cases.

The discovery of an accurate test was seen as a major breakthrough, giving authorities worldwide a chance to track the virus. Only later would the risks of using a test that could be tuned to find tiny amounts of virus become clear. But by then, PCR testing had become standard worldwide, despite its flaws.

The publication of the genome also allowed researchers to create detailed models that demonstrated what Sars-Cov-2 and its spike proteins looked like.

Nucleotides are clumped in groups of three, each clump telling our bodies to produce a specific type of amino acid. While the nucleotides in RNA and DNA contain the *information* necessary for life, the amino acids that they tell our bodies to produce are life itself. They form the basic structures of proteins that come together to make up not just viruses but all life on earth, including human beings.

All that complexity comes from combinations of just twenty different amino acids, each with a different chemical structure. The acids have names like arginine and lysine. Scientists represent each one with a different letter of the alphabet, such as R for arginine or K for lysine.

Three nucleotides are needed to code for each amino acid. So scientists knew the thirty thousand nucleotides in the virus's genome meant the virus itself consisted of nearly ten thousand amino acids. (A few of the nucleotides were junk that did not produce any amino acids.)

But unlike the thirty thousand nucleotides in the RNA of the virus, the ten thousand amino acids were not all linked together in one single structure. The nucleotides were sorted into different genes, and each gene coded for a different piece of the virus, such as the spike proteins that studded its shell.[4]

Those pieces were built one by one out of amino acids. The pieces then came together to make the entire virus. To understand how the virus would look and work, scientists had to figure out the shape the amino acids would make when they folded together to make the pieces. Then they needed to figure out how the pieces would come together to make the complete virus.

A generation ago, those questions were basically unanswerable. As the American Society for Biochemistry and Molecular Biology explains, "All proteins with the same sequence of amino acid building blocks fold into the same three-dimensional form, which optimizes the interactions between the amino acids. They do this within milliseconds, although they have **an astronomical number** of possible configurations available to them" [emphasis added].

But with the help of massive computing power, researchers have made great progress in predicting what the amino acid chains will look like when they fold together. Thus knowing the exact genome of Sars-Cov-2 enabled the scientists to model the structure of the entire virus—and most important, the spike proteins that stuck to its surface.

They almost immediately realized that the novel coronavirus was a serious threat. Its spike proteins merged with a receptor found on the surface of many human cells. The receptor was called ACE-2 (angiotensin-converting enzyme 2), which plays a role in regulating blood pressure. Physicians prescribe drugs called ACE inhibitors to help reduce blood pressure.

Scientists knew that lung cells had many ACE-2 receptors, a fact that helps explain why both the original SARS and Sars-Cov-2 did so much damage to the lungs. So did other cells, including the walls of blood vessels, called the endothelium.[5]

The widespread distribution of ACE-2 receptors meant that both SARS and Sars-Cov-2 could invade many different cells. Worse, scientists quickly learned that the Sars-Cov-2 spike protein bound to ACE-2 in a way that meant it could not be easily displaced.

In a paper published online on February 19, 2020, researchers at the University of Texas reported that the novel coronavirus "binds at least 10 times more tightly than the corresponding spike protein [of the original SARS]...to their common host cell receptor."[6] Equally worrisome, antibodies that helped neutralize the original SARS did not work against Sars-Cov-2. Other researchers would cite the paper more than four thousand times, an indication of its importance.

Researchers also quickly discovered that the virus's uncanny ability to bind with the ACE-2 receptor was no accident. To merge with human cells, the spike needed to change shape from a "pre-fusion" to a "post-fusion" structure.

But the spike protein couldn't change its shape on its own. It needed help from an outside source, a human enzyme called furin, located in the very cell it was attacking. The spike got that help by showing the furin enzyme a password of sorts. The "password" consisted of a specific group of four amino acids—called RRAR—in the spike. The RRAR password caused the furin enzyme to cut the spike and allow it to open.

Researchers realized the RRAR "password" on the spike protein, which they called the "furin cleavage site," was positioned nearly perfectly, at least as far as the virus was concerned.[7] The cleavage site opened the spike in a way that allowed the virus to attach to the ACE-2 receptor and merge with the cell and dump its RNA inside. Getting the RNA into our cells was the next step in the virus's process of copying itself.

They also realized that other coronaviruses in the same family as Sars-Cov-2 did not have a similar password, much less one positioned so well. That finding raised the question of why Sars-Cov-2 did.

A few scientists speculated openly whether the virus had been designed or modified in a laboratory. But most dismissed those questions as irrelevant, if not outright conspiratorial.[8] They insisted that the virus must have jumped to humans from a bat or some other animal—and that the "zoonotic host" would be identified soon enough.

"We stand together to strongly condemn conspiracy theories suggesting that COVID-19 does not have a natural origin," twenty-seven research scientists wrote in a letter to *The Lancet* in February 2020, not even two months after the virus had emerged.

Instead of worrying about the unusual features of Sars-Cov-2, scientists should simply "stand with our [Chinese] colleagues on the frontline." The letter chilled debate about the origins of the virus, tainting any scientist who raised questions as an anti-Asian conspiracy theorist.

In any case, once the virus had put its RNA into the cell, its work was nearly done. The viral RNA then hijacked a piece of cellular machinery called a ribosome. The ribosome translated the nucleotides in the viral RNA into the amino acids that would join together into new coronaviruses. As Thomas Rivers had realized almost a century before, viruses can't reproduce themselves. But they don't need to. Their hosts do the work for them.

Thus within months of the virus's emergence in China, researchers understood exactly how it replicated itself, as well as the importance of the spike protein, which became an immediate target for companies developing a vaccine.

But those gains did not translate into immediate help for Covid patients. Knowing *why* the spike protein was so dangerous did not mean physicians could stop its deadly work.

Patients came under attack in several ways. Many had problems breathing and needed supplemental oxygen or ventilator support. Others had more problems with blood clots, suffering deadly strokes or embolisms that blocked the flow of blood in their lungs.

The clots appeared to be one culprit behind a frightening aspect of Covid. Patients would appear to be improving, then sicken around the eighth day after being infected.[9] (Reliable statistics on how often the "second-week crash" occurred were hard to come by. But the media eagerly reported on the phenomenon, probably because it made Covid seem especially dangerous.)

Still other patients saw their immune systems go into overdrive, with a severe inflammatory response that caused even more damage to their lungs and other organs than the virus itself.

In response, doctors tried dozens of therapies. The first to gain wide attention was an anti-malarial drug called hydroxychloroquine, or HCQ. In 2005, researchers had found that chloroquine, a related compound, inhibited the original SARS in laboratory tests. It appeared to reduce SARS's ability to fuse with the ACE-2 receptor.[10]

That finding led physicians to offer Covid patients both chloroquine and HCQ, a closely related but less toxic compound. As early as February 19, Chinese doctors reported that chloroquine had shown "apparent efficacy in treatment of COVID-19 associated pneumonia."[11]

Other doctors were less convinced. They warned that chloroquine and HCQ could cause heart irregularities, making them particularly unsuitable for treating Covid patients.

Then President Trump became involved, repeatedly speaking positively of HCQ's potential. The drug suddenly became a pawn in the larger battle between Trump and the media over Trump's response to the coronavirus.[12] Because Trump had supported it, a shocking number of reporters and scientists seemed almost to *want* the drug to fail.

In May 2020, *The Lancet*, a top medical journal, published a paper that purported to show HCQ not only did not work but might actually be dangerous. "Antimalarial drug touted by President Trump is linked to increased risk of death in coronavirus patients, study says," the *Washington Post* reported.[13]

Independent researchers quickly raised questions about how researchers could have gotten access to the patient databases that supposedly formed the core of the study. Less than two weeks later, *The Lancet* was forced to retract the report after its authors could not prove that their data actually existed.[14]

Nonetheless, the controversy about HCQ, and the lack of clear evidence that the drug helped, soured many physicians on it. The next supposed magic bullet was remdesivir, a potent anti-viral drug originally developed as a treatment for hepatitis C. While hydroxychloroquine helped block the coronavirus from attaching to the ACE-2 receptor, remdesivir worked against the virus by directly attacking its RNA strand.

Remdesivir was not yet approved for any use in early 2020. And it could be given only to hospitalized patients because it carried a risk of serious liver damage.

Still, Fauci and other federal officials considered remdesivir promising enough that they immediately fast-tracked it for a clinical trial.[15] In April 2020, the National Institutes of Health reported that the trial had shown remdesivir "accelerates recovery from advanced COVID-19."[16] Patients given remdesivir and standard treatments were hospitalized for eleven days on average. Those given only the standard treatments were hospitalized for fifteen.

An excited Fauci told reporters that remdesivir would become the new "standard of care" for coronavirus patients. "What it [the study] has proven is a drug can block this virus," he said.[17]

But when the full results were published weeks later, they showed that Fauci had overestimated the drug's value. Although remdesivir might help some patients, the findings made clear the drug would neither slow the epidemic nor significantly reduce deaths.[18] Even in the United States, remdesivir wound up being given to only about half of all hospitalized Covid patients.[19]

Still, the treatment turned into a bonanza for Gilead Sciences, its maker. Gilead earned over $4 billion from remdesivir in the first nine months after it began selling the drug.

Besides looking for medicines to attack the virus directly, physicians tried drugs intended to reduce the "inflammatory cascade" that killed many patients.

Our immune systems try to defeat viruses by destroying the cells in our body that they have invaded. Unfortunately, aggressive immune responses can sometimes do more damage than the original virus. To tamp the immune system, doctors gave patients "monoclonal antibodies" such as tocilizumab, which binds to proteins active in the immune system and helps to negate their effects.

As with so much else around Covid research and treatment, monoclonal antibodies stood at the edge of a medical frontier that hardly existed a generation ago. Traditional pharmaceutical drugs such as aspirin are small, simple chemicals. They can be made cheaply in factories and taken in pill form.

Monoclonal antibodies are different. They are grown in specially engineered cells and must be given as infusions because they are much larger molecules. They are often far more expensive than traditional small-molecule drugs, and they can have serious side effects. But they can also help treat previously untreatable diseases. And the theory of giving patients immunosuppressive drugs made sense.

So doctors had high hopes for tocilizumab and similar antibodies.

But they proved to be another disappointment, rarely helping patients. A paper published in early 2021 showed that patients treated with tocilizumab were just as likely to die as those who did not receive the treatment.[20]

Along with the antibodies, physicians tried injectable steroids, which are broad and potent anti-inflammatories. And on June 16, 2020, a large British trial called RECOVERY reported that an old and inexpensive steroid called dexamethasone had reduced deaths in patients on ventilators by 36 percent—an amazing finding.[21]

Including other groups of patients, dexamethasone cut mortality by 17 percent—saving one person out of every six who received it. The finding made it the first drug to be proven to save the lives of Covid patients. The news was cause for cheer.

Yet even the dexamethasone report came with an asterisk. While the United States had more Covid cases and deaths than any other country, the dexamethasone trial not been conducted here. Large clinical trials such as RECOVERY could efficiently try several different treatments at once and had no inherent bias towards newer, more expensive medicines. But the United States instead had hundreds of trials competing for patients, mostly run by drug companies focused on finding expensive new treatments.

Fauci could have encouraged the National Institutes of Health to focus on examining older off-patent medicines such as HCQ—or even more basic interventions, such as encouraging people to take vitamin D. Instead, he focused on finding shiny new drugs such as remdesivir.

Without a silver bullet that could defeat the virus, physicians were reduced to offering "supportive care." In essence, they managed patients' symptoms, trying to keep them alive until their bodies could defeat the virus on their own.

Ventilators—machines that breathed for patients who could not—quickly became a crucial tool in the fight. Physicians in China used ventilators aggressively. By early March, physicians in Italy had followed suit.

As a letter to a journal published by the Society of Critical Care Medicine would later explain, "Experts from China, Europe, and the United States supported a strategy of intubating patients early under the premise that early intubation allowed for more controlled circumstances and would provide superior lung protection.[22]

The heavy use of ventilators, which were in limited supply, was one crucial reason that Neil Ferguson and other modelers became so concerned that coronavirus patients might overrun hospitals. Even the best-equipped hospitals do not keep huge numbers of ventilators in

reserve. And using ventilators properly requires highly trained pulmon-
ologists, nurses, and respiratory specialists.

But the early use of ventilators wasn't meant to help only the patients.

Medical staff weren't immune from the panic sweeping the world.
Doctors didn't know exactly how transmissible the virus might be, or
how dangerous. Even if the virus's risks were concentrated among the
elderly, it had sickened and killed some people treating it. On March 18,
an Italian physician died only days after warning that Italy was short on
protective gear.[23]

The specter of health system collapse also loomed, if too many
physicians and nurses were sickened or died—or became too afraid to
work. In a grim piece titled "We're Failing Doctors" in *The Atlantic*
(more to come on *The Atlantic*, which would soon take a unique position in the American coronavirus media ecosystem), an emergency room
physician warned,

> No one is so fearless or stupid as to discount all risks. Physi-
> cians fled epidemics in ancient Greece, the black death in
> Europe, and the great influenza pandemic of 1918....
> At some point, the system could break, and we will all
> be gone.[24]

Medical staff knew that ventilators could help protect them. Intu-
bated patients no longer coughed. They also did not need to be treated
with nebulizing masks that put even more virus-filled droplets in the air.
And in addition to doing the patients' breathing for them, ventilators
could deliver doses of aerosolized steroids and other drugs.

A March 27, 2020, statement from the Food and Drug Administration offered a revealing look into the agency's priorities: "FDA takes
action to help increase U.S. supply of ventilators and respirators for
protection of health care workers, patients."[25]

Two days earlier, a young physician in New York had explained
exactly what the FDA meant, writing that her hospital was intubating

patients quickly "to avoid aerosolizing procedures to protect staff."[26] (She would later delete the tweet.)

Unfortunately, the overly aggressive use of ventilators backfired. Intubation should be a last-resort procedure. Ventilated patients are at high risk for bacterial lung infections. Most must be sedated with powerful opioids because ventilation is uncomfortable and painful. But those drugs carry their own dangers. And because sedated patients cannot move, they are at risk of developing bedsores.

Worse, many early Covid patients received high-pressure ventilation. The goal was to keep their lungs inflated, but the high pressure appears to have destroyed the lungs of some patients.

As early as April 8, only weeks after American hospitals began to see large numbers of Covid patients, Stat News reported:

> Some critical care physicians are questioning the widespread use of the breathing machines for Covid-19 patients, saying that large numbers of patients could instead be treated with less intensive respiratory support....
>
> The question is whether ICU physicians are moving patients to mechanical ventilators too quickly.[27]

Two weeks later, on April 22, the *Journal of the American Medical Association* published a stunning report from Northwell Health, a major hospital system in the New York City area.

Only 38 out of 1,151 patients who had been put on ventilators during the first Covid wave had been discharged, while 282 had died. The rest remained in the hospital, their prognosis grim. In other words, for ventilated patients for whom an outcome was available, almost 90 percent had died.[28] For patients under 65 years old, ventilation appeared to be especially likely to lead to bad outcomes.

The Northwell study sped the end of overly aggressive ventilation tactics, which were already going out of favor. But we may never know how many people—especially in New York City in March and April

2020—died because they were put on ventilators when they didn't need to be.

So it was that for nearly the entire first year of the pandemic, the two biggest treatment advances turned out to be a sixty-year-old steroid and "proning"—in other words, laying patients on their stomachs so they could breathe more easily.

Medicine is hard. The human body is wondrous and complicated. Truly rapid advances are rare. Worse, new treatments often turn out to have side effects that become obvious only with time.

But in March 2020, the desperation for a quick fix was palpable. Outside the laboratories and research centers, the world was panicking.

8

The Star of New York

A ndrew Cuomo's daily coronavirus briefings began on March 2, with a bland announcement: "Governor Cuomo Announces State Is Partnering with Hospitals to Expand Novel Coronavirus Testing Capacity."

That briefing began an amazing run for Cuomo, the fifty-sixth governor of New York. He would give press conferences for more than one hundred days straight, often wearing a polo shirt as he delivered the grim news of the day.

At age sixty-two, Cuomo had a deeply lined face, a full head of hair, and a well-earned reputation as controlling and misanthropic. In 2015, the *New Yorker* had opined, "It's sometimes said of certain politicians that they love humanity but hate people; Andrew Cuomo does not appear especially fond of either."[1]

In weeks, that reputation melted away. Cuomo, a Democratic governor in a highly liberal state, became a hero to reporters and many Americans. CNN and other networks carried his conferences live. He jousted openly with Trump and warned, "I operate on facts." By late

April almost 80 percent of New York voters approved of his performance, his highest rating ever.[2] Chelsea Handler and other celebrities
began referring to themselves as "Cuomosexuals."[3]

Yet the panic in New York City and its suburbs only grew as March
wore into April.

It is hard to overstate the importance of the fact that when the coronavirus arrived in the United States, it hit New York first and hardest.
The city and its suburbs held almost 20 million people, the richest and
densest population center in the United States. And New York was the
global media capital, home to broadcast and cable news networks and
the world's most important newspaper.

Cuomo briefly fought a New York City lockdown even after the
Imperial College report became public. "That cannot happen," he said
on March 17. "It cannot happen legally."[4]

Two days later, on March 19, he was equally emphatic: "I'm not
going to do it."[5]

The next day, March 20, he reversed course, announcing a statewide
"stay-at-home" order—as most governors preferred to call the lockdowns. Along with the California lockdown, a huge increase in the
number of new coronavirus cases in his state had forced Cuomo's hand.

The number of positive tests had risen from seven hundred to almost
eight thousand *in less than a week*. The state had nearly half of the cases
in the entire United States. Most were in New York City or its suburbs.

In its article reporting the lockdown, the *New York Times* sounded
an alarm:

> For weeks, as the coronavirus has spread across the globe,
> New York officials have warned that a surge of cases could
> overwhelm the state's health care system, jeopardizing thou-
> sands of patients.
>
> Now, it seems, the surge has arrived...the sharp increase
> is thrusting the medical system towards a crisis point, offi-
> cials said.[6]

That was Friday.

Two days later, on Sunday, March 22, Cuomo had even grimmer news. The number of people hospitalized in the state for Covid had *doubled* over the weekend, to more than two thousand. Most were in the city. And the projections were growing more dire by the day.

"April is going to be worse than March," New York City mayor Bill de Blasio told *Meet the Press*. "And I fear May will be worse than April."[7]

■   ■   ■

New York was the eye of the storm, but the fears that hospitals would be overwhelmed reached throughout the country, with the Associated Press reporting on March 13 on the "tremendous strain" hospitals were facing: "U.S. hospitals are setting up circus-like triage tents, calling doctors out of retirement, guarding their supplies of face masks and making plans to cancel elective surgery as they brace for an expected onslaught of coronavirus patients."[8]

Few readers of panic-inducing reports like this were likely to know that triage tents were a standard feature of public health planning, utilized in bad flu years as recently as 2018. In fact, a January 18, 2018, *Time* magazine article on the bad flu that year is eerily similar to the March 13, 2020, Associated Press Covid story: "The 2017–2018 influenza epidemic is sending people to hospitals and urgent-care centers in every state, and medical centers are responding with extraordinary measures: asking staff to work overtime, setting up triage tents, restricting friends and family visits and canceling elective surgeries, to name a few."[9]

When some noticed a gap between the alarmist reports in the press and the reality at their local hospitals, there was a brief fad of posting photos and videoclips of empty hospital parking lots and deserted-looking emergency room entrances on social media. The hashtag #FilmYourHospital got enough traction that the fact-checkers at PolitiFact felt the need to declare, "No, empty hospital beds do not indicate COVID-19 is 'fake crisis.'"[10]

Covid victims were seemingly everywhere, feeding the panic. When the *New York Times* reported on March 27 that Alan Finder, a former reporter for the *Times*, had died of Covid at seventy-two,[11] the subtext was hard to miss. *It could have been one of us; it could have been you.*

The same day, the playwright Terrence McNally died at eighty-one of complications from Covid in Florida. "Rage for Terrence McNally," thundered the headline of the obituary in the *New Yorker*, which focused on McNally's role as a chronicler of gay life and HIV. "Another decade, another plague. McNally deserved better. So do we all."[12] It would fall to other publications to note that McNally had suffered from lung cancer and chronic obstructive pulmonary disease.[13]

In densely populated neighborhoods in Brooklyn and Queens, hundreds of people lined up outside hospitals for coronavirus tests. Inside, emergency rooms and intensive care units filled to capacity, and sometimes past. The city's municipal hospitals, which functioned as safety-net facilities for poor New Yorkers, faced the most stress.[14]

On Friday, March 25, the *Times* carried a dire report focused on one of those hospitals—Elmhurst, in Queens. "13 Deaths in a Day: An 'Apocalyptic' Coronavirus Surge at an N.Y.C. Hospital," the headline ran. (Putting the word "apocalyptic" in quotation marks was an old headline writer's trick. It meant someone in the article had used the word, so the *Times* was not taking responsibility for it.)

The article portrayed a hospital and an entire system on the edge of collapse:

> In several hours on Tuesday, Dr. Ashley Bray performed chest compressions at Elmhurst Hospital Center on a woman in her 80s, a man in his 60s and a 38-year-old who reminded the doctor of her fiancé. All had tested positive for the coronavirus and had gone into cardiac arrest. All eventually died....
>
> Earlier this week, 60 coronavirus patients had been admitted [at Elmhurst] but were still in the emergency room. One man waited almost 60 hours for a bed last week....

Like other hospitals, Elmhurst has come perilously close to running out of ventilators several times; other hospitals have replenished its supply.

Pulling back to the broader crisis, the article warned that all 1,800 intensive care beds in New York City would be full within days. The report did have one positive note, though. Although the number of Covid patients hospitalized in the city had topped 3,900, the rate of increase had slowed sharply from the previous weekend—from doubling every two days to every five.[15]

By March 30, though, the *Times* was painting an almost hopeless picture. A quote from a nurse in a piece headlined "Nurses Die, Doctors Fall Sick and Panic Rises on Virus Front Lines" captured the tone: "'I feel like we're all just being sent to slaughter,' said Thomas Riley, a nurse at Jacobi Medical Center in the Bronx, who has contracted the virus, along with his husband."

(Only much later in the article did the reporter note that Mr. Riley and his husband began to recover from their Covid infections within days of becoming ill.)[16]

The last paragraph of the article—what reporters call the kicker, often a pithy summary—quoted a nurse saying, "We all think we're screwed."

By then, the *Times* and other media outlets were focused on the desperate shortage of hospital beds and ventilators New York was supposedly about to face. "As many as one million patients could need to use one of the machines over the course of the outbreak," the *Times* reported on March 25. Hospitals in New York "are already on the verge of running out, Gov. Andrew Cuomo said this week."[17] That day, he forecast a potential need for thirty thousand ventilators.

The next day, the *Times* reported that New York–Presbyterian, one of the city's most prestigious hospitals, had begun sharing ventilators between patients. The story carried a stunning headline: "'The Other Option Is Death': New York Starts Sharing of Ventilators." It called the move "a desperate measure that could help alleviate a shortage of the critical breathing machines."[18]

Only near the end of the article did the *Times* acknowledge the reality that "the hospital has not yet run out of ventilators." In fact, the hospital had used the shared ventilators *as an experiment* to see if sharing would be possible. A total of six patients were placed on three ventilators for two days each.[19]

The panic worsened further on March 27, when Cuomo raised his estimates of the shortage to *40,000* ventilators. That figure dwarfed the available supply not just in the state but nationally. The entire federal emergency reserve of ventilators totaled only about 12,700 in mid-March.[20]

"All the predictions say you could have an apex needing 140,000 [hospital] beds and about 40,000 ventilators," Cuomo told reporters that day in Manhattan. "I don't operate here on opinion. I operate on facts and on data and on numbers and on projections."[21]

On Thursday, April 2, Cuomo warned that New York's stockpile had fallen to 2,200 ventilators, which might last only 6 more days.

Reporters warned the coming shortages might lead to rationing, forcing physicians to decide which patients would have a chance to live and which would face certain death. "Ventilator Shortages Loom as States Ponder Rules for Rationing," National Public Radio explained April 3. "The specter of rationing is most imminent in New York City, where the virus is spreading rapidly and overwhelming hospitals with patients....If there are not enough ventilators...hospitals in New York would need to begin making excruciating decisions."[22]

If the news in the *Times* and other outlets was grim, the tone on Twitter—especially in tweets from people living in New York City—was far worse.

On March 24, Molly Jong-Fast, a Brooklyn writer with hundreds of thousands of followers, predicted that between 2 and 7 percent of Americans, or twenty-three million people, would die of the virus. (She has since deleted the tweet.)[23]

Dr. Tom Frieden, the former head of the Centers for Disease Control, wrote on March 29, "I hear sirens in NYC all day.... Words & tears cannot express the tragedy."[24]

The peak of the Twitter panic arguably came on April 6, when Mark Levine—who wasn't just a New York City councilman but the *chair of the Health Committee*—warned that the city was about to bury corpses in its parks.

"Soon we'll start 'temporary interment.' This likely will be done by using a NYC park for burials (yes you read that right)," he tweeted.[25] "Trenches will be dug for 10 caskets in a line."

Other city officials quickly responded that Levine was wrong. The tweet was "totally false," Mayor de Blasio said. Levine walked back his tweet, saying that using parks for burials was merely a contingency plan. Still, even the false specter of parks being turned into graveyards led to another wave of articles with headlines such as "New York City Has Contingency Plan for Temporary Burials of COVID-19 Dead."[26]

New York seemed to be spiraling out of control.

Local, state, and federal governments hastily built field hospitals across the city to cope with the expected tsunami of patients. The largest was at the Jacob Javits Convention Center in Manhattan. It opened March 30 with the capacity to care for 1,200 patients and the ability to quickly expand to almost 3,000 beds.[27] On the same day, the U.S. Navy brought a 1,000-bed hospital ship, the USNS *Comfort,* to New York. A private charity called Samaritan's Purse even opened a small field hospital in Central Park, near Mount Sinai Hospital.[28]

"The hospitals are overrun and in desperate need of extra capacity," the charity's press release reported.

Not just in New York but around the country, the political-journalistic class all knew who was responsible for the unfolding disaster: Donald John Trump.

By late March, the fear and anger were aimed as much at Trump as the virus itself. The narratives were intertwined. The virus will devastate us. The president has failed us. The most apocalyptic predictions nearly all came from people on the left. Some of them had warned against anti-Chinese hysteria in January and February and downplayed the threat of the virus. Now they felt differently.

On March 23, Steve Schmidt—a one-time Republican strategist who had left the GOP to found the anti-Trump Lincoln Project—tweeted: "Trump is incompetent, dishonest and profoundly indecent. His staggering incapacity for moral leadership in this unprecedented moment is hard to overstate. His empty boasting, dishonesty, blame gaming, lack of empathy and fragile ego are a deadly combination of traits right now."[29]

Schmidt had more than 1 million followers; the tweet was liked or retweeted more than 115,000 times.

On March 29, Florida senator Marco Rubio chided journalists for their apparent "glee & delight" in the rising coronavirus case count. Michelle Goldberg, a *New York Times* opinion writer with over one hundred thousand followers, fired back: "Journalists are concentrated in cities that are being ravaged by a plague that could have been better contained with a competent president. They're lonely and scared and reporting while homeschooling their kids. No one feels glee or delight. Some of us feel white hot rage."[30]

The next day, a professor at Medill, a top journalism school, tweeted to his tens of thousands of followers that he had attended an online funeral for someone who had died of the virus. He went on: "Fuck all of this. Fuck COVID-19. Fuck Trump letting it rip thru our most vulnerable."[31]

■   ■   ■

Trump did not do himself any favors, of course. He repeatedly made foolish and sometimes false statements about Covid.

"It's going to disappear," he said on February 28. "One day, it's like a miracle, it will disappear." A week later, he promised that "anyone who wants a test can get one," a patently false statement. And he repeatedly promoted hydroxychloroquine.[32]

But his most embarrassing gaffe came at an April 23 press conference, when he suggested rather incoherently that ultraviolet light or a disinfectant might cure Covid:

> Whether it's ultraviolet or just very powerful light...supposing you brought the light inside the body, which you can do either through the skin or in some other way, and I think you said you're going to test that, too. It sounds interesting. And then I see the disinfectant, where it knocks it out in a minute. One minute. And is there a way we can do something like that, by injection inside or almost a cleaning. Because you see it gets in the lungs, and it does a tremendous number on the lungs.[33]

Media outlets around the world wasted no time ridiculing the suggestion that injecting a disinfectant might cure the coronavirus.

"Outcry after Trump Suggests Injecting Disinfectant as Treatment," the BBC reported.[34]

Not Trump's finest moment, to be sure.

Yet on the most important point of all, Trump was right—right from almost the very beginning.

In a March 4 phone interview with Sean Hannity of Fox News, Trump said he believed the death rate from Covid would be "a fraction of 1 percent," as opposed to the 3 or 4 percent being reported at the time:

> This is just my hunch, but based on a lot of conversations with a lot of people that do this, because a lot of people will have this and it is very mild....
>
> So if, you know, we have thousands or hundreds of thousands of people that get better, just by, you know, sitting around....
>
> But again, they don't—they don't know about the easy cases because the easy cases don't go to the hospital, they

don't report to doctors or the hospital in many cases...personally, I would say the number is way under 1 percent.[35]

The usual suspects jumped on Trump for his prediction.

"Trump floats his own coronavirus hunches," *Politico* reported. "The president contradicts public health experts' statements on death rate, contagion."[36]

The *Washington Post* thundered, "Trump's habit of fudging inconvenient numbers enters dangerous territory."[37]

But Trump's optimistic view would be borne out. The Covid death rate turned out to be well under 1 percent. Further, Trump was not just right; he was right for the right reason.

Data from Italy and elsewhere showed that most people infected with Sars-Cov-2 recovered without any medical treatment, even a doctor's visit.[38] In other words, Trump had intuitively understood the crucial distinction between the "infection fatality rate"—deaths compared to the overall number of people who were infected with the coronavirus—and the "case fatality rate"—deaths compared to people who became sick enough to be counted as Covid cases.

But reporters never acknowledged when Trump was right, only when he was wrong. They also understood by late March that the coronavirus had become a political disaster for him.

Though his reelection was hardly a lock, Trump had been in a strong position in early 2020. Betting markets viewed him as a favorite to be reelected.[39]

At the time, the Democratic Party was suffering through a center left vs. hard left split. Its progressive wing viewed Joe Biden, the presumptive nominee, as out of touch. Republicans, in contrast, had come together around Trump.

Meanwhile, strong economic growth was helping Trump among independents. Not only was the stock market at an all-time high in February 2020, but the U.S. unemployment rate had fallen to 3.5 percent, its lowest level in more than fifty years. Unemployment among

African Americans and Hispanics had reached the lowest levels ever recorded.[40]

The coronavirus crashed the economy overnight. By mid-March, the question was not whether the United States would face a recession, but how deep and how long it would be. Unemployment soared to 14.8 percent in April. Suddenly more than one in seven Americans could not find work, the highest unemployment rate since the Depression. Trump's economic advantage had vanished.

Further, the coronavirus crisis could not have been more ill-suited to Trump's personality. Contrary to what the left insisted, Trump did have strengths as a leader—notably, a willingness to trust his instincts and take bold action.

But he had serious weaknesses too—narcissism, a lack of empathy, and a failure to master details. The United States and world needed reassurance in March 2020. Trump could be entertaining. He was never reassuring. He didn't know how to be. Instead, he resorted to his usual bluff and bluster and picked pointless fights with reporters—all of which was increasingly out of touch with the nation's mood, a mood the media eagerly fed.

Thus, while governors such as Cuomo benefited from the equivalent of a wartime bounce and saw their approval ratings reach the high seventies or even the eighties, Trump's approval ratings rose only slightly in mid-March and then faded.

And so, whether because they genuinely feared the virus, believed it was kryptonite to Trump's chances of reelection, or both, reporters attacked Trump relentlessly. Meanwhile, they held up Fauci as the real hero of the epidemic.

"How Anthony Fauci Became America's Doctor," the *New Yorker* explained in its April 10 edition. "At White House briefings, it has regularly fallen to Fauci to gently amend Trump's absurdities, half-truths, and outright lies."

Fauci was supposedly nonpartisan. Elevating him gave the attacks on Trump an apolitical gloss. And on those rare occasions when the media credited the federal government for doing something right, Fauci, not Trump, received the credit.

In late March, the attacks centered on the supposed ventilator shortage. Reporters pilloried Trump for failing to invoke the Korean War–era Defense Production Act to force manufacturers to build ventilators immediately.

"Trump Resists Using Wartime Law to Get, Distribute Coronavirus Supplies," NPR reported on March 25.[41] Six days later, the *New York Times* said, "Wartime Production Law Has Been Invoked Routinely, but Not with Coronavirus," part of a trend for coverage to skirt the line between news and opinion.[42]

Yet even as the media shrieked, physicians were warning that a shortage of the devices wasn't the problem. Even if the ventilators were needed, and it was not clear they would be, the bottleneck would be in training enough doctors, nurses, and respiratory therapists to run them safely.

The *Times* based its March 25 estimate of 1 million Covid patients needing ventilators on a study from the Society of Critical Care Medicine, which used a worst-case figure of 960,000 based on 5 million hospitalized Covid patients. Yet the same study reported that hospitals nationwide could handle only an extra 26,000 to 56,000 ventilators on top of their existing stockpile of 200,000. "The rate limiting-feature is the absence of the requisite number of respiratory therapists to manage the ventilators," the study found.[43]

In other words, no matter how many ventilators Trump ordered manufacturers to make, without trained staff, they would be nothing but furniture.

Within weeks, it would be clear that the ventilator shortage was mythical. By April 5, states on the West Coast offered to send extra ventilators to New York—a step their governors would never have taken had they believed their own hospitals might need the machines.[44] By April 15, *New York itself* was shipping out ventilators to other states.[45]

A week later, the bombshell Northwell Health study in the *Journal of the American Medical Association* showed that ventilators had not only not been lifesavers but had also likely killed some patients.

But news organizations simply ignored the fact they had been wrong about ventilators. When the ventilator shortage didn't materialize, they moved on to bash Trump over backlogs in coronavirus testing.

Over and over, they claimed that Trump's failures had caused tens or even hundreds of thousands of preventable deaths.

Yet the anti-Trump narrative was largely untrue.

Not because Trump has much to brag about in terms of his early response to the coronavirus. He could have done more to ready the United States for Covid in February. His only aggressive action, the travel ban from China, made at most a minor difference. The virus had already reached American soil by then. In any case, in an age of worldwide travel, banning travel from China—while allowing it from Europe—hardly mattered.

So why was the narrative wrong?

In part because Trump's powers were surprisingly limited. One hundred and sixty years after the Civil War, American federalism remained strong. Unless Trump declared martial law, he could not have locked down the entire country even if he had wanted to. Individual governors had that power.

A similar dynamic would play out in the debate over school re-openings, where Trump was unequivocally in the right, but where he turned out to be almost powerless.

But more important, the critics never clearly explained what Trump should have done in February or March, or how he could realistically have contained the virus. Many of them had *opposed* the Chinese travel ban. They said Trump should have encouraged the CDC to make tests more widely available in February. Those steps might have helped on the margins.

But studies of blood donors would later show the coronavirus had reached the United States by December 2019, even before the Chinese sounded their first public alarm.[46] Given the speed with which the virus could spread when conditions favored it, that fact strongly suggests that any efforts to test and trace infections would have been hopeless. European countries where lockdowns began sooner and were stricter had even *more* deaths than the United States in the spring of 2020.

In fact, by summer 2021—more than a year after the epidemic began—overall coronavirus death rates in the United States had turned out to be nearly the same as those of big Western European countries, with the exception of Germany. The death rate in the United States was slightly lower than in Italy, slightly higher than in Britain, Spain, or France.

Those countries had slightly older populations. But the United States had higher rates of morbid obesity, a major risk factor. The death rates suggested that Trump's policies hadn't made much difference either way.

Most important, Trump's instincts about the virus were *right*. As he told Hannity in March 2020, death rates from the coronavirus appeared much higher early on than they were.

This problem is common when epidemiologists estimate risks. Knowing how many people recover without help is crucial to estimate the dangers of a new disease. But that fact can be very difficult to know.

Sars-Cov-2 generally killed people who were either over seventy-five, severely ill, or both. Finding healthy people under fifty who have died of Covid is rare. Finding such people under the age of thirty is nearly impossible. The flu is more dangerous. In reality, the virus posed only a minor risk to most people. Covid wasn't truly a threat to *society*—as opposed to a danger to some elderly and vulnerable people.

But Trump never figured out how to explain those facts without sounding callous. When he talked about having prevented two million deaths, he only called attention to the deaths that *had* occurred. When he bragged about the wonderful job he had done, he seemed foolish and out of touch, as if he didn't care about the people who had died. And whenever he made a mistake, the media made sure everyone heard about it.

Even as they attacked Trump, media outlets lionized Democratic governors such as Cuomo, despite the massive death toll in New York. Over time, the media's negative picture of the federal response, even as reporters largely ignored the failures in Democrat-run states, would appear increasingly calculated—and effective.

9

Twisting the Kaleidoscope

I can't remember exactly when I first read about the mysterious virus plaguing Wuhan.

It had to have been mid-January 2020, though. By the time China locked down Hubei province on January 22, I'd developed a healthy (or unhealthy) curiosity about what was happening.

Why? I had decent excuses. I'd covered the drug industry for several years during the aughts as a reporter for the *New York Times*. Along the way, I had learned a fair bit about medical research. I'd always been interested in epidemics and bioterrorism, too. My first novel, published in 2006, featured a detailed look at how terrorists might use a plague against the United States.

But really, why did any of us get interested, when the virus was so far away, the videos so hard to trust? If we're being honest, it was for the same reason we read about the Black Death or watch movies about asteroids hitting the earth.

The prospect of mass sickness, societal collapse, and ultimately human extinction—no matter how far-fetched—concentrates the mind.

End-of-days cults exist for a reason. It's so much more exciting to believe you'll see the apocalypse firsthand than to face the harsh reality that, in the words of Charles de Gaulle, the cemeteries are filled with indispensable people. Sooner or later you, too, will be one of them.

So I read everything I could. And I waited for the world to panic. And waited.

Near the end of January, with the Chinese building field hospitals in Wuhan, I asked a retired hedge fund manager I knew why big investors didn't seem more concerned. He pointed out that the original SARS had petered out after generating frightening headlines. The 2009 swine flu had come and gone without a trace. Most people expected the same this time, he said. Panic rarely paid off.

Fair enough. Still, I was concerned enough about the virus that I considered postponing that mid-February trip to New Zealand. I was in a hotel near the southern end of New Zealand's South Island—a long way from the rest of the world—when I heard that Italy had suddenly locked down towns near Milan. The news struck me as world-changing. *Italy? Weren't we supposed to be worried about South Korea and Japan?*

We had obviously lost any chance to contain the virus within China. Like Neil Ferguson, I feared the worst.

On February 22, I tweeted this warning:

> Coronavirus is coming. It's highly infectious. It doesn't have a cure or a vaccine. It badly sickens 1 in 5 people who get it. It kills—well, we don't know, maybe 1 in 50. And we can't contain it. It is going to roll around the globe in waves.[1]

Five of the seven sentences in this prediction would prove correct.

But the two that were wrong, the two in the middle, mattered far more. Coronavirus didn't "badly sicken" 20 percent of the people who got it. It didn't kill 2 percent. On a worldwide basis, both estimates were off by a factor of almost ten—the difference between a pandemic that could rock the world and a very bad but manageable flu season.

At the time, though, the numbers seemed to be in line with what the data from China showed. If anything, I thought I was being conservative. And even a 1 percent death rate would mean that more than 3 million Americans and 80 million people worldwide might die.

When I got back from New Zealand, I loaded up on non-perishable food, basic first aid gear, and cleaning supplies for our family. In the back corner of a Walmart, I found a few precious N95 respirators and snapped them up.

My wife Jackie, a psychiatrist, viewed my growing alarm with some amusement. (Like all psychiatrists, Jackie is a fully trained medical doctor.) She had been born in Canada and lived there during the original SARS epidemic. She remembered how quickly SARS had vanished. She had also just started a tough new job running an inpatient ward at a big hospital. Taking care of real patients with real problems left her little time to indulge in Covid fantasies.

After March 11, though, neither of us could ignore the fact that Covid was about to upend our lives. School closures appeared imminent. Our nannies were about to quit, leaving me to watch over our infant and two school-age kids. (I feel compelled to explain that one nanny worked two days a week and the other three—we did not have two full-time nannies.)

I should have panicked that week, as Europe shut down and the virus came to New York. Instead, as I watched the fear grow, I went the other way.

Journalists fall into two categories. Inside reporters are good at getting powerful people to talk to them. Outside reporters prefer to dig up facts those people would rather not discuss at all. I had always been an outside reporter, naturally contrarian and cynical. I was comfortable poking through databases and papers and reaching my own conclusions.

And I started to wonder: Did shutting the economy really make sense? What would happen to people forced to stay in tiny apartments as the weather warmed up? Everything I had read suggested that kids weren't at huge risk, so why were we in such a rush to close schools? My skepticism ramped up day by day.

On March 16, the Imperial College report, Neil Ferguson's masterpiece, came out. I read it that night. Reread it. Reread it again. I kept coming back to the table on page 5, the one that had estimates of the infection fatality ratios by age.

At the top of the table:

Age 0–9, 0.002%—2 deaths in 100,000 infections.

Age 10–19, 0.006%—6 deaths in 100,000 infections.

(Both of those estimates were probably high.)

At the bottom:

Age 80+, 9.3%–9,300 deaths in 100,000 infections.

I had known the elderly were more vulnerable to Covid than the young. I hadn't had any idea how *much* more. This gold-standard report said the oldest people were *thousands* of times as likely to die as the youngest.

I could almost feel the scales dropping from my eyes.

I'd had similar experiences as a reporter before. In 2004, investigating the stun guns called Tasers for the *Times*, I discovered a document showing their manufacturer had researched the full effect of its electrical charges on only one pig and five dogs before decreeing the weapons "non-lethal."

What? You're telling police officers these can't kill people on the basis of experiments on six animals?

In 2017, after Jackie repeatedly told me to read the scientific research about cannabis and mental illness, I finally did. I found that the National Academies of Sciences, Engineering, and Medicine (NASEM) had said in a five-hundred-page report, "Cannabis use is likely to increase the risk of developing schizophrenia and other psychoses; the higher the use, the greater the risk."[2]

NASEM was chartered to offer the federal government advice on complex scientific questions. *So as the United States moved to legalize cannabis, how come no one had even heard about this report, much less read it?*

Both times, those documents didn't mark the end of my research. They came closer to the beginning. But they twisted my internal kaleidoscope. They helped me *see*.

So did the Imperial College report.

As I read it, I wondered why the media weren't explaining that Sars-Cov-2 was far riskier to older people than everyone else. Why we weren't focusing on protecting the old rather than locking down the young. And how a virus that posed at most a minor threat to anyone healthy under fifty could really be the worldwide menace we'd been told.

I had learned firsthand that the media couldn't be trusted to tell the truth if it was ideologically inconvenient. When Simon & Schuster published *Tell Your Children*—my book about the psychiatric health risks of cannabis—in 2019, I expected the marijuana industry to pummel me.

But I felt confident that major news outlets would give the book a fair hearing. After all, *Tell Your Children* drew on evidence from the world's most respected medical journals. And I thought the investigative work I had done at the *Times* would give me credibility. I was no right-wing apologist. I even acknowledged that one could understand the risks and still favor legalization.

Further, just before the book appeared, Malcolm Gladwell drew on it at length in a *New Yorker* article about cannabis. He said that I had a "reporter's tenacity, a novelist's imagination, and an outsider's knack for asking intemperate questions" and that my findings were "disturbing," even though he didn't necessarily agree with them.[3]

That take struck me as fair. I assumed that other reporters would have a similar response. Instead, top media outlets—including the *Times*—either mocked or ignored *Tell Your Children*. NPR stations scheduled and then canceled interviews. They were unwilling even to discuss the potential dangers of cannabis.

The response surprised and disappointed me. When I had worked at the *Times*, it had leaned left. But it had been committed to accuracy and truth-telling above all. Now it seemed to have abandoned any pretense of being non-partisan.

I could already see Covid coverage falling into the same trap.

■   ■   ■

On March 25, Neil Ferguson spoke to the British Parliament's Science and Technology Committee. Ferguson gave his testimony remotely. He was actually infected with the coronavirus at the time; he had contracted it a week before and was recovering.

"It was like rather bad flu," he told the committee. "For a couple of days it was quite unpleasant, but I think I am basically on the mend now."[4] (The world would subsequently learn just how "on the mend" he had been.)

But Ferguson's firsthand report on Covid was the *least* interesting part of his testimony.

Nine days before, his Imperial College paper had warned that, without immediate action to shut society, the coronavirus would kill more than a half-million Britons. Worse, even *with* school closings and social distancing, hospitals would be overwhelmed through at least mid-May. Mitigation measures would have to last at least three months, then cycle on and off. Still, a quarter-million people were likely to die. Only "suppression" could keep deaths down. Only a vaccine could permanently solve the crisis.

Ferguson's report had used clear, direct language:

> The interventions need to remain in place for as much of the epidemic period as possible....
>
> Given that mitigation is unlikely to be a viable option without overwhelming healthcare systems, suppression is

likely necessary in countries able to implement the intensive controls required.[5]

But on March 25—with the United Kingdom having entered lockdown only days before—Ferguson offered very different predictions. The British hospital system would *not* be overrun. The number of patients in intensive care would peak and begin to fall within three weeks, he said.

Ferguson had changed his view on lockdowns, too. "We clearly cannot lock down the country for a year," he told the committee. In fact, "in three or four weeks' time" he expected "to replace the current regime [lockdown]."

But even without a prolonged quarantine, Ferguson now predicted the number of people who would die from Covid in Britain "would probably be unlikely to exceed about 20,000." Up to two-thirds of those people were so sick they might have died by the end of 2020 in any case, he said.[6]

Not 500,000.

Not 250,000.

Not 100,000.

Twenty thousand.

Ferguson had just reduced his death estimates for the coronavirus— the same estimates that barely a week before had shocked the world into lockdowns—*by more than 90 percent.*

The testimony generated a few articles in British newspapers. "UK has enough intensive care units for coronavirus, expert predicts," the *New Scientist* reported.[7]

"Two thirds of coronavirus victims may have died this year anyway, government adviser says," the *Telegraph* explained.

But no one in the United States seemed to notice or care about what Ferguson had said.

Until the morning of March 26, when I linked to the *New Scientist* article and tweeted, "This is a remarkable turn from Neil Ferguson...."

I'm not exaggerating when I say that tweet—actually a "thread" of five linked tweets—changed my life.

Over the next day it went viral. Elon Musk, the founder of Tesla, retweeted it. So did Donald Trump Jr. More than six million people saw it. Suddenly I was part of the political and scientific wars exploding over the coronavirus and lockdowns.

What I found so strange about the response to my thread was that I wasn't saying anything Ferguson hadn't said himself. Ferguson had seen new evidence about the coronavirus, evidence that it was spreading faster than he'd previously believed.

He said in his testimony that he believed the virus had an R of 3, meaning that each newly infected person went on to infect three other people. His previous estimates had been in the range of 2 to 2.5.

"What we have been seeing, though, in Europe...is a rate of growth of the epidemic that was faster than we expected from early data in China," he told the committee.

The difference may seem small, but even a small-seeming difference in the infection rate has large implications for a respiratory virus with a short infection cycle. Over a month, a single infection with an R of two can become fifty infections—but *five hundred* for a virus with an R of three.

And paradoxically, from the point of view of dangerousness, a higher R may be good news. Why?

To make the math simple, imagine that ten people are hospitalized with Covid over a month. If only *fifty* people are infected that month, the coronavirus has put one in five people of the people it infects in the hospital. But if *five hundred* have been infected, the virus has only caused one in fifty to be hospitalized.

More infections means the virus is *less* dangerous per infection.

Thus Ferguson had updated his prediction, as serious scientists should when they get new information. (Of course, they also have a responsibility to colleagues and the public to be transparent about the changes they're making.) His revised forecast was *good news*. When I retweeted it I expected people would be pleased.

I was wrong.

The only happy people were either conservatives such as Trump Jr. or coronavirus skeptics such as Musk. In the next few days, journalists from the *Financial Times* and elsewhere defended Ferguson. They claimed—with his support—that he had not changed his prediction, that the new forecast was consistent with the original March 16 Imperial College report.[8]

This argument was nonsense. Again, the original report had said that even a short-term lockdown would not reduce British deaths below 250,000.

I wish I didn't have to spend so much time on Neil Ferguson and his forecasts. They may seem like inside baseball. They aren't, though. And not just because Ferguson's initial report was so crucial to lockdowns, both in Britain and worldwide.

At the time, I didn't know much about Ferguson, including his long history of failed predictions. But I knew he was a crucial voice. The way reporters circled the wagons around him made clear to me that in spite—or maybe because—of Covid's importance, journalists would not be honest in reporting about it.

Health authorities had gone all in on efforts to stoke coronavirus hysteria, as the March 22 SAGE paper would reveal when it was ultimately released. Reporters were working hand in glove with government agencies to stoke fear in people at low risk, no matter if they had to lie to do so. They would attack anyone who offered facts that didn't fit their preferred narrative. They would even rewrite history, *history that was only ten days old*.

■   ■   ■

I could tell you I had to decide in March 2020 if I was ready to fight. I could tell you I carefully weighed the cost of potentially angering Simon & Schuster, and the personal hate I could already see I would face.

But I didn't.

In 2006, as a *Times* reporter, I was given access to files from Eli Lilly, a big drug company. They showed that Lilly's medicine Zyprexa caused terrible weight gain and even diabetes in many people who took it. Zyprexa was a drug given to the severely mentally ill—among the most vulnerable people around.

I wasn't supposed to have those documents. They were sealed under federal court order. I didn't care. I had a story that people needed to hear, facts they weren't getting elsewhere, facts that could help patients and doctors make better choices. The *Times* didn't care either. "Eli Lilly Said to Play Down Risk of Top Pill," read our front-page headline on December 17, 2006.[9]

The federal judge who had sealed the documents later called me "reprehensible" for my role in breaking the seal.[10]

It may have been my proudest moment at the paper.

March 2020 was no different.

Reporting wasn't a choice. It was an instinct.

10

My Father and Me

Yeah, I felt compelled to speak out. And I did.

Within weeks, Twitter had taken over my life.

The situation was not without its darkly comic side. The schools were closed in New York as everywhere else. Our kids were home. Our nannies—healthy women in their thirties who had worked for us for years—had given days of notice and disappeared.

And in late March, I found myself unwell. I had fever and shortness of breath that lasted more than a week. I had gone to a large party in Brooklyn in mid-March, as the virus swept through New York City. As a rule, I don't get sick—a three-day flu I had in 2019 stands out to me because I hadn't been laid up for years.

Whatever it was, this new bug stuck around. I lost ten pounds before I finally shucked it. To this day I don't know if I had Covid. I took an antibody test in late April and was shocked when it came back negative. But antibody tests are not always reliable.

Meanwhile, Jackie was working harder than ever. Her hospital had opened a unit for psychiatric patients infected with Covid—double winners in life's lottery. She volunteered to run it. I was proud of her fearlessness. But she seemed to get home later every day.

So it was that I found myself chasing three kids around the house, cleaning up the messes made by Callie, our seventy-pound semi-trained puppy, cooking more quesadillas than anyone should, wondering if I too had come down with coronavirus—all the while reading every paper I could find about hospitalizations, viral transmissibility, and epidemiology. I spent a lot of time with the baby in one hand and my phone in the other.

The situation was...not ideal. One fine spring afternoon I decided to put the baby in the stroller to get some air. I'd walk Callie too, multi-tasker that I was. Who needed a leash? We lived on a dead-end dirt road.

I made it maybe a hundred yards before Callie saw a neighbor walking her own dog up the road. Did I mention Callie was unleashed? I locked the stroller in place and chased the dog down the hill. No one was happy, not Callie, not the baby, and not our neighbor.

Luckily, after a couple of weeks, we found a new nanny, one no more concerned about catching Covid than we were. With her arrival, I could focus full-time on what seemed to have become my new job: investigating everything from Neil Ferguson's history of failed predictions to data about Florida hospital beds, then reporting it to anyone who would listen.

In other words, tweeting.

Jackie didn't like any of it. She thought I was wasting my time, that Twitter ranked somewhere between useless and embarrassing. I couldn't convince her otherwise.

Not even after Maggie Haberman, who covered Trump for the *New York Times*, reported on April 5 that my tweets were "making their way around the White House among some senior officials."[1] In weeks, I had become among the most prominent lockdown skeptics.

I had a model to thank.

No, not Gigi or Kendall or any of the runway walkers.

The IHME model.

IHME stood for Institute for Health Metrics and Evaluation, "an independent population health research center" at the University of Washington. Like Imperial College and many other coronavirus players, IHME took lots of money from the Bill and Melinda Gates Foundation. In 2017, the foundation had given the institute a $279 million grant, the largest donation in the history of the University of Washington.[2]

Now IHME was playing the same role in the United States as Imperial College had in Britain. On March 26, IHME began releasing hair-raising forecasts about the number of coronavirus patients who would be hospitalized, need intensive care, or die.

Other epidemiologists and private companies also made local and national forecasts. But IHME's were the most important. They were publicly available, covered every state, and were updated frequently. The White House coronavirus task force used them, as the *Washington Post* reported on April 2: "The peak of the outbreak would come in the middle of April, task force member Deborah Birx explained. She showed a graph using modeling from the University of Washington's Institute for Health Metrics and Evaluation (IHME). The projected peak would come on April 15, with 2,214 deaths on that day."[3]

New York also relied heavily on the IHME models, which showed the city and state would soon be desperately short of hospital beds.[4] On March 30, IHME forecast that the state would have a shortage of almost sixty thousand hospital beds, including ten thousand intensive care beds, *within ten days.*[5]

What no one seemed to notice as these terrifying reports flooded out was that IHME's predictions were wrong. *Completely* wrong.

I am not exaggerating. I wasn't exaggerating then, and I'm not exaggerating now. I wasn't guessing, either. I don't mean that at the end of March I could somehow see into the future and know the IHME model for New York—or any state—would be wrong in a few days.

Here's what I mean: The model's predictions looked like a curve on a graph. Each day's projections were a point on the curve. And the curve didn't start a week or a month in the future. It started in the *past*, before running through the current day into the future. I apologize if this explanation seems obvious. It's necessary because what comes next is so mind-blowing.

I, or anyone, could compare the *actual* number of hospitalizations or ICU patients for the *current* day in New York—which Governor Cuomo reported at his daily press conferences—and for other states as well, with the model's projections *for that day.*

In other words, I was not trying to outguess the model's future predictions. I was just comparing the IMHE's "predictions" for the *current* day with the actual statistics for that current day, to make sure the IMHE model correctly represented reality at the moment.

It didn't.

Over and over, I found massive discrepancies between the number of hospitalized patients Cuomo reported on a given day and the number *for that day* in the model. For example, on April 3, 2020, IHME said that on April 3 (that same day) New York would have 61,000 hospitalized Covid patients, including 11,500 in intensive care. In reality, the state had 14,810 coronavirus patients, including 3,731 in intensive care.

In other words, the IHME model was reporting the number of people hospitalized in New York on April 3 at *four times* the actual number of patients. And remember, IHME hadn't made this model years or even months earlier. It had released the model barely a week before.

Yet in those few days, the model had completely failed. (*Why* the model was so wrong is a crucial question, and I promise to come back to it shortly. But for now, simply understand that the *fact* of its failure was inarguable. Anyone who looked at the numbers could see it.)

I began to highlight these discrepancies on Twitter, comparing the real numbers each day with those in the model. On April 2, I tweeted:

> Update on the @IHME_UW model versus reality in New York State: reality is still winning. 56,000 hospitalizations and 11,000 ICU beds projected for April 2; 13,400 hospitalizations

and 3,400 beds used. Reminder: this model was released one week ago.[6]

Each day, I made similar updates. As shocking to me as the model's errors was the fact that IHME did not seem to care. The errors piled up day by day. The modelers supposedly drew on real-world data to make their predictions—so how come they couldn't even get the *actual* numbers right?

In their world—the alternative reality of their model—more than fifty thousand coronavirus patients had *already* overrun New York's hospitals by early April. Each day the tide of untreated patients grew. In the real world, the hospitals were stressed but coping. The field hospitals remained nearly empty.

The fact that New York had locked down didn't explain the model's failure, either. The model had been released *after* the lockdown began, and it explicitly took the effects of social distancing into account in its predictions.

The final straw for me came on April 5. IHME had promised it would revise its model by Saturday, April 4. The revision didn't come. I assumed the institute was making drastic changes after its failures. And when IHME finally put out its new version late Sunday night, it did show significantly lower estimates of deaths and hospitalizations for future dates.

But the current-day numbers were *still wrong.* The revised model said New York had about twenty-four thousand hospitalized patients that day, when the real number was under sixteen thousand. The modelers were still making basic errors. How could we possibly trust their predictions if they did not care enough to get the known facts right?

But then the media didn't seem to care either. Reporters parroted the empty predictions of hospital collapse as if they had some basis in reality.

Worse, officials were still relying on the models to make public policy. On April 6, the *New York Times* reported that New York governor Andrew Cuomo had referred to predictions by the institute for Health Metrics and Evaluation at the University of Washington, known as IHME....

The models serve a purpose, and Governor Cuomo has spoken of their importance to leaders amid a pandemic. "I follow data," he has said. "I don't have instinct. I don't have a gut. It's not about emotion."

(The article did not make the exact date of that quotation clear, but it would appear to have been at some time in the week leading up to April 6.)[7]

Meanwhile, academics on Twitter were worried not that the IHME models were too pessimistic but that they were too *hopeful*. "My personal impression [of the model] is that it's extremely optimistic," Carl Bergstrom, a biologist at the University of Washington, tweeted on March 28.[8]

So I had the field of pointing out the gap between reality and the dreadful forecasts more or less to myself. A handful of right-leaning reporters noticed, most notably Brit Hume, Fox News Channel's senior political analyst, a pundit whom even liberals respected.

Hume repeatedly retweeted me to his million followers, amplifying my reach hugely. The rest of Fox followed. Producers for Tucker Carlson, Sean Hannity, and Laura Ingraham were soon inviting me on.

To be clear, no one at Fox *ever* suggested what I should say during interviews. In fact, I clearly made Hannity uncomfortable when I told him on April 10 that "kids, children, almost anybody under 30 is at no risk from this, no serious risk from this virus," before quickly adding, "I'm not saying it can never happen."

Yes, the public health misinformation campaign to hide the real age-stratified risks of the virus had been so successful that even *Sean Hannity* believed it.

Similarly, I had no special relationships in the White House. Over the entire course of the epidemic, I spoke a couple of times to people there. I met Robert O'Brien, the national security adviser, once. No one ever asked me to write anything. I don't remember their ever giving me any useful information either. I prided myself on my independence and tried to keep it, though more and more I found myself labeled a Trump apologist, a Covid denier, a conspiracy theorist, a grifter, and a liar.

If my wife was unhappy with my sudden star turn on Fox, my father liked it even less.

"I saw you on *Tucker Carlson*," he emailed in early April. "You are very articulate and I believe wrong. You want to do an experiment that all of the experts say is dangerous."

I didn't argue with him. He was desperately afraid, I knew. Afraid of the leukemia gnawing his bone marrow, afraid that after two and a half years the doctors had nothing left to offer him. He had jumped from oncologist to oncologist, from New York–Presbyterian to Memorial Sloan Kettering to Dana-Farber.

But his leukemia wasn't interested in medical brand names. It didn't care my dad had been healthy his whole life. It was out for blood, hardee-har.

In truth, my father's quest for a cure had already nearly killed him. In March 2019, one of the fancy doctors gave him an extra round of chemotherapy to feed his long-shot hope of a stem-cell transplant. Then my dad talked the doctor into sending him home early. Days later he went into septic shock and collapsed.

He spent almost three weeks on a ventilator, in a propofol- and fentanyl-induced coma. His kidneys and lungs failed. His skin turned papery and tore. The ugliest fluids imaginable bubbled through tubes hidden under his sheets. The breathing tube in his throat and plastic mouthpiece stuffed between his lips meant he couldn't speak.

Sitting at his bedside felt like looking out an airplane window at a forest fire glowing in the night, the horror vivid but unreachable. A few times during those weeks he seemed to wake up while I was there. His eyes grew wide and frantic. He twisted his head side to side and grunted hopelessly.

This has to be worse than death, I thought. *Death would be a relief.*

Yet he beat the infection. He was a tough old man. His lungs recovered. He came off the vent. He didn't seem to remember any part of those weeks, his horror least of all. Propofol's a hell of a drug.

As soon as he could, he hopped back on the treatment treadmill. He didn't want to die. Not dying was job one. Through 2019 and the winter of 2020, he shuffled from hospital to hospital, focusing his energy on finding a miracle. The new doctors happily accommodated him with new drug combinations, fourth- and fifth- and sixth-line treatments. Nobody did anything wrong. Insurance paid for all of it.

Do something, anything, anything must be better than nothing, I've worked my whole life, paid my taxes, gone easy on my health insurance, my turn now. No one seemed willing to tell him that his odds were slim to none and slim had left the building. I'm not sure he would have cared if they had. He didn't want a good year or two, a descent into hospice. He didn't want to hang out with his grandkids and sit in the backyard.

He wanted to *live*.

When the coronavirus came to town, he didn't want to die of it either. If that meant locking down the world, so be it. He made clear he didn't care how long he or society had to stop living, as long as he stayed alive.

I wanted him to live, too. But I knew he wouldn't. And I knew the truth was that the coronavirus wasn't what would kill him, even if he died of it. He'd been strong his whole life. The Polish Bull, we called him. A strong, angry, impatient man. Now he had nowhere to hide from the disease that lurked in his very bones.

I couldn't help thinking his desperation to escape death at any price embodied our society's myopia. He had always liked to ride his bike through Central Park, walk the streets of Manhattan. He'd been born in Oregon but had moved east for college and never gone back. After fifty years, he was a New Yorker through and through.

But he seemed ready to give up those pleasures indefinitely. Did he plan to stay inside all spring? All summer? All year? He had five grandchildren. Did he intend never to see them again? Did he think they should be denied school? And for how long?

I never said anything like this to him, of course.

But I knew I wouldn't stop talking about the failed models and the lack of evidence for lockdowns, no matter how much he wished I would.

I hoped Covid wouldn't be what killed him.

It wasn't.

He was hospitalized one final time at the beginning of May. He tested negative for the virus. We couldn't see him, because no one could visit anyone in the hospitals in New York.

The doctors stabilized him. Then they gave him the mercy of sending him home to die. On the morning of Wednesday, May 13, he did. Of leukemia, not Sars-Cov-2. We mourned him that Friday night with a Zoom ceremony that was more touching than I expected it would be, a couple of hundred people from all over the country telling stories about Harvey. Then I got back to work.

I'd like to think that by the end my father was proud of me for fighting the lockdowns, fighting for the truth.

But since we're talking about the truth, the truth is: I'm pretty sure he wasn't.

11

Locked Down

The world panicked in March.

But April was the month when the grim reality of lockdowns set in. Europe, the United States, South America, and much of Asia came to a near total halt. Businesses and schools shut. Elective surgeries were canceled. Our diversions vanished. No professional sports. No restaurants or movies or haircuts.

What we were missing was obvious. Commerce and forward motion define American life. That energy can come at the expense of taking pleasure in the quiet joys of the everyday. Western Europeans treasure their vacations. Americans prefer to work hard, for better or worse.

So the stereotype goes. Plenty of data backs it.

But the pandemic left us paddling in circles. It worsened our addiction to screens and transformed our frantic energy into panic. Out of fear, sheer boredom, or an urge to virtue-signal, many Americans seemed overcome with the urge to tattle on their neighbors. They called 911 to report backyard parties[1] and people who weren't wearing masks.[2] Los

Angeles County sheriff's deputies arrested a man for ignoring the state's stay-at-home order—while he was paddleboarding alone on the ocean.[3]

An April 7, 2020, article in the *Tampa Bay Times* captured the madness: "They called the police on homeless people standing outside a Mobil in Gibsonton, and because they saw people shake hands at Petrol Mart in Thonotosassa. Someone called the cops on a Michael's craft store for being open, and on employees at a jewelry store on Dale Mabry not standing six feet apart. Someone called about a lone man selling flowers on the side of the road. Another said that a neighbor had opened his home gym up to the neighborhood."

Worse, although the police for the most part did not want to be involved, politicians encouraged the trend. Cities and states set up tip lines and websites, asking people to inform on one another and on businesses that tried to stay open.

"Snitches get rewards," Los Angeles mayor Eric Garcetti told his city's residents. "We want to thank you for turning folks in."[4]

Of course, even the strictest American rules were less harsh than those in European countries, much less those in China. In France and Italy, police routinely ticketed and fined people for being outside. Ireland and the United Kingdom enforced strict limits on the distances people could travel from their homes.

American constitutional protections and a tradition of freedom meant that lockdowns in the United States focused more on businesses than individuals. Although people were told to stay home, police checkpoints were essentially nonexistent. I left our house almost every day and never came across one. My wife had the same experience on her commute to work.

Anyone who was stopped could simply say he was an essential worker or was going for groceries. A low point came when authorities in Rhode Island and some other states briefly announced constitutionally dubious efforts to discourage New York residents from traveling to their states. Rhode Island actually set up a license plate checkpoint on I-95, the main highway on the East Coast, so that state police could stop people with New York plates. It also sent National Guard members to knock on doors "to inform any New Yorkers who may have come to the state that they must self-quarantine for 14 days."[5] But after sharp criticism, most states pulled back from strict enforcement efforts.

American governors relied instead on closing retailers, schools, bars and restaurants, and public spaces such as parks and libraries. Their explicit goal was to keep everyone home by giving them nowhere to go.

Exceptions included grocery stores, gas stations, and, of course, Target and Walmart, which wound up with a huge advantage over smaller retailers that had to close. Liquor stores were generally also allowed to stay open, in recognition of the grim reality that withdrawal could be lethal for late-stage alcoholics.

Of course, police officers, firefighters, and prison guards stayed on the job, as did physicians, nurses, and other hospital workers—along with everyone who worked in food supply and logistics, and many construction and factory workers.

Still, for the most part, the lockdowns were effective.

In an early April 2020 survey, only about 10 percent of Americans said they had gone to a restaurant, someone else's house, or church or community gathering in the previous week.[6] They were telling the truth. The iPhone mobility data for early April showed that movement in the United States had plunged about 60 percent compared to a few weeks before. That drop wasn't quite as much as the 80 percent decline in Italy, but it was still unprecedented.[7]

Government rules were only part of the reason people stayed home. Media outlets at every level did everything possible to stoke fear.

"Can Coronavirus Survive in Your Refrigerator?" the San Francisco NBC affiliate asked on April 1, in a story that was not intended as an April Fool's parody. "Here's What a Renowned Scientist Told Us....Before you put the latest round of groceries in your refrigerator, take a few minutes to disinfect all items."[8]

On April 2, the *Today* show warned people that they should not visit friends or family members "even if you and your loved one aren't exhibiting symptoms, you've all been diligently quarantining and you maintain social distance."

Further, people should not gather in groups of more than two, even outside, an expert explained. "If you want to go for a walk or another outdoor activity with someone you are not isolating with, that's okay as long you can keep a distance of six feet," Dr. William Schaffner—the medical director of the National Foundation for Infectious Diseases—said on the show.

On April 6, the public health director of Los Angeles County suggested residents avoid even going out for groceries. "If you have enough supplies in your home, this would be the week to skip shopping altogether."[9] That day, the county reported 420 new coronavirus cases among its 11 million residents.

Newspapers and cable networks focused relentlessly on the deaths of people from Covid.

On March 27, the *New York Times* began a series called "Those We've Lost," which would last more than a year. After September 11, the *Times* had run a series called "Portraits of Grief," with the goal of memorializing everyone who had died in those attacks. It ultimately covered more than 2,400 people. "Those We've Lost" aimed to give the same treatment to Covid victims.

Even the *Times* acknowledged that covering a respiratory virus like a terrorist attack didn't make much sense: "This time there was no finite number of the dead. No geographical point united them. Their backgrounds were of infinite variety. They did not die all at once on a bright blue morning."[10]

Nonetheless, the *Times* decided to move forward, hoping "to convey the human toll of Covid-19" in a way it had never done for any other illness or cause of death—not drug overdose or suicide or heart disease or cancer. It would run obituaries of people who had died of the coronavirus, not for a day or a two, but forever.

The effect was both to privilege people who had died of Covid, making their deaths more meaningful than others, and also to make the epidemic seem far worse than it was. More than ten thousand Americans die every week of heart disease. If the media reported all of their stories, fears of cardiac death would surely skyrocket.

On Twitter, the tone was even more hysterical.

"We're literally all in hiding," Dr. Craig Spencer—the director of Global Health in Emergency Medicine at Columbia University Medical Center—wrote in mid-April. "From a virus. That will kill many of us. If it finds us. In a shop. Or on a beach. In NYC. Or Oklahoma."

The relentless fearmongering stoked the perception that the coronavirus was a real-life version of Captain Trips—the fictional "superflu" in *The Stand* that kills more than 99 percent of the people it infects.

An online tracking poll from the University of Southern California showed how out of touch with reality people's fears had become. The poll surveyed nine thousand Americans who were chosen to represent a good demographic match for the entire country.

By early April 2020, Americans said they believed they had a 25 percent chance of dying from the coronavirus if they were infected. That was about one hundred times their actual risk.[11] While their perceived risk fell slightly over time, it remained around 12 percent until the poll ended in June 2021. Women, who were less likely to die than men, believed their risk was higher.

Even more stunning, people under forty said they believed their risk of death was about one in five. For most of them, that estimate was off by a factor of at least ten thousand. Healthy people under thirty had a risk of death from the virus that was almost too low to measure. Even in their thirties, people who were not seriously overweight had a risk significantly less than 0.01 percent, or one in ten thousand, according to a peer-reviewed paper that examined Covid outcomes in a group of seven million British people in 2020.[12]

(The Centers for Disease Control offered an estimate of one death per two thousand infections for people from eighteen to forty-nine.[13] But that figure included people in their forties, who were at higher risk. More important, it included people with morbid obesity, uncontrolled diabetes, and other serious health problems, who made up a huge proportion of the people under fifty who died from Covid.)

But the media's insistence on hiding these facts meant almost no one knew the real odds. Some people seemed to lose their minds to fear. They refused to leave their homes for any reason. They sprayed disinfectant over their mail. They wore masks and gloves even when they were alone.

Worse, parents behaved in ways that would have qualified as abusive before March, refusing to let their children play outside for months, kicking out college-age kids who had left their houses to meet friends.

The days are long, but the years are short, the old saying goes. But in 2020, the minutes, the days, and the months all seemed to stretch on forever.

With no distractions, every day became Blursday. Only the Covid death counts changed. Driven by a surge in New York City, deaths in the first wave peaked nationally in mid-April at around 2,200 a day (based on the 7-day average, which smooths out reporting lags on weekends).

Just as individuals came under extraordinary pressure to stay home, the handful of states that had not yet shut by late March faced a torrent of criticism from reporters. Not coincidentally, they all had Republican governors. Florida took the most criticism, even after its governor Ron DeSantis imposed a lockdown, effective April 1.

On that day, Jennifer Rubin, a *Washington Post* columnist, published a piece headlined "We Must Hold Politicians Responsible for Deaths They Could Have Prevented." Because DeSantis had delayed closing his state, he would be "morally—if not legally—responsible for hundreds if not thousands of preventable deaths," Rubin wrote.[14] She went on to blame Trump for failing to impose a national lockdown (again, a step he could not have taken without imposing martial law).

The *New York Times* thundered, "Florida, Finally," in an April 2 piece by David Leonhardt: "The state will go on lockdown, far too late."[15]

Internationally, Sweden faced similar pressure. Unlike nearly every other country in Western Europe, the Swedes refused to impose hard lockdowns or close schools.

A Swede who had returned home in April wrote, "What I quickly noticed during the ride to my Stockholm apartment was how things seemed exactly normal for this time of year." He was not happy about what he saw. "Sweden's citizens…have gone along with policies leading to large-scale death."[16]

So the lockdowns, first sold to the public as a temporary emergency measure to protect the hospital system—a.k.a. "fifteen days to flatten the curve"—were extended through April and May in the United States and Europe. Most people were so frightened that they willingly went along.

I saw how deep the fear ran when I traveled into New York City to visit my father. My eeriest visit came in mid-April, a month after the crisis began. The day was bright and sunny. Manhattan should have been packed, its streets jammed with tourists and office workers.

Instead it was empty. Times Square—the crossroads of the world—had a few cops hanging around. No one else. I could stand in the middle of the intersection of Forty-Fifth Street and Seventh Avenue and take photos. There were almost no cars. (The photo showing a deserted street just west of Times Square on the cover of this book was taken on that trip.)

The rest of Manhattan was equally deserted. The subways were empty. The streets were empty. A giant mall near the World Trade Center had a single person walking through it.

The strangest thing was the quiet. The sirens that had supposedly defined the first days of the pandemic were gone. Nothing had replaced them. New York is never silent, not even at 4:00 a.m. Drunks stagger home from bars, shouting. Dogs bark at rats. Cabs race up the avenues, gunning their engines as they search for fares.

The city can be quiet, but it's never silent.

Now it was. In New York in April, the world truly seemed to have ended. I had lived in Manhattan's East Village on September 11—close enough to smell the burning rubble of the World Trade Center for weeks. The emptiness was, without doubt, worse.

In retrospect, I wish I had taken many more photos. But no matter, the deserted city will stay with me forever.

Nearly as disturbing as the city itself, though, was the response I received on Twitter when I posted the pictures I had taken. "My city in ruins," I wrote, a reference to a Bruce Springsteen song about September 11 (its actual title is "My City of Ruins.")

The full tweet:

> My city in ruins: here is New York, empty and stricken and silent, not merely from a virus that has killed a tiny fraction of its citizens—mostly, sadly, elderly and frail—but from the panic that came before and continues.[17]

Come on, rise up, come on, rise up, Springsteen sings.

■   ■   ■

But the liberal intelligentsia who set the tone on Twitter disagreed with that message. They lit into me for suggesting that the largest city in the United States needed to begin to live again.

"Fuck you, you weasel," wrote Angus Johnston, a professor at the City University of New York with almost seventy thousand followers.[18] Chase Mitchell, a writer for Jimmy Fallon, crowed of the empty city: "best it's ever looked."[19]

Mitchell was not alone in his bizarre view that New York was somehow *better without people*, especially in Times Square. Many commenters responded that the area was a consumerist, tourist wasteland. They scorned the idea that anyone might take pleasure in the square's energy or the skyscrapers where thousands of people worked. "Who will go to the Olive Garden now?" one commenter wrote mockingly.

The Times Square comments reflected a powerful impulse on the far left to use Covid not just to hurt Donald Trump's reelection chances but to press for broad societal changes. The desire was evident from the beginning of the crisis. No one expressed it more clearly than Gregg Gonsalves, an associate professor at Yale University, epidemiologist, and AIDS activist. On March 23, Gonsalves tweeted: "As a friend of mine said this weekend: 'There are no natural or social laws preventing us from remaking the economy for the next 18 months, the next 18 years, or forever.... There are only political and cultural barriers, barriers we must overcome....'"[20]

Similarly, Michael Hiltzik, a left-leaning columnist for the *Los Angeles Times*, wrote in May that the coronavirus could boost plans for universal basic income—government-provided welfare payments for all.[21] (In October, actress and liberal activist Jane Fonda would express an even blunter take: "I just think Covid is God's gift to the left."[22])

Of course, for the threat of Covid to justify the wholesale remodeling of American society, Covid had to be very dangerous.

The woke left had put itself in the odd position of rooting for disaster.

The irony didn't end there. Some of the world's largest and most profitable companies also had reason to hope that lockdowns continued. Giant chains such as Walmart profited from government-mandated shutdowns of their competitors.

But even those gains paled compared to the riches won by big technology and social media companies—Apple, Facebook, Google, Microsoft, and especially Amazon. Even before the pandemic, those companies had become the world's most important. They were the Information in the Information Age. They were all among the world's largest companies in terms of market value, and enormously profitable, with more than $150 billion in earnings in 2019.

Now they had an almost unthinkable advantage—a world in which people had to rely on the internet to connect socially, for work, and to shop. Wall Street figured this dynamic out very quickly. Shares of Amazon and the other tech giants fell in February and early March along with other stocks. But they rallied sharply by late March, even as the media focused on the apparent catastrophe in New York.

Within days, the tech companies had put their might behind lock-downs. By early April, they were running aggressive advertising campaigns to normalize social distancing and quarantines.

"We're never lost if we can find each other," a Facebook ad proclaimed.[23] "There is so much peace to be found in people's faces. I love people's faces"—especially if those faces were viewed on a Facebook page, presumably.

An Apple ad called "Creativity Goes On" featured a hand holding a cupcake up to a screen where a man opened his mouth to eat it—virtually. As piano music played softly in the background, Oprah proclaimed, "The pandemic has the possibility to bring us together in ways none of us would have been able to predict or expect."[24]

Google took a more direct approach in an ad called "Thank You Healthcare Workers." As the usual images flowed—a mother and young child pressing their faces to either side of a glass door, people clapping from balconies to show their support—the company proclaimed, "To everyone sacrificing so much to save so many, thank you. Help save lives by staying home."[25]

All three ads made sure to meld use of their companies' products with the supposedly charitable and apolitical stay-at-home messaging. "More than ever, people are searching," the Google ad opened, before "How to help" was typed into a Google search bar. The message was clear: depend on us to get through this.

Played over and over on social and conventional media, the ads proved extraordinarily effective. Support for lockdowns stayed high through April, not just in the United States but worldwide.

An Associated Press poll released on April 22, 2020, showed 61 percent of adults believed that restrictions "to prevent the spread of coronavirus are about right."[26] Another 26 percent believed they should be tightened even further. Only 12 percent, including only 22 percent of Republicans, thought they should be loosened.

The findings highlighted the fact that for at least the first six weeks of lockdowns, the partisan gap over whether they made sense was small.

Into early May, nearly as many Republicans as Democrats believed the coronavirus was a danger to their families that required aggressive federal intervention.

A relative handful of people did try to protest in April, after governors announced they would extend lockdowns into May or beyond. But the protests gained little traction.

The fiercest early protests came in Michigan, where Governor Gretchen Whitmer attracted scorn on April 10 when she ordered stores to stop selling plants, seeds, paint, and carpeting.[27] And grocery stores weren't allowed to take bottle returns.

Viewed one way, Whitmer's order actually made sense. She was trying to restrict big-box retailers to selling groceries and other staples. She wanted to keep them from selling goods that their closed competitors could not. Yet the logic of her order revealed the profound illogic of stay-at-home orders generally. Unless the United States planned to lock everyone up and have the military deliver food to shut-ins, people were going to need to go out to shop. Whitmer also told people they could not travel to their in-state vacation homes, a provision that was probably unconstitutional.

Whitmer's overreach inspired residents to organize against the lockdowns. On April 15, they came together in Lansing, the state capital, in the first major anti-lockdown protest, "Operation Gridlock." Several thousand people drove slowly through Lansing's streets, waving American flags and holding signs with slogans such as "Liberty once lost is lost forever." They blocked traffic but otherwise stayed calm and orderly.[28] The fact that most protestors remained in their cars—and thus did not violate rules against gathering in large crowds—underscored the mildness of the protest.

But the media who covered the rally were less than sympathetic. "Scores ignored organizers' pleas to stay inside their vehicles," NBC News reported breathlessly. "At least two Confederate flags were spotted."[29]

In contrast, Whitmer's claim that the protest would cause Covid to spread received uncritical coverage. "This demonstration is going to come at a cost to people's health," she said. "We know that when people gather that way without masks...that's how Covid-19 spreads."[30] Even people who stayed in their cars in Lansing might have spread the virus if they touched gas pumps to fill up along the way, she said.

The protest did apparently encourage Whitmer to loosen her April 10 restrictions. On April 24, she allowed the sale of gardening supplies again. But the core of the lockdown remained. And when protestors returned on April 30 and entered the capitol itself, they faced even harsher criticism, especially since some were armed. Michigan law permitted them to carry weapons openly, but reporters and Democratic lawmakers raised the specter of an armed takeover of the building.

The story was the same elsewhere. Efforts in Illinois and New York to organize protests largely fizzled. Many cities declared that lockdown protestors could be arrested since protesting might spread the virus.

"There should not be protests taking place in the middle of a pandemic by gathering outside and putting people at risk," New York police commissioner Dermot Shea said.[31] A month later, the city would take a very different stance.

So as April turned to May, no one could doubt which side had the upper hand. Lockdowns rolled on in most of the United States—not just with no end in sight, but with no end even over the horizon.

12

The Perfect Storm

Yet a few of us looking closely at the data—not at what public health authorities or governors or reporters were saying about the data but at *the data itself*—could see two crucial facts emerging as early as the first week of April 2020.

First, Covid was far less threatening than it had originally seemed.

Yes, it could be deadly, especially to the elderly and people with severe comorbidities such as kidney disease. But it would *not* overwhelm the medical system, much less all of society.

Second, the lockdowns, at least as the United States and Europe conducted them, were useless, if not counterproductive.

How did we on what I came to call Team Reality decipher these counterintuitive truths despite the high-octane fear the media pumped every day?

We grew to understand that one single datapoint mattered most in charting the epidemic: the number of people *hospitalized* with Covid each day, not the number of new cases or deaths.

Why?

Reported positive cases varied with testing policies. Were tests hard or easy to get? Were only very sick people being tested, or was everyone? (Later we would learn the way the tests were conducted made a crucial difference, too. But at the time only a few insiders understood how federal regulators had set up testing rules to inflate the case count.)[1]

Hospitalizations were a better metric than cases. Decent physicians wouldn't admit patients without good reason—especially in April in the Northeast, where many hospitals were close to capacity.

Hospitalizations mattered for another reason, too. *The potential stress Covid posed to the hospital system was the reason governments had imposed lockdowns in the first place.* Remember, "flattening the curve" did not mean that Covid would necessarily infect or kill fewer people. Sars-Cov-2 would still be out there. Flattening the curve meant *lengthening* the time period over which the crisis occurred, so that hospitals could handle it without being overwhelmed.

But if hospitals weren't overwhelmed, much of the rationale for lockdowns disappeared. So tracking hospital admissions especially closely made sense.

What about deaths? Weren't they an even more important indicator than hospitalizations?

No.

As I tweeted repeatedly in April 2020, *deaths lag*. The number of reported deaths was a trailing indicator, a sign of where the epidemic had been, not where it was going.

Why?

Covid turned out to be a relatively predictable disease. It followed a course much like the flu. Many people never developed symptoms after being infected. Those who became sick usually did so about four or five days after being exposed.

Most of the ill recovered quickly after a few days of coughing and fever. But some worsened and wound up hospitalized—usually about a week after first showing symptoms. The unlucky few who died usually did so within a week to ten days of hospitalization.

Not every case was the same, of course. Very old and frail people tended to die even more quickly, often without ever being hospitalized at all. Younger and healthier people could hang on longer. Still, on average, the coronavirus killed roughly three weeks after infection.

One final time lag followed. Hospitals and medical examiners could take days or weeks to certify deaths to the state health authorities, which then reported them to the public. As a result, reported deaths could rise well after an epidemic had peaked and passed.

But hospitalizations generally occurred less than two weeks after infection. And hospitals reported bed counts on a daily or even hourly basis. They had to, in order to know whether they had room for new patients.

Thus hospitalizations were a far better real-time indicator than deaths. And by April, many states—including New York—reported hospitalizations publicly, making them easy to track.

You already know the Institute for Health Metrics and Evaluation (IHME) forecasts for the number of hospitalized patients were far too high for New York.

Understanding the reason why is crucial.

Governor Cuomo had announced the lockdown on March 20. It took effect on March 22.[2] The IHME and other forecasters predicted new hospitalizations would surge at least until early April, about two weeks after the lockdown began. By then, according to the models, New York hospitals would be admitting up to 10,000 new Covid patients a day—on their way to an unthinkable total of 140,000 patients, far more than the state could handle.[3]

Instead, new hospitalizations rose much more slowly after March 25. After April 2, they plunged.

The *total* number of patients in hospitals rose for several days more, because most patients were hospitalized for several days before being released. But the peak in new admissions in New York at the beginning of April signaled that deaths would fall later in the month.

Sure enough, deaths peaked on April 13, when the state's seven-day moving average of deaths reached 957 a day.[4] (Again, I use the seven-day average to smooth out weekend reporting fluctuations.) The rising deaths led to a new wave of media hysteria. But the reality was that the peak of the epidemic had already passed in New York.

Hospital-level data also offered a crucial window into the situation in states that had locked down later than New York or not at all, especially Florida. Despite its reputation for zaniness (Florida Man!), Florida has excellent open-records laws and responsive state agencies.

In early April 2020, Florida began reporting in real time how many hospital and intensive care beds it had available. At the time, nearly every public health expert believed the state faced impending doom. On April 2, a South Florida television station featured dire warnings:

> Dr. Terry Adirim…senior associate dean for clinical affairs at Florida Atlantic University's Charles E. Schmidt College of Medicine, said she's worried about the number of available hospital beds….
>
> "We're just not going to have enough ventilators or ICU beds," Dr. Adirim said in an interview with Contact 5, noting modeling shows COVID-19 cases will peak locally in three to four weeks.[5]

Dr. Scott Gottlieb, a former Food and Drug Administration commissioner who was rapidly becoming very widely quoted on Covid, also warned that Florida's lockdown had come too late. "'I don't understand why those governors have not acted more forcefully right now,' Gottlieb said before DeSantis issued his stay-at-home order. 'Especially when you look at a state like Florida. Florida has a very large epidemic underway. There's multiple hot spots, they were probably seeded in early February. Now they have large clusters.'"[6]

DeSantis issued the lockdown order on April 1.

And the IHME model predicted that Florida's epidemic would worsen dramatically by mid- to late April. Its April 7 forecast predicted a peak on April 21, with 242 Covid deaths in Florida that day.

The model also predicted Florida would have about 13,000 Covid patients hospitalized on that date, with 2,500 needing intensive care and 2,100 on ventilators. Its hospitals would be short 769 intensive care beds when demand peaked.[7] The gap was not as large as those predicted for New York or the Northeast, but still, it meant the hospital system would need help.

But the actual data on the state's Agency for Health Care Administration website presented an entirely different picture.

As of April 3, Florida's hospitals had about 25,000 beds and 2,200 intensive care beds available. Hospitals were about 60 percent full—*below* their typical occupancy rates. In the next couple of days they emptied further, as Florida's hospitals readied themselves for a surge of Covid patients.

The surge never came.

On April 12, the hospitals had *more* space available than they had had on April 3—28,000 empty beds and 2,300 ICU beds. On April 16, the figures were almost exactly the same.[8]

The plateau as of April 16 was crucial, because at that point Florida was more than two weeks past the start of its lockdown. If infections had really spread in late March, before the lockdown, the hospitals and ICU wards would have filled by April 16. Instead, they were almost half empty.

How wrong were the predictions?

Florida's cases peaked around *April 8*—at 1,132 a day. *Cases.* Not hospitalizations or deaths. As for deaths, on April 21, the state had 42, about one-sixth the number IHME had predicted for that day. Further, deaths did *not* rise steeply and fall, as the IHME had predicted, but instead remained mostly flat for months.

By early May, even mainstream reporters could not ignore the fact that Florida had escaped the doom they'd predicted. Vox, the *Wall Street Journal*, and other outlets published articles with puzzled headlines such as, "Why the Worst Fears about Florida's Covid-19 Outbreak Haven't Been Realized (So Far)."[9]

Inevitably, the stories gave Florida's lockdown credit for the good results.

"Every expert I talked to cited social distancing, first and foremost," Vox's Dylan Scott wrote. The *Wall Street Journal* reported that "people [in Florida] began hunkering down in mid-March."[10]

Of course, at the beginning of April, reporters *had said exactly the opposite.*

On April 2, the *New York Times* had run a story using location and movement data to show that people in a band of counties from central Florida north through Virginia and west to Texas had been the last to reduce their travel.

Even after March 26, the counties—denoted with an ominous red—still had an average trip of at least two miles. (Two miles may not sound like much. But the average trip in Seattle, which had locked down early and hard, fell from four miles to *sixty-one feet.*) "Where America Didn't Stay Home," the *Times* headline read. The article explained how DeSantis's lockdown order had come too late:

> Florida waited so long to shut down travel that it will struggle to control local outbreaks even if people immediately change their behavior significantly, said Thomas Hladish, an infectious disease modeler at the University of Florida. People who now sequester themselves at home still risk having brought the virus home to their families, he said....
>
> "In order to really have a big effect with social-distancing measures, you would have had to move it back in time."[11]

Hladish was wrong, of course. Florida had no problem controlling local outbreaks. It had no surge of hospitalizations. Its late lockdown did not seem to have mattered at all.

And it wasn't just Florida.

Outside a handful of northeastern states, hospitals had patient counts well below normal in April 2020. Few Covid patients were being hospitalized. Elective surgeries had been postponed. And some people were too scared to go to emergency rooms even if they had chest pains or other signs of heart attacks. Without patients, hospitals laid off or furloughed tens of thousands of employees, including nurses and other medical staff.

Some hospitals even closed.[12]

Yet news organizations based in New York and Washington seemed completely unaware of what was happening in the rest of the country. On April 13—the same day *Becker's Hospital Review* carried fourteen separate articles on hospitals furloughing workers[13]—the *Times* ran an article headlined "Foreign Doctors Could Help Fight Coronavirus. But U.S. Blocks Many."[14]

Back in New York, the situation was different. The state's crisis was real and undeniable. Still, its surge did not track the doomsday predictions. New York had locked down hard and relatively early, on March 22. The crisis that followed did not rise to the level forecasters had predicted—but it also lasted longer than they had expected.

The pattern was more complicated than in the rest of the country, but the takeaway was the same. New York's lockdown probably hadn't mattered. It may even have done more harm than good.

The proof was in the failures of the models. In making their predictions, forecasters had overestimated the impact lockdowns would have.

Remember, hospitalizations rose extraordinarily fast in mid- to late March, as the epidemiologists made their predictions for April. Between March 16 and March 25, new hospitalizations in New York State rose 13-fold, from 91 to 1,248.

A 13-fold increase in 9 days was terrifying on its own. But it was even more worrisome *because of the 2-week lag from infection to hospitalization*. Those March 25 hospitalizations mostly resulted from people who had been infected before March 12.

When they made their predictions, the modelers could not know how many people had been infected from March 12 through March 20. They assumed infections had risen exponentially in mid-March, just as they had in early March.

To understand exponential growth, imagine a gambler who never takes his money off the blackjack table but just allows it to double with each win. If he starts with one dollar and wins five straight times, he'll have thirty-two dollars. If he wins five more, he'll have over one thousand dollars.

Each "win" is equivalent to a viral infection cycle. And respiratory viruses have short transmission cycles, only four or five days in the case of the coronavirus. As a result, the number of infections can grow extremely fast. In a month of exponential growth, one infection can become one thousand. In another month, those thousand cases will become one million.

From one infection to one million in two months.

That's roughly what the models predicted for New York in March and April.

But in reality, exponential growth suddenly stopped in mid-March, a week before the lockdown went into effect on March 22. That's why additional hospitalizations in New York City slowed so quickly after March 25.

We still cannot be sure why infections slowed so suddenly. But the one thing we can know for sure is that lockdowns do not deserve the credit. The slowdown occurred *before* they could have had any impact.

But the models were wrong in another way about New York, as well. According to their predictions, new hospitalizations and deaths should have fallen as quickly as they rose. Instead they lingered on into May.

Why?

Because infections remained stubbornly high well into April, instead of crashing after the lockdowns were imposed.

That fact may seem counterintuitive.

But on March 4, 2020, the British SAGE committee was warned that general "social distancing"—a soft lockdown that shut most schools and businesses—would actually *increase* infections inside households by 25 percent. The harsher alternative of "whole household isolation" could cause those infections to double.[15]

In this case, SAGE's analysis proved prescient.

Less than three weeks later, the British moved ahead with an extremely strict lockdown, the functional equivalent of "household isolation" for the entire country. And the United Kingdom did *not* see a quick end to its crisis. After peaking around 950 daily in mid-April, deaths in Britain remained above 400 a day a month later (again, using the seven-day average). Italy, France, and Spain had similarly strict lockdowns and similarly long first waves.

In the United States, the rules were less strict. Still, media-stoked fear kept many people in self-imposed "household isolation" for months—especially in New York City. And in New York, like Western Europe, the epidemic dragged on.

In reality, lockdowns likely *worsen* intrafamilial transmission in the short run. They force younger people who may have been infected to stay home with parents and grandparents, who are at greater risk.

On March 30, at a press conference in Geneva that should have received far more attention than it did, Dr. Mike Ryan explained the dynamic clearly. Ryan, the epidemiologist who led the World Health Organization's Covid team, warned that lockdowns simply moved the spread of the coronavirus into homes and apartments: "At the moment in most parts of the world, due to lockdown, most of the transmission that's actually happening in many countries now is happening in the household at family level. In some senses, transmission has been taken off the streets and pushed back into family units."[16]

Ryan then went a step further, advocating for the forcible removal of people infected with Covid from their homes even if they had no symptoms: "Now we need to go and look in families to find those people who may be sick and remove them and isolate them in a, in a safe and dignified manner."

Only countries that removed and isolated people with Covid could "transition from movement restrictions and shutdowns and stay-at-home orders," Ryan said.

Ryan and other epidemiologists wanted Western countries to follow the approach that Harvard biostatistician Xihong Lin had suggested in his March 12 briefing—aggressively isolate infected people, as China had done.

"Centralized quarantine worked!" Lin had proclaimed. "Infected patients, suspected cases and close contacts were less likely to infect others (reduce transmission). Patients received medical care immediately."

But though Americans and Europeans would accept lockdowns, the first part of the Chinese attack on the coronavirus, they would not even consider the second. It was anathema to Western traditions of individual rights and government restraint. Even the far-fetched suggestion that governments might separate family members provoked furious backlash, forcing governors such as Ohio's Mike DeWine to deny any plans for medical camps.[17]

As a result, the United States and Europe chose arguably the worst possible path—lockdowns that damaged their economies, shut schools, and made many people depressed and fearful while *increasing* in-home transmission. By late spring, the results in countries such as Spain and states such as New York had made clear that Western-style lockdowns that did not include forcible isolation of the infected would work only slowly, if at all.

Maybe the most stunning example of the gap between policymakers' understanding and reality came on May 6. At his daily press conference, Governor Cuomo reported that a survey of a thousand newly hospitalized coronavirus patients in New York over a three-day period had found that two-thirds of them had been infected at home.

Cuomo sounded genuinely baffled by what had happened. "Sixty-six percent of the people were at home, which is shocking to us," he said. "We thought maybe they were taking public transportation...but actually no, because these people were literally at home." Eighty-four percent stayed home almost every day.

"Were they working?" Cuomo said. "No. Only 17 percent were working." The rest were retired or unemployed. "They're not working, they're not traveling."

Cuomo went on to engage in a bit of victim-blaming. "Much of this comes down to what you do to protect yourself," he said. "**Everything is closed down**, government has done everything it could, society has done everything it could, now it's up to you. Are you wearing the mask, are you doing the hand sanitizer? . . . But it comes down to personal behavior" [emphasis added].

Next to him, a slide explained, "Stay home/protect the vulnerable."

Neither Cuomo nor anyone else appeared to recognize the irony.

Another major source of infection was what scientists call "nosocomial," in hospitals or nursing homes. Lockdowns did little or nothing to slow those infections, either, as a fascinating March 2021 paper from Scotland's National Health Service showed.

Scotland had a harsh and long-lasting lockdown. It also aggressively encouraged people at high risk from Covid because they had serious illnesses such as cancer to stay home.

But the paper showed that those people were eight times as likely to develop severe Covid as people without risk factors.[18] And about one in three of their infections came from hospital visits. Lockdown or not, people with chronic illnesses had no choice but to go to the hospital for treatment. But going exposed them to Covid.

"Mitigating the impact of the epidemic requires control of nosocomial transmission," the paper's authors wrote.

Lockdowns did not change that dynamic, and they may even have increased hospital transmission in the short run. The media hysteria around them sent people to emergency rooms, putting people who didn't have the coronavirus in close contact with those who did.

Worst of all, by early April 2020 we had strong evidence the coronavirus essentially did not spread outdoors—and thus that making people stay inside was not just pointless but counterproductive.

On April 7, 2020, Chinese researchers published a paper tracking more than 7,300 Covid cases in China—about two-thirds of all the cases outside Hubei province in January and early February. They pinpointed 318 "outbreaks," which they defined as 3 or more related cases, totaling 1,245 infections. Almost 80 percent of the outbreaks occurred in homes, while one-third took place on buses or other transport. (The numbers totaled more than 100 percent because some outbreaks spread in more than one location or could not be determined.)

Only *one* proven transmission out of the 7,324 cases took place outside, the authors wrote.

Given the large number of cases tracked, this paper should have put to rest any serious concerns that outdoor transmission would be a major infection route for Sars-Cov-2.

Theoretical work also backed the findings. Ultraviolet light, which is far stronger outdoors than inside, kills most viruses, including the coronavirus. A June 2020 paper found that winter-strength "simulated sunlight" killed 90 percent of coronavirus particles within twenty minutes. Summer-strength sunlight did so within eight minutes.[19] Simple common sense suggested that outdoor transmission could hardly be frequent, given that a minimum number of viral particles is necessary for infection and that even the slightest breeze will disperse them.

By May 2021, even the *New York Times* acknowledged, "There is not a single documented Covid infection anywhere in the world from casual outdoor interactions, such as walking past someone on a street or eating at a nearby table."[20]

Yet the efforts to shame people into staying home continued through 2020 and even into 2021. The state of Oregon warned: "Don't Accidentally Kill Someone. Stay Home. Save Lives."[21] In a series of videos, Chicago mayor Lori Lightfoot strummed a guitar and sang, "Stay home, save lives," then told a friend, "You're not bored, you're saving lives."[22] On Twitter, Jimmy Kimmel told his millions of followers, "#StayHome" and proclaimed, "#JimmyKimmelLiveFromHisHouse."[23]

The campaigns were not confined to the United States. In November 2020, a comedic German ad featured a man telling viewers, "The fate of this country lay in our hands. So, we mustered all our courage and did what was expected of us, the only right thing. We did nothing....Our couch was the frontline and our patience was our weapon."[24]

Two months later, the United Kingdom took a more emotional approach. Its ad asked, "Can you look them in the eyes and tell them you're helping by staying at home?"[25]

Those European ads, at least, took place in the fall and winter, when people were less likely to spend time outside if they left home. But those ads, like the "stay home" messaging generally, made no distinction between indoor and outdoor activities. Intentionally or not, they encouraged viewers not to leave their homes at all.

On Twitter and social media, the shaming went much further. On May 3, a blue check named Bess Kalb tweeted to her hundreds of thousands of followers:

> If you are lucky enough to make it off a ventilator (the equivalent exertion required for that is running a marathon without training), you will likely get put on dialysis and a feeding tube next. It's a nightmare. It's hell. It's what you're risking on your beach day....[26]
>
> Send this thread to any idiot fucker who posts an Instagram at the beach or a crowded park. Tell them my dad says see you later.[27]

Kalb's father was a retired physician who had supposedly seen a raft of terrible coronavirus cases in the previous few days, including "young people" who were "talking one minute, stroking out the next."

He lived in New York but saw coronavirus intensive care patients via telemedicine in southern New Jersey and Louisiana, according to Kalb. Taking care of seriously ill patients via telemedicine is very rare except in extremely rural areas; when I tried to confirm that Kalb's father had actually done so, I was unable to.

Nonetheless, Kalb's tweet thread was liked or retweeted hundreds of thousands of times. It was part of a much bigger trend on Twitter. Unverified second- and third-hand horror stories were regularly retweeted tens of thousands of times, especially if they included information about young people becoming ill and dying. Many of those stories would later be proven false, but far fewer people saw the retractions or corrections.

■　　■　　■

In many states, especially those with Democratic governors, efforts to curb outdoor activity were not merely suggestions.

Even as its nursing homes were turning into abattoirs, New Jersey closed its state and county parks on April 7. "We are seeing far too many instances of people gathering in groups in our parks, erroneously thinking that since they're outside social distancing doesn't matter," the state's governor said.[28]

Los Angeles County closed *golf courses and tennis courts* for much of the spring, though it was hard to imagine two sports where people were less likely to transmit Covid.[29]

States such as New York and Massachusetts kept their beaches closed through Memorial Day, and then insisted on discouraging restrictions. New York ruled even after beaches opened: "No active sports will be allowed, picnic areas and playgrounds will be closed, and CDC 6' social distancing measures must be adhered to. Concession stands will also be closed."[30]

Worst of all were the closed playgrounds. With schools shut, denying kids playtime outdoors added insult to injury. Police tape cordoned off swings and slides. Basketball hoops were removed. In Venice Beach, California, the Los Angeles Department of Parks and Recreation filled the ramps and half-pipes at a skateboard park with sand.[31]

Snitches made sure the rules were enforced. My wife and I saw the insanity first-hand when we took our kids to a park near the Hudson

River whose swings and slides were cordoned off with tape. It was a beautiful spring day—but we were the only family present.

Enough, Jackie said. She tore down the tape.

A car was parked in the lot at the edge of the playground. A woman sat in it. She lowered her window and yelled that she would call the police. And she did. Within minutes, a police officer drove up and threatened to arrest Jackie. Jackie hated backing off, but she didn't want to be arrested in front of our kids. We left.

The next time, we found another playground, one that didn't have police tape.

So the lockdowns went on. Stupid laws, stupidly enforced, with just enough flexibility and loopholes that open rebellion seemed more trouble than it was worth. Why be arrested when you could just find another playground? Why get thrown out of a Walmart when you could just hold a cup of coffee and pretend to drink it and wear your mask around your chin while you looked for paper towels for the thousandth time?

It could have been worse. It always could be worse. So the rebellions fizzled, as Michigan's experience proved.

If reporters had taken a hard look at the data around lockdowns, public opinion might have shifted. But they didn't. Throughout the spring of 2020, major news organizations never considered the possibility that lockdowns might have failed or even been counterproductive.

They barely even mentioned the failure of the models to predict hospitalizations. They ignored the reality that hospitals were half empty almost everywhere—and that even in New York the field hospitals had gone mostly unused.

Only at the end of April did the *Times* and other outlets face reality and acknowledge that the peak of the epidemic had passed in New York.

A fair appraisal at that point would have begun with one crucial fact: New York's experience had proven that, whatever its dangers, Sars-Cov-2 was a manageable threat. New York City in March was perhaps the worst possible place for Covid to hit: a densely packed metropolis of nine million people, heavily dependent on mass transit, in the middle of flu season, at a time when physicians had little idea how to treat Covid and were overusing ventilators.

And while the city had some world-class hospitals, millions of its poorer residents depended on municipally run facilities that struggled to deliver competent care at the best of times. In one infamous 2014 incident, a fifty-three-year-old man fell into a coma and died after waiting in the emergency room of Lincoln Hospital in the Bronx for nine hours.[32]

The mismanagement and poor care went back for generations. A scathing 1988 report about *the same hospital* had found that emergency room patients were waiting as long as *six days* to be treated or admitted.[33]

Further, New York's strategy of forcing nursing homes to accept transfers of Covid patients from hospitals caused unnecessary deaths.

This decision may have been the most important policy mistake that resulted from the IHME predictions. Because the IHME and other forecasts vastly overestimated the number of Covid patients who would need hospitalizations, New York wanted to make sure that recovering patients were quickly moved from hospitals to make room for new patients—so the state forced nursing homes to accept them. But nursing homes were ill-equipped either to treat Covid patients or to prevent them from infecting other residents.

Newsday, a newspaper on New York's Long Island, explained the problem on March 29, only days after the state put the policy in place:

> New York State's nursing homes cannot reject newly released hospital patients solely because they tested positive for the novel coronavirus, a new state directive says.
>
> The order raised concern in an industry whose elderly and frail residents have the lowest survival rate for the disease....
>
> Hospitals are under pressure to discharge patients, including ones stricken with the coronavirus but who don't need ventilators, to open up beds for what **Gov. Andrew M. Cuomo says will be a surge of thousands more cases in the next two to four weeks.** However, nursing homes, whose

workforce is struggling with problems like those in hospitals—arranging child care and managing a shortage of supplies like protective garb—fear their facilities will be overwhelmed [emphasis added].[34]

The industry's fears were correct. A study would later find that in New York "COVID-positive new admissions…were associated with several hundred and possibly more than 1,000 additional resident deaths."[35] On May 10, New York reversed its order and prohibited hospitals from sending Covid-positive patients to homes. But by then the damage had been done.

Other states, including New Jersey, followed New York's lead—and they, too, suffered terrible outbreaks in nursing homes. In a single large nursing home in New Jersey, seventy residents died in weeks—with seventeen of the dead stuffed in body bags and left in a storage room until police found them.[36] In all, almost eight thousand nursing home residents and staff died in the state, the worst per capita death total anywhere.[37]

In contrast, Florida and some other states always prohibited hospitals from sending elderly patients back to nursing homes until they tested negative for Covid. Florida even created National Guard "strike teams" to provide frequent Covid testing for nursing home residents. It transferred residents who tested positive to hospitals or a handful of nursing homes that had been dedicated to treating Covid patients. Florida suffered far fewer nursing home deaths per capita than the northeastern states.

All the factors that led to the singular crisis in New York City in March and April 2020 were visible at the time. The city's density, subways, and large apartment buildings offered the perfect environment for viral spread—especially in winter, when the weather kept people inside.

On April 23, New York State released a study showing that 21 percent of New York City residents had already developed antibodies to the virus. In other words, more than 1 in 5 New Yorkers, or 1.8 million people, had already been infected with and recovered from the disease. That number may well have significantly underestimated the true prevalence. But even at 21 percent, New York's infection rate was likely far higher than anywhere else in the United States at the time.[38]

Precise estimates do not exist because the federal government—bizarrely—never conducted proper random antibody sampling to track the spread of the coronavirus (more on this later). But the United States as a whole probably had an overall infection rate in the low to middle single digits in April. It did not hit a 20 percent infection rate until the fall.

In other words, New York suffered several months' spread in a matter of weeks. The ultimate proof of how hard New York had been hit in the spring of 2020 came almost a year later, in the winter of 2021, when the city suffered relatively few infections and deaths even as another major coronavirus wave hit the United States.

So New York had far more than its share of infections in March 2020. Meanwhile, ventilator overuse, badly run hospitals, and nursing home transfers led to thousands of preventable deaths among the infected.

The combination of high infection rates and preventable deaths caused New York City to have among the highest per capita Covid death rates anywhere in the world early on.

By April 14, more than ten thousand city residents had died—40 percent of all the deaths in the United States at the time.[39] By the end of the month, the total topped seventeen thousand, about one in five hundred New Yorkers. At that point, New York City had nearly as many deaths as France, which had a population eight times as large and was itself among the world's hardest-hit countries.

What happened in New York City in the spring of 2020 was a tragedy.

But Covid was only part of the reason for it. Over time, the city would revert much closer to the mean. Its death counts didn't rise much, as the rest of the nation and world slowly caught up.

But New York's importance as a media center meant that its problems were broadcast all over the world, cementing the perception that Covid was exceptionally dangerous. The fact that the city's hospitals were never overrun received far less attention.

In this sense, New York played the same role in April 2020 it did on September 11, 2001. Its experience caused Americans to overestimate a risk that—although real—was smaller than it seemed.

And that mistake fueled the lockdown fire.

13

How Deadly?

For journalists, dramatizing stories about the coronavirus could be difficult, especially as the epidemic dragged on.

Hospitals offered limited access because of privacy rules and concern about infections. The early Chinese videos notwithstanding, no one was dropping dead in the street. Essential government services such as policing continued to function. Celebrities who announced they had been infected nearly all recovered quickly at home.

Villains—especially Donald Trump and Republican governors—were easy to pillory. But finding heroes turned out to be tricky. As much as journalists lionized Dr. Fauci, he wasn't actually *treating* anyone.

Physicians, nurses, and medical staff cared for patients in grueling and difficult conditions, and they garnered deserved praise. But those stories could only be written so often.

Researchers attacked the virus in labs worldwide, making slow progress on unlocking its secrets. But no scientist had beaten the virus with an unexpected and brilliant drug combination.

For a while, news outlets tried to personalize the crisis.

On CNN, first Chris Cuomo and then Brooke Baldwin told their tales of infection first-hand. Those would-be horror stories turned out to be unintentionally ironic. Cuomo complained to viewers that he'd chipped a tooth. Baldwin wrote she "was fighting constant body aches," needed to take hour-long baths for a few days, and sometimes took "two extra-strength Tylenol." (Her story was titled "How Fighting Coronavirus Taught Me about the Gift of Connection.")[1]

The *New York Times* and other outlets produced more lyrically written versions of the same story: *I (or my significant other) had a cough, spiked a fever, didn't go the hospital, was afraid, felt lousy for a few days, and got better.* They contained a surprising number of paragraphs like this, from a *Times* magazine piece in March 2020:

> The nurses, in masks, check T's vitals. He has a slight fever, just over 99 degrees, but that may be lowered because of the recent ibuprofen and acetaminophen in his system. His blood pressure is fine. His pulse is fine. His oxygen saturation is fine...he is not wheezing. He is not having breathing problems. He can keep being treated at home.[2]

Over time, the media largely stopped running these first-person stories, perhaps recognizing they were less compelling than they seemed to the authors.

Instead, reporters focused more attention on the overall death toll from the coronavirus. CNN and MSNBC added death counts to their screens, with total cases and deaths for both the United States and worldwide. The death tickers inched relentlessly higher, hour after hour, day after day. They were cumulative and never reset.

They proved amazingly powerful.

Yet they were, at best, a weak approximation of reality.

As the epidemic in the United States accelerated in March, the Centers for Disease Control muddied the rules for counting Covid deaths.

The CDC explicitly told medical examiners and physicians to use loose criteria when they labeled deaths as Covid-related.

On March 24, 2020, the CDC issued a one-page bulletin introducing a new International Classification of Diseases (ICD) code for Covid deaths.

All death certificates contain basic information on the manner of death—whether someone has died from a homicide, suicide, accident, or natural causes. The certificates also contain the cause of death, such as a heart attack or cancer. Those causes are represented by ICD codes.

The codes begin with a letter to represent the broadest category of disease, followed by numbers representing specifics. For example, ICD categories A and B are infectious and parasitic diseases. Within the general category of infectious disease, A00.0 is the code for cholera in particular.

The codes are largely the same worldwide. The standardization helps governments and researchers in different countries compare death rates from different illnesses. Hospitals, physicians, and insurance companies also use ICD codes on treatment and billing records. ICD codes are the universal language of medicine.

In its March 24 bulletin, the CDC said the new code for Covid cases would be U07.1. (The U code was used for "provisional assignment of new diseases.") But the CDC didn't just introduce a new code for a new cause of death; the Centers for Disease Control specifically encouraged people who coded death certificates to use the U07.1 code in any case where they suspected Covid. A confirmed laboratory test for the illness was not necessary.

"The rules for coding and selection of the underlying cause of death are expected to result in COVID19 being the underlying cause more often than not," the alert explained. It went on to make clear that deaths of people who did *not* have a positive Sars-Cov-2 test could be reported as Covid-related:

> Should 'COVID-19' be reported on the death certificate only
> with a confirmed test?
>
> COVID-19 should be reported on the death certificate for
> all decedents where the disease caused or **is assumed to have
> caused or contributed to death** [emphasis added].[3]

The Centers for Disease Control had created a double standard
for Covid death coding—a double standard that most states quickly
adopted.

Medical examiners and states had the discretion to call deaths
Covid-related *without* positive tests. As the state of Virginia explained,
a case investigator could classify a death as due to Covid "through
medical record review, talking with the patient's healthcare provider, or
talking with their family."[4]

At the same time, a positive test for Sars-Cov-2 meant a death would
be counted as Covid-related, even if the death certificate did not mention
Covid. To make sure they caught all cases, states matched death certificates to registries of people who had had positive Covid tests. Any person
on both would be added to the list of Covid deaths.

In some states, the death had to occur within a month of the test. In
others it could be two months or more. For example, Arizona included
anyone "who died of a heart or lung condition who received a positive
COVID-19 test within 60 days," according to the public health director
of the state's largest county.[5]

The rule led to absurdities. Some states, such as Arizona, at least
tried to ensure that they screened out victims of suicide, homicide, or
drug overdoses[6] who had had positive Covid tests.[7] Other states included
even those in their count of Covid deaths. Younger people were especially
likely to be misclassified as dying from Covid, the CDC reported in a
March 2021 paper.[8]

Still, the obvious mistakes made up only a small fraction of the total
reported Covid deaths. In its 2021 review, the CDC put the number at
3 percent.

A second issue around the coding for Covid deaths was larger, and nearly impossible to fix. It was the reality—so rarely discussed in the media—that the vast majority of Covid victims were very old, very obese, very unhealthy, or all three.

In the United States, the median age at which people died of the coronavirus was seventy-eight.[9] (The median age is the point at which half of people are older and half are younger.) In European countries, it was even higher, typically in the low eighties. In Canada it was eighty-five.[10] About 65 percent of the people who died of Covid in Canada were over eighty. Fewer than 2 percent were under fifty.[11]

Even compared to other people the same age, those who died of the coronavirus tended to be very sick. In the United States, about 35 percent of all coronavirus victims lived in nursing homes and other long-term care facilities, even though they made up less than 1 percent of the population.[12] Nursing homes generally house the frailest of the elderly. A 2010 study found that 53 percent of residents died within six months of being admitted.[13]

In Italy, which had more deaths per capita than any other big European country, the Italian National Health Institute examined hospital records of Covid patients to see how sick they were. It found that the average Italian who died from Sars-Cov-2 had nearly four serious pre-existing conditions. As of April 2021, almost one in three had diabetes, one in four had dementia, one in six had had a recent case of cancer, and nearly as many were in heart failure.[14] About 10 percent of all the people who died of Covid were hospitalized for conditions that appeared to have nothing to do with the virus, such as cancer or cirrhosis.

Only 281 of the 118,000 Italians who died were under 40 years of age. Of those, only 41 did not have serious preexisting conditions such as kidney disease. Italy has about 24 million people under 40, so the odds that people under 40 and healthy would die of Covid in the first year-plus of the illness were less than 1 in 500,000.

The United States had somewhat more young people die of Covid than other wealthy countries for the worst possible reason—Americans are more likely to be morbidly obese and have other chronic conditions.

Those were the aggregated statistics.

The details of individual cases offered a closer and sadder view. They were available on death certificates, which some medical examiners released online with names removed. The Milwaukee County coroner's office was one.[15] The deaths it reported looked like this, for case 21-4084:

Age	69 Years
Gender	Female
Race	White
Mode	Natural
Cause A	Complications of infection with novel Coronavirus (COVID-19)
Cause B	
Cause Other	Diabetes mellitus, chronic obstructive pulmonary disease, bipolar disorder

Or this, for case 20-06169:

Case Number	20-06169
Case Type	Body Released
Date of Event	
Date of Death	9/3/2020, 12:00 PM
Age	90 Years
Gender	Female
Race	White
Mode	Natural
Cause A	Complications of chronic congestive heart failure
Cause B	
Cause Other	Chronic renal failure; infection with novel Coronavirus (COVID-19)

Or case 20-06158:

Case Type	Body Released
Date of Event	
Date of Death	9/2/2020, 11:10 PM
Age	84 Years
Gender	Male
Race	Black
Mode	Natural
Cause A	Hypertensive and atherosclerotic cardiovascular disease
Cause B	
Cause Other	Prostate cancer, dementia, infection with novel Coronavirus (COVID-19)

Those were reported as Covid deaths. And Covid may well have been the last straw for the victims. But as the Canadian Broadcasting Corporation had noted in a 2012 article about the way Canada counted deaths from flu: "Death can be complicated. If someone already extremely fragile with heart or lung disease is tipped over the edge with a flu infection, is that a flu death, or a heart death or a lung death? Which database gets to claim it?"[16]

In March 2020 testimony to the British Parliament, Neil Ferguson estimated half to two-thirds of coronavirus deaths might have occurred in people who would have died within nine months. That guess was probably high. In September 2020, Service Corporation International, the largest American funeral home operator, reported that about one-third of all the funerals of people who had died of Covid would have occurred in 2020 in any case. Another one-third or more would have happened in 2021, the company said.

Covid victims with dementia, Alzheimer's disease, or cancer accounted for over 100,000 of the dead in the United States through late spring 2021. For those people, it could be impossible to distinguish between dying *from* Covid and dying *with* Covid.

But they were all counted as Covid deaths.

That said, Covid clearly did kill hundreds of thousands of Americans in 2020. The reason we can be so sure is that about a half-million more Americans died in 2020 than 2019. A total of 2,854,000 Americans died in 2019,[17] compared to 3,358,000 in 2020.[18]

The difference between the two years—roughly half a million more deaths in 2020—was generally reported as the number of "excess deaths." In reality, the excess was probably slightly lower. The number of deaths rises over time as the population grows and ages. Improvements in medical care can only keep people alive for so long. Between 2009 and 2019, deaths in the United States rose about forty thousand per year on average.

We will never know how many people would have died in 2020 if Covid had not existed, of course. The CDC used a relatively low baseline, assuming that deaths would not have increased much over 2019. In reality, the "natural" year-over-year increase could have been as high as 100,000 deaths in 2020, to make up for relatively small increases in deaths in 2018 and 2019. In that case, a better baseline would be 2.95 million American deaths, not the 2.85 million the CDC used.

Further, part of the 2020 increase came from deaths caused by lockdowns. Deaths of despair surged. Rising overdoses were the most obvious example. The number of Americans who died from overdoses rose by at least twenty thousand in 2020, to nearly one hundred thousand, the highest total ever. Homicides and traffic deaths also rose.

Other deaths occurred when people delayed medical care because they feared going to hospitals and catching the virus—though those are much harder to quantify. (In April 2020, the chief medical officer of Ontario, a Canadian province with fourteen million people, reported that thirty-five people had died in the month after Ontario's lockdown began from delayed cardiac surgeries alone.[19] That figure would have translated into almost one thousand unnecessary cardiac deaths in the United States for the month. But it was only a single datapoint.)

Still, lockdown deaths accounted for only a fraction of the 2020 surge in deaths. The United States reported about 378,000 Covid deaths in 2020. Even if aggressive coding rules mean that 20 percent to 30 percent of those deaths occurred "with" rather than "from" Covid, the only reasonable conclusion is that Sars-Cov-2 caused the majority of the overall increase in American deaths in 2020.

But just as reporters almost never discussed who really died of Covid, they almost never put those death figures in the context of overall mortality. Even in the United States and the hardest-hit European countries, and even forgetting about the "with" versus "from" problem, Covid deaths accounted for at most 1 in 8 of all the people who died in 2020.

Worldwide, the ratio was far lower. About 1.9 million deaths were attributed to Covid out of nearly 60 million deaths total. In other words, Covid killed roughly 1 out of every 30 people who died in 2020.

That number probably somewhat underestimated the real toll, because in some countries—such as Russia—overall deaths rose far faster than the number of reported Covid deaths. In those countries, Covid deaths may have been undercounted for political reasons or because tests were not widely available—the opposite of the situation in the United States.

Still, Covid was far from the world's leading killer. It would have ranked sixth in 2019, coming in just ahead of lung and other smoking-related cancers. (Heart disease was first, killing almost 9 million people; stroke killed another 6 million.)

Journalists also chronically overestimated the death rate from the coronavirus—the odds that it would kill someone it infected.

By mid to late March, scientists understood that the early Chinese estimates that the virus might kill 3 to 4 percent of the people who got it were far too high. They quickly cut their estimates to roughly 1 percent.

The 1 percent figure became a common benchmark in the media. In May, *USA Today* reported that Dr. Fauci had "testified to Congress in March that the mortality rate may be as low as 1%."[20]

Similarly, the Associated Press said in August 2020 that "scientists have estimated that fewer than 1% of all COVID-19 infections result in death." The AP then provided two estimates of around 0.7 percent.[21] In November 2020, Reuters reported that "social media users...[say] the disease itself has a survival rate of 99%."[22]

The 1 percent mortality rate figure became widely used in part because 1 percent seems relatively easy to understand. It also seems relatively low, helping most people understand why they personally did not know anyone who'd died. At 1 percent, one person out of every one hundred infected with the coronavirus would die, while ninety-nine of them would survive.

But as the articles that used the 1 percent figure usually went on to explain, a 1 percent death rate, when multiplied by the United States' population of 330 million, meant the virus could kill 3.3 million Americans. Worldwide, that 1 percent rate would translate into *80 million* deaths. Those numbers were high enough to justify strict restrictions.

But the real coronavirus rate was *not* 1 percent. It was much lower. What was it?

To find out quickly, governments should have run large-scale and randomized antibody tests. Our immune systems make antibodies to fight off viruses or bacteria. A positive antibody test shows someone has already recovered from infection. Researchers can then compare the antibody results to the number of positive PCR tests, which find people who are actively infected.

The difference matters immensely. Before we can know the true risk of the coronavirus, or any virus, we need to know how many people it has infected. In the risk equation, the number of people who die is the numerator (the top figure). But we also need the denominator (bottom figure)—the number of infections.

Deaths are relatively easy to track. Every death is recorded. But not every infection is, especially if people recover on their own without seeing a doctor or even feeling sick.

So a national randomized antibody screen should have been a top priority for the United States in 2020. But for reasons that remain unclear to this day, federal authorities did not run one in the spring of 2020, when the answers would have mattered most.

Still, some states and cities performed their own, as did other countries.

In the spring of 2020, those studies consistently found that up to 50 times as many people had antibodies as the number of infected people that that PCR tests had identified. For example, Miami-Dade County reported in April 2020 that its tests showed 165,000 people had positive antibody tests, compared to 10,000 who had positive PCR tests—a ratio of 16.5 total infections for every 1 reported.[23]

Los Angeles County said its tests had found an even bigger gap—between twenty-eight and fifty-five to one.[24] "Early Results of Antibody Testing Suggest Number of COVID-19 Infections Far Exceeds Number of Confirmed Cases," the county reported in a press release. Tests in Santa Clara County found the difference might be as high as eighty-five to one.[25] A survey in Boston in May found the ratio was more like seven to one.[26]

Along with individual antibody tests, sewage monitoring offered another way to track community-wide transmission and caseloads. The feces of infected people contained a detectable and predictable amount of Sars-Cov-2. So counting the number of viral particles in wastewater allowed researchers to estimate infections.

For example, monitoring of a sewage plant that served a county in Delaware revealed about 15,200 infections in mid-April. At the time, the county had reported 974 infections. That ratio—16 to 1—was remarkably similar to that Miami researchers had found at the same time, using a very different method to find cases.[27]

The gap between the actual number of cases and the reported number resulted both from a relative lack of tests early in the epidemic and because so many people were never tested—because they had few or no symptoms. In all, the tests pointed to massive undercounting in the spring. Perhaps as many as twenty to twenty-five cases were missed for every one that was caught. (Later in the year, as PCR testing became wider and caught more infections, that multiple would drop. Still, it remained in the range of three to five. For example, a paper published by the *Journal of the American Medical Association* estimated about 47 million Sars-Cov-2 infections as of November 15, at a time when the United States had 11.5 million cases.)[28]

In late April 2020, the reported death rate for the coronavirus was about 6 percent—about sixty thousand deaths had been reported out of one million cases.[29]

In other words, based on PCR test results, six out of one hundred people who were infected with the virus were supposed to be dying. That figure was terrifying, even higher than the Spanish flu.

But it *didn't* represent the real death rate. It wasn't close. The twenty-to-one ratio of antibody tests to PCR positives suggested that the real mortality rate was one *twentieth* as high as that 6 percent figure. In other words, 6 percent divided by twenty—or 0.3 percent.

If the ratio was twenty-five to one, the real risk was roughly 0.24 percent.

That figure equaled not six deaths out of every one hundred infections, but one death out of every three to four hundred infections.

At that rate, the coronavirus was far less dangerous than the earliest estimates had suggested, and significantly less dangerous than the 1 percent figure that journalists used as shorthand. It was perhaps three to four times as deadly as an average flu strain.

But the flu was *relatively* more dangerous to children and teens than Sars-Cov-2. A paper in *The Lancet* would later suggest that in big Western European countries, about one in *one million* teenagers had died of the coronavirus through February 2021, the entire first year of the epidemic.[30]

A separate paper in the *British Medical Journal* on children and teenagers who had been hospitalized for the coronavirus found that they made up only about 1 percent of all patients in Britain through May

2020. Six children died, the authors reported. All six were profoundly ill with conditions unrelated to Covid.[31]

Most of us, if pressed, would admit that although all deaths are terrible, not all are equally tragic. The death of a child with her whole life ahead of her hurts more than the death of an eighty-five-year-old who has already led a full life.

Economists and epidemiologists have a way to quantify this idea: "life-years lost." They measure "life-years lost" by figuring out how many years the average person had left to live when he died of a certain disease. Then they multiply that figure by the number of overall deaths.

Traffic accidents and drug overdoses and AIDS, which kill mostly younger people, account for a disproportionate number of life-years lost. COVID ranks on the opposite end of the scale, because it kills the old and infirm far more than anyone else. In the United States in 2020, life-years lost to overdoses were likely significantly higher than those lost to Covid.

But to say that truth aloud, or even hint at it, was to risk being called callous, a grandma-killer. The author of one bizarre piece published in *The Atlantic* in September 2020 appeared to be shocked by this finding: "Globally, people don't value elderly lives as much as they do young people's, research shows. When it comes to deciding who lives or dies, there's a disregard for the elderly, even *among* the elderly."[32]

How could this research surprise anyone? If the question were posed the other way—*Should the young be sacrificed to benefit the old?*—the answer would clearly be no.

Yet our inability to discuss the risks of Covid honestly and explicitly meant that we were making that choice day after day, as the lockdowns stretched on.

14

Hitting Bottom

T he coronavirus's effect on government spending was as extraordinary as everything else about it.

By May 2020, the federal government was spending hundreds of millions a week on PCR testing alone. Extra federal payments to hospitals came to more than $3 billion a week *for over a year.* They totaled almost $200 billion.[1]

As big as those expenses were, they were dwarfed by the spending to mitigate the economic cost of lockdowns.

As the panic accelerated in March 2020, the American and world economies appeared close to collapse. Smaller stores and travel and hospitality businesses such as hotels and restaurants faced immediate crises. Some kept their doors open with dramatically smaller workforces. Others shut basically overnight.

New unemployment claims, which typically total 200,000 to 250,000 a week, rose to an unthinkable 6.9 million in the last week of March. By the end of April, almost 30 million Americans—one-seventh of the working-age population—had filed for unemployment. The jobless rate rose from 3.5 percent in February to almost 15 percent in April, the highest level since the Great Depression.[2]

Briefly, food and energy supply chains appeared to be at risk of real disruption.

In late April, the price of oil for near-term delivery fell *below* $0 a barrel—and kept falling, all the way to minus $37.63.

In other words, storage tanks were so full that traders who had promised to buy oil but didn't have space to store it had to pay other traders who had a place to put it. The space was more valuable than the oil.

"In the age of coronavirus...the world's most important commodity is quickly losing all value as chronic oversupply overwhelms the world's crude tanks, pipelines, and supertankers," Bloomberg News said in a story about the crisis.[3]

Toilet paper, paper towels, and cleaning products disappeared from stores. Fresh fruit was hard to find. So were staples such as rice and flour. After big meatpacking plants shut due to outbreaks, processing companies claimed they could not guarantee grocery stores would remain supplied with meat. "The food supply chain is breaking," Tyson Foods warned in a full-page ad in late April.[4]

Those reports were exaggerated. The shortages had more to do with panic buying than any real disruption on the manufacturing side. The people who died of Covid were mostly retired, not in the workforce. Meatpacking plants did have more than their share of outbreaks because they were poorly ventilated and crowded. Even so, the vast majority of workers were asymptomatic. In one pork processing plant in Missouri, *not a single one* of the 370 workers who tested positive for Covid had symptoms.[5]

Still, the empty shelves were frightening. Full stores and cheap food had been the American way since at least the end of World War II.

In spring 2020, shoppers queued up in long, frigid pre-dawn lines outside Walmarts, under the wary eyes of police. I remember those mornings well. I was one of those shoppers, and those lines felt dystopian.

Maybe humbling is a more accurate description. We stamped our feet to stay warm and looked at each other in profound disbelief. But we were there, waiting our turn to shop, making sure our families wouldn't have to worry about food. In weeks, the United States had somehow become barely recognizable.

The financial system also briefly came under tremendous stress.

Between Valentine's Day and March 20, when Cuomo announced New York would lock down, the Standard & Poor's 500 Index lost almost one-third of its value. Indexes of market volatility spiked to levels not seen since the 2008 financial collapse.

With unemployment soaring, banks faced the risk of defaults on mortgages so severe that even the extra cash they had raised after the 2008 financial crisis might not save them. Stocks of big banks such as Wells Fargo were even harder hit than the overall market, with some banks losing more than half their value.

In response, the Federal Reserve—the central bank of the United States—and the federal government offered unprecedented financial support.

The Fed made essentially unlimited cash available to banks and financial companies. It also began to buy corporate debt—directly supporting big companies, a step it had never taken before.[6] As the *New York Times* explained on March 23, "The Fed is throwing its full weight at confronting the economic fallout from the coronavirus, which poses a severe threat as factories shut down, people lose jobs and the economy grinds to a halt."

Days later, Congress passed a $2 trillion economic aid package—more than $6,000 in new spending for every American—that seemed to have free money for almost everyone. Unemployed people received an extra $600 a week in addition to their state benefits. Many people wound up being paid more to stay home than they had been when they were working.[7]

Airlines, hotels, and travel companies received $25 billion in federal cash and another $25 billion in loans.[8] State and local governments were given $150 billion in cash.[9] Hospitals and health care received massive Covid payments, of course. Other businesses benefited from the "Paycheck Protection Program," which allowed them to receive ultra-low-interest loans that most would never repay.

Local, state, and federal employees continued to be paid too, whether they worked or not. I found no reports of any government employees laid off during the spring or summer of 2020 because of Covid budget cuts.

The biggest federal borrowing binge in history paid for the spending. The wave of borrowing raised the national debt to almost $27 trillion as of September 2020. The figure was an all-time high compared to the size of the American economy, even more than the previous peak during World War II. Every American would have to work for an entire year to pay off the debt.

Economists call what the Federal Reserve did "monetary" stimulus. Basically, the Fed was trying to keep prices stable or rising and help the financial system by pumping money into it. They call what the federal government did "fiscal" stimulus—borrowing money and giving it to companies, local governments, and ordinary people.

Never before had the United States used so much monetary and fiscal stimulus so quickly. The Federal Reserve's balance sheet, which had risen by about $1 trillion after the 2008 financial crisis, soared by $3 trillion in spring 2020. The $2 trillion in federal spending dwarfed President Obama's $831 billion stimulus package after the 2008 financial crisis.[10]

The effects were immediate.

Within months, the economy had not just stabilized but turned up. Pressure on supply chains dissipated. The prospect of meatpacking shortages vanished after the government said plants should stay open even if workers tested positive.[11] Oil prices stabilized too. (For some reason, paper towels and cleaning products remained in short supply for most of 2020.)

After soaring in April, unemployment turned down in May. Overall, the United States economy shrank about 10 percent in the spring. Though that was its worst performance since the Great Depression, it was far better than big European countries such as France and Britain that had locked down harder.

The extra unemployment payments saved millions of Americans from poverty. After plunging 30 percent in late March, consumer spending rapidly came back. In fact, low-wage workers were actually spending *more* on average by early summer than they had been spending in February. (Wealthier people still spent about 10 percent less, in part because they were eating out and traveling less.)

Over the summer, the V-shaped American recovery accelerated, with the United States regaining strength nearly as quickly as it had lost it in the spring. By the end of the year, the United States unemployment rate had fallen to 6.7 percent—about twice its level before the epidemic began, but within the range of normal. States where lockdowns had been less severe, such as Florida, performed even better. Florida's unemployment rate was 6.1 percent at the end of December, while California's was 9 percent.[12]

Overall, the American economy shrank 3.5 percent in 2020.[13] The European Union had a harder fall, shrinking more than 6 percent.

All those outcomes were positive, and fair. Ordinary Americans did not cause the Covid epidemic, so why should the government allow lockdowns to bankrupt them? Yet by blunting the economic hardships of lockdowns, policymakers reduced the pressure to end them quickly.

The effects on the stock market and financial system were even more stunning—and harder to defend. March 20 was the bottom. Stocks reversed course *even before the lockdowns began*. Hedge funds and big investors took a cold-eyed look at the data around hospitalizations and deaths. They realized the media hysteria was wrong and the United States could easily weather the coronavirus.

But the money the Federal Reserve poured into the system also fueled the fire. In the spring of 2020, even bold companies and entrepreneurs had few ways to make real capital investments. A significant portion of the cash went into the stock market instead, pushing prices higher.

No one benefited from the rally more than technology companies. After falling less than the overall market in early March, shares in

Amazon almost doubled between March and August. Facebook had a similar run.

Smaller internet-centric companies gained even more. The value of Pinterest rose seven-fold in the eleven months after its March lows. Zoom gained five-fold from March to October.

The majority of Americans own no or almost no stocks. They gained little from the rally. Instead, trillions of dollars in wealth went to the top 10 percent, the top 1 percent, and especially the tech executives at the very apex of the wealth pyramid.

The gains made billionaires of many of them—and supercharged the already vast fortunes of titans such as Facebook's Mark Zuckerberg and Amazon's Jeff Bezos. Suddenly the tech elite had both extra ammunition and extra motivation to support the lockdowns. They could live in comfort in their second or third homes, with food and everything else they wanted delivered, watching their fortunes mount day by day.

They had no reason to want anything to change.

15

Apocalypse Not

B y May, the epidemic's first wave had waned, not just in New York but nationally.

Led by Georgia and Florida, big Republican-run states eased their lockdowns. The change prompted forecasts of doom from the same media outlets that had breathlessly counted deaths in New York.

"Georgia's Experiment in Human Sacrifice," a headline in *The Atlantic* called it on April 29. "The state is about to find out how many people need to lose their lives to shore up the economy."[1] By then, *The Atlantic* was distinguishing itself as the most hysterical elite media outlet of all—no small feat.

Eight days before, Dana Milbank of the *Washington Post* had written that "Georgia Gov. Brian Kemp...has a bold plan to turn his state into the place to die."

He added, "Several Republican governors, with Trump's encouragement, are racing to reopen during the pandemic, using their constituents as lab rats to see what happens when you relax virus containment."[2]

Beyond being in fantastically bad taste, Milbank's predictions were wrong. Georgia saw no increase in cases for more than a month after its lockdown ended.

But the national media continued to fan panic. On May 4, the *New York Times* highlighted an outdated federal forecast predicting the United States could suffer three thousand Covid deaths a day by June 1. "Models Project Sharp Rise in Deaths as States Reopen," the headline read. The article starkly warned, "The numbers underscore a sobering reality: The United States has been hunkered down for the past seven weeks to try slowing the spread of the virus, but reopening the economy will make matters worse."

The article predicted daily deaths would rise more than 50 percent during May.[3]

In fact, they *declined* about 50 percent, from just under two thousand deaths on May 7 to just over one thousand three weeks later. Yet the *Times* never updated the prediction or acknowledged the mistake, just as it had largely ignored the failure of its predictions about ventilators and hospital overrun.

Meanwhile, Trump's squabbles with reporters worsened, especially after his comments about injecting disinfectant became comic fodder. "Trump Wanted a Coronavirus Victory Event," the *Washington Post* said in mid-May. "It Ended When He Stalked Off after Clashing with Two Female Reporters."[4]

The more contemptuous journalists became of Trump, the more they fawned over Anthony Fauci. "Dr. Fauci's firm adherence to science makes him a profile in courage," a *Minneapolis Star-Tribune* columnist wrote on May 5.

Throughout the spring, Fauci gave a stunning number of interviews—not just to the *New York Times* and CNN and NPR, but to celebrities such as Steph Curry, the star Golden State Warriors guard. Curry hosted a podcast where Fauci appeared in March.

By early May, the White House was trying to wind down the federal coronavirus task force, an obvious attempt to lower Fauci's profile.[5] Like so many of the president's attempts to restore normality in 2020, the move backfired. Within hours, he was forced to reverse course.[6]

The move was yet another of Trump's self-inflicted wounds. Even many Republicans simply did not trust Trump to lead the fight against the coronavirus. The skeptics turned instead to governors such as DeSantis, whose briefings had the seriousness and attention to detail that Trump's lacked.

Through the spring and summer, Trump and the White House found no way to counter the narrative that he and the United States had failed. The media and public health experts ignored the reality that most Western European countries had per capita Covid death rates similar to the United States'.

When the government corrected one supposed failure, the doom-sayers moved their attention to another. We lacked ventilators. We lacked masks and gloves for medical staff. (This narrative persisted for months, even after hospitals and states began reporting vast stockpiles of personal protective equipment.)

We needed more tests, more contact tracers, more warnings.

Most of all we needed more patience, more time in lockdown.

We needed more, always more. If the government could do more it would save us.

No matter how the president or his aides tried to respond, the death counts overpowered them. Thirty-five thousand, sixty thousand, ninety thousand, they ground inexorably higher, and the media excitement as they approached one hundred thousand was palpable. Excitement is an ugly word, but nothing else properly describes the tone.

"When Will US Reach 100,000 Deaths? After a Horrific April, Grim Milestone Could Hit in May," *USA Today* predicted on May 1.[7] Some outlets added a dash of anti-Trump seasoning. "Trump, Maskless, Goes Golfing as Coronavirus Death Toll Nears 100,000," *Vanity Fair* observed. "Determined not to let a pandemic ruin his holiday weekend, the president was seen golfing with three partners."[8]

On Saturday, May 23, determined to ensure no other outlet would get credit for calling the milestone first, the *New York Times* jumped the gun. The paper devoted its entire front page to a list of one thousand Covid victims. The headline read, "U.S. DEATHS NEAR 100,000, AN INCALCULABLE LOSS." The words were emotionally arresting—and profoundly illogical. After all, what was the death count if not a *precise calculation* of the loss?

Somehow, the article did not mention the more than one million Americans who had died from other causes in the first five months of 2020. Their deaths didn't matter.

And the sixth person on the *Times*'s list hadn't died of Covid at all. Twenty-seven-year-old Jordan Driver Haynes was a homicide victim. He was found dead March 12 in a car parked along an Iowa interstate,[9] a fact that anyone at the *Times* could have learned by simply Googling his name. Haynes's inclusion proved an unfortunate reminder that many young people who were supposedly Covid victims had actually died of other causes.

Before the real cause of Haynes's death came to light, I had predicted a death like his would be included high on the *Times* list. Just after the article appeared online, I tweeted:

> Serious question: anyone wonder how far down the list one would have to go to find the first "gunshot wound" or "alcohol poisoning" death? I'm not going to bother, but unless these names were vetted very carefully (unlikely—the job would be huge), probably not too far.[10]

Needless to say, tweets like these did not endear me to my former employer or the people who worked there.

16

Musk, Bezos, and Me

T hen I decided to write something longer.

By May, people were asking me if I could compile information from my tweets into a longer form. I had tweeted thousands of times. Finding specific information from my feed could be difficult, even for me. And I wanted to create something more lasting than Twitter threads.

Also, as my wife had begun to remind me, all those tweets weren't paying the bills. Of course, we were in no financial danger. Jackie was working. I had saved money from my book contracts.

Still, I felt like I should find a way to make some money from the work I was doing—and I no longer doubted it was work. People on Twitter liked to call me a grifter, as if reporters at the *Times* and elsewhere weren't paid for their writing. Some followers had offered to donate, but I didn't want to take money directly. Ditto with the hedge funds that had tried to hire me to consult.

I considered a podcast. I even bought a microphone and recorded a couple of episodes. They were okay. But a real podcast required professional production and lots of time. I wasn't sure if anyone would want to hear me.

No, I was a writer. I would write a booklet about the epidemic and see if anyone wanted it. I could self-publish it through Amazon's Kindle Direct Publishing platform. The economics were straightforward. As long as I priced the ebook between $2.99 and $9.99, Amazon would charge a 30 percent fee for access to its self-publishing platform. I would keep the remaining 70 percent (less a few cents for the cost of the download). For the paperback booklet, I'd pay the costs to print the book plus a 40 percent distribution fee. I would make about $2 on each $2.99 ebook, a little less on each $5.99 pamphlet.

I had no idea how interested my Twitter audience would be and whether I would sell two hundred, two thousand, or twenty thousand booklets. I figured anything over five thousand copies would be gravy, for what I hoped would be only a couple of weeks' work. At the least I'd show my wife I wasn't just wasting time on Twitter.

The booklet wound up taking longer and being longer than I expected. I needed to make sure it was airtight, every fact triple-checked. To keep its length manageable, I dropped the idea of offering a broad look at the crisis. Instead I focused on the issue of how the United States tracked and reported Covid deaths, as well as the real death rates from the virus. The timing made sense because of the hundred-thousand-deaths milestone.

As I was writing, I held myself to the same standard I had as a reporter for the *Times*. Maybe higher. I didn't have an editor to back me or a libel lawyer on call if someone sued. As with this book, I included citations to primary sources so readers could judge them first-hand.

I did have excellent informal editing help from other anti-lockdown journalists who read it and offered suggestions, which I gratefully accepted. I finished my final edits June 3. The booklet was about six thousand words in all, the equivalent of a long magazine article, meaty but not overwhelming. Or so I hoped.

I ended the booklet with a prediction that Covid might kill as many as six hundred thousand Americans. I figured publicizing that number might upset some readers, since it was almost six times the death count at the time. But it was what my estimate of the infection fatality rate suggested, and I was resolved to report it—even if doing so would raise questions about my general anti-lockdown stance.

Because the booklet took me longer than I had expected to finish, I worried that I had missed my window. What if the news cycle was leaving Covid behind? In retrospect, I know that idea seems ludicrous. But in early June 2020 the Black Lives Matter protests were receiving around-the-clock coverage. Covid deaths were falling. Still, I had done the work. I figured I might as well post the booklet and see what would happen.

I had planned to call the booklet the *Essential Guide to Covid-19 and Lockdowns*. At the last minute I decided to change the title to *Unreported Truths about Covid-19 and Lockdowns*. I thought *Essential Guide* sounded too much like a handbook for backpackers. *Unreported Truths* captured my goal more accurately.

On the afternoon of June 3, I uploaded the Word file to Kindle Direct Publishing. I put together a simple cover, black type on a grey background, and made sure the booklet looked okay. (It looked okay. Not great. It looked self-published, for sure.) I set the price and clicked through to start the publishing process. I expected to see the booklet for sale that night, or the next day at the latest.

Instead, the next morning, Amazon emailed me that it had rejected *Unreported Truths*.

> Your book does not comply with our guidelines. As a result we are not offering your book for sale.
>
> Due to the rapidly changing nature of information around the COVID-19 virus, we are referring customers to official sources for health information about the virus. Please consider removing references to COVID-19 for this book. Amazon reserves the right to determine what content we offer according to our content guidelines.

Oh? All I needed to do to get my book about Covid printed was remove all references to Covid?

Got it.

The rejection offered no way to appeal. I couldn't even ask what Amazon had found offensive in the booklet. Since the note made no reference to anything specific I had written, I suspected Amazon was blocking almost all self-published books about Covid. Was the censorship automated? Given the thousands of books writers uploaded each day to Kindle Direct, I imagined it had to be. (I later asked Amazon but did not get a straight answer.)

Nor was Amazon alone in suppressing opinions about Covid that contradicted whatever the preferred public health and government narrative was at the moment. In April, YouTube had taken down a press conference downplaying the dangers of the coronavirus given by two California physicians. The fact that *a local ABC affiliate* had aired the conference didn't matter.[1]

Later, YouTube would pull a talk given by Dr. Scott Atlas, a Stanford physician.[2] (This censorship was particularly stupid. At the time, Atlas was advising President Trump on Covid. Everyone needed to hear his views even if—or especially if—they were outside the medical mainstream.)

Facebook wasn't just suppressing videos or posts. It erased entire groups organizing anti-lockdown protests, most notably a Michigan group that had 400,000 members.[3]

With the world depending on them for information and virtual communities, technology and social media companies had become something close to utilities, if not monopolies. The law had not caught up to their power.

The censorship was particularly galling because of the way big tech companies were benefiting from the lockdowns. No company or person gained more than Amazon or its founder, Jeff Bezos.

Under the circumstances, I thought Amazon and Bezos had an obligation to allow debate over Covid. In the past, Amazon had generally allowed people to publish whatever they wanted on Kindle Direct, even neo-Nazi pamphlets. As ProPublica had reported in April 2020,

It takes just a couple of minutes to upload one's work to Kindle Direct Publishing (KDP), Amazon's self-publishing arm; the e-book then shows up in the world's largest bookstore within half a day, typically with minimal oversight. . . .

Interviews with more than two dozen former Amazon employees suggest that the company's drive for market share and philosophical aversion to gatekeepers have incubated an anything-goes approach to content: Virtually no idea is too inflammatory, and no author is off-limits.[4]

But the tolerance Amazon offered neo-Nazis didn't extend to books that might hurt its business.

Amazon's rejection left me with only a handful of choices, none appetizing. I could try to sell the booklets through my own website. But I'd have to set up my own payment, printing, and fulfillment. The more booklets I sold, the harder staying on top of those pieces would be.

I could make the booklet available for free downloads and ask people to donate. But I wanted to have physical copies available. And, again, I didn't want to be dependent on donations.

I could try to find an independent or conservative publisher who would publish the booklet. I knew at least one was interested. But that publisher had told me that the process would take several weeks, while Amazon could begin printing and shipping booklets within forty-eight hours and make ebooks available for immediate download. And I would have to give up at least half of what I made, with no guarantee that Amazon wouldn't censor the booklet, even from the publisher.

Or I could take try to a run at Amazon—make a public fuss and hope the company relented. Of course, that option was a long shot, at best. Amazon did what Amazon wanted. As a shoe company executive had said in a 2019 *New Yorker* piece, recounting his struggles with Amazon, "We're just one company, and there's millions of companies they deal with every day. . . . You have to swallow what they give you and you can't complain."[5] The piece was called "Is Amazon Unstoppable?"—and it had been written *before* the pandemic.

I wasn't even a shoe company. I was a troublemaker who went on *Tucker Carlson* every so often.

Still. It couldn't hurt. At 9:06 a.m. on June 4 on Twitter, I posted Amazon's email to me, with three furious sentences. "Oh fuck me. I can't believe it. They censored it." I followed up:

> THEY CENSORED IT! It is based entirely on published government data and scientific papers. It doesn't say coronavirus isn't real or doesn't kill people (in fact, the worst-case death toll is likely to be striking to people). And Amazon won't run it.[6]

Privately, I emailed journalists I knew, asking them to speak out.

A few did, including Glenn Greenwald, the lawyer-turned-journalist who had helped Edward Snowden publicize documents about the National Security Agency's spying. Greenwald wrote that he had found my anti-lockdown stance "reckless, but book banning by corporate tech giants is a far worse danger than whatever threats his book supposedly presents. If you like this because you hate him, a book you like will be next."[7]

Andrew Sullivan, a longtime *New York* magazine columnist, was pithier: "I think this guy is nuts. But denying him access to Amazon because of the content of his book is appalling."[8] Mainstream conservative journalists, including Brit Hume, offered more unqualified support.[9]

To my disappointment, my former colleagues at the *Times* were silent. On Twitter, some people even said they thought Amazon, as a private company, had every right to censor me—ignoring Amazon's overwhelming power in the book industry and its stated commitment to allowing a broad range of views.

By noon, I worried Amazon would simply ignore me. The news cycle is relentless. If I didn't succeed in forcing Amazon's hand with the first wave of publicity, the odds that I ever could would drop fast. I started to feel like a fool. How exactly had I planned to force Amazon's hand, anyway?

Then Elon Musk stepped in.

With Steve Jobs gone, Musk was the world's best-known chief executive. He had founded PayPal, SpaceX, and, of course, Tesla, the pioneering electric vehicle company. Tesla's rocketing stock had pushed Musk from mere deci-billionaire status into a race with Bezos to be the world's richest person. His personal life was also the object of some fascination—he had dated actresses and rock stars and smoked cannabis during a podcast with Joe Rogan. His brilliance, wealth, and edgy weirdness had earned him tens of millions of followers on Twitter.

More important, at least from my point of view, Musk was a coronavirus skeptic who had somehow come across my March tweets about Neil Ferguson. Musk and I had been in touch since early May—I had asked him if he might finance an investigative reporting project around Covid. He agreed. I even talked to several potential hires.

But ultimately we decided against moving ahead. I was not sure how I could possibly set up a virtual newsroom in the midst of the pandemic, especially since I had never hired another reporter in my life. I also worried that taking money from Musk might make it seem as though I was doing his bidding in my reporting—though that concern didn't seem to apply to liberal journalism nonprofits that took money from the super-wealthy.

I told Musk what Amazon had done. A few minutes later, he tweeted his (at the time) thirty-million-plus followers, "This is insane @Jeff Bezos."[10] (The @ sign meant Musk was sending the message publicly and directly to Bezos's Twitter account.)

Musk quickly followed up, "Time to break up Amazon. Monopolies are wrong!"

The two tweets were liked or retweeted almost sixty thousand times. Less than an hour later, Amazon emailed me to say the company would publish *Unreported Truths*. The censorship had been a mistake, Amazon told reporters. The company never gave me any reason for what it had done, but I can only assume that Musk's tweet forced its hand.

The story had a happy ending, at least from my point of view. The publicity from the aborted censorship was rocket fuel for the booklet. The *Wall Street Journal* published two articles about the controversy. The coverage of the attempt to censor me was the only decent publicity I had received outside conservative media since March. Even the *Washington Post*—which Amazon founder Bezos owns—ran an article on the controversy. (The *New York Times* ignored it, apparently viewing the attempted censorship of a former *Times* reporter as unworthy of note.)

That Thursday night, a few hours after Amazon reversed course, I appeared on Fox News with Tucker Carlson to talk about the censorship. In an hour, the booklet sold ten thousand copies.

That weekend, it would briefly be the top-selling book on Kindle. It and several follow-up booklets I wrote would go on to sell hundreds of thousands of copies. Even more people than I had realized were desperate for unbiased and well-sourced information about Covid.

For better or worse, the booklet's success cemented my role as a voice against lockdowns, mask rules, and other government overreach.

From then on, I would straddle what I considered an uneasy boundary between reporter and activist. In truth, though, supposedly mainstream journalists at the *New York Times* and other top outlets had reached this boundary years before, as Twitter helped erase the boundary between news and opinion.

For example, when movie producer Harvey Weinstein was charged with assault and rape on May 24, 2018, *Times* reporter Jodi Kantor—who was reporting the Weinstein story for the *Times*—tweeted:

"One phone call and you're done."
"I have eyes and ears everywhere."
"I'm Harvey Weinstein, you know what I can do."
Not anymore.[11]

Her tweet did not *exactly* cheer Weinstein's arrest, but it came close. Was Kantor's job to report the case, or prosecute it?

In November 2020, *New York* magazine reported on the *Times*'s increasingly open political and social stances, especially on issues of race, in an article headlined "In the Trump Years, the New York *Times* Became Less Dispassionate and More Crusading, Sparking a Raw Debate over the Paper's Future."[12]

So I felt that whatever I was becoming was thoroughly in keeping with the new principles of journalism. *One man's terrorist is another's freedom fighter*, the saying goes. In an age of social media, one man's incendiary tweeter may be another's crusading investigative reporter.

17

Attention Citizens!

In February 2020, when I first tweeted about the Covid-19 pandemic, I had about seven thousand followers.

They remembered me from my years as a reporter for the *New York Times* or knew me from my spy novels, or they had found me because of *Tell Your Children*, my book about the mental health risks of cannabis use. I was a verified user, a so-called "blue check" with a confirmed identity. The check gave me slightly more credibility than the average Twitter user.

But slightly more than zero wasn't much. And a few thousand followers wasn't many, not in a world where Kim Kardashian had tens of millions.

After a year of using Twitter to debate cannabis, I was used to swimming against the tide of public opinion. At its best, Twitter lets independent journalists reach large audiences. At its worst, it is a forum for ugly fights that too often turn personal. It can be dangerously addictive, too. The feedback loop is as real as a drug.

But at the time Twitter was my only real outlet. I didn't work for the *Times* anymore (and they would hardly have run stories questioning the panic when they were doing as much to promote it as anyone). Twitter it would be.

I had started asking questions.

With so few people willing to stand up publicly to the panic, I quickly grew louder and bolder. I developed my own Twitter vocabulary. On one side, Team Apocalypse—the media outlets and public health experts who reveled in the crisis. On the other, Team Reality—skeptics like me, who insisted the situation was more complex and lockdowns less useful than the media would admit.

I updated my Twitter backdrop with images from Orwell's work, such as the cover of *Animal Farm* and the INGSOC flag—letters that stand for "English Socialism," the ruling ideology in *1984*. I sent satirical tweets from "Your Dept. Of Pandemia" that began and ended, "Attention citizens!"

The message that defined my tone on Twitter—for better or worse—came early, on April 6:

> Attention citizens: Your Dept. Of Pandemia requires 10,000 New York citizens to report to hospitals. 2,000 of you will be fortunate to receive intensive care. If the model cannot adjust to reality, reality must adjust to the model. We'll solve this together. Attention citizens![1]

At a time when hundreds of New York City residents were dying each day of the coronavirus, this joke was probably in bad taste. Check that. It was in bad taste. Especially the line about being "fortunate to receive intensive care."

But I was doing everything possible to point out that the models had failed. I believed the danger of hysteria far dwarfed the danger of the coronavirus. With the entire media—led by the *Times*—in a blind panic, a sharp satirical voice seemed a necessary corrective.

Or maybe I was just being a jerk, as plenty of people on Twitter and off were happy to tell me. Including my wife.

Journalists who were friends told me to stop fighting the mainstream narrative. They warned me I was relegating myself to right-wing irrelevance. Some turned to attacking me publicly. On April 7, the day after that original Dept. of Pandemia tweet, Michael Powell—a *Times* reporter I'd had dinner with more than once—wagged a finger at me for being "appallingly obnoxious…in a moment of maximum pain for so many people. There is a path to raise questions and there's another to be an asshole."[2]

Other friends of mine retweeted his comments, and similar ones. Apparently they weren't my friends anymore.

People I didn't know were even more cutting. Media blue checks with tens or hundreds of thousands of followers promised to bully me into being quiet. They called me a "ghoul"—and a "stupid insane ghoul,"[3] a "fucking ghoul,"[4] and a "death ghoul" who should "eat shit."[5] (As opposed to a life ghoul who shouldn't?)

My worst night on Twitter came on Saturday, May 2, when I tangled with a guy named Jamelle Bouie, a *New York Times* op-ed writer with 300,000 followers. Bouie had complained weeks earlier about Georgia's decision to end its lockdown.

I tweeted at him that I wished I lived in Georgia because I needed a haircut.

"This pandemic killed my grandfather but yes, I am sorry you have not been able to get your haircut," Bouie replied.[6]

Oh no.

I didn't know about his grandfather. Obviously, if I had, I wouldn't have said anything. Doing so would have been not just nasty but foolish. What followed was predictable. Bouie's tweet was liked or retweeted sixty-five thousand times. Hundreds of his followers and friends attacked me—telling me that they hoped I died, threatening to fight me.

On Twitter, this phenomenon is called dogpiling. It usually happens to people who have offended the left. It can have real-world consequences.

In June 2020, James Bennet, the editorial page editor of the *New York Times*, would be forced to resign his job. Bennet wasn't forced out because of anything he personally had written, but because he had published a column *by a United States senator* that sparked anger on Twitter.

Fortunately, I didn't have a job at the *Times* to lose. My readers were my employers. As long as they liked my writing, I could support my family. And I knew the hate was virtual.

Still, having strangers call me a liar or diagnose me as sociopath wasn't much fun.

There wasn't much I could say in response to Bouie. I wrote only:

> Very sorry to hear about your grandfather. My grandparents died of brain cancer, Alzheimer's, a heart attack, and lung cancer. I suspect they were all about the same age as yours (not my dad's father, he was 53). The world didn't stop for them either.[7]

Perhaps I shouldn't have included that last sentence. Perhaps it was too raw a comment to someone still in mourning.

But, in truth, I wanted to go further. I wanted to point out that *Bouie* was the one who had brought up his grandfather publicly to score political points. I NEVER talked about my father or his leukemia on Twitter, never mentioned the fact his illness didn't seem to matter to the world because it wasn't Covid.

I kept those thoughts to myself. Even what I saw as a relatively restrained effort to defend myself riled Bouie's followers, such as David Slack, a screenwriter with almost thirty thousand followers. Slack tweeted, "Hey Alex. Fuck you, you complete piece of shit." He followed up by telling me, "If you're ever in Los Angeles, let's meet up to discuss this comment and your character in person. I feel like you have too many teeth."[8] (Yes, this is the level of discourse on Twitter a lot of the time.)

Within a couple of days the controversy quieted, of course. Online anger can be overwhelming, but it fades fast. That was especially true for me, since I didn't have a job to lose. When blue checks realize they can't get their targets fired, they get bored and move on.

Over time, I learned how to use Twitter for maximum advantage:

Punch up, not down. Don't waste time arguing with people who have few followers—unless they are making a good point that needs an answer.

If users—even users with many followers—libel you by calling you a liar or a grifter or repetitively make annoying comments about your tweets, block them. Otherwise ignore them. Twitter works best as a broadcast medium, not a social medium.

To that end, argue on your own terms. Make your points and move on. If someone is desperately baiting you to respond, he's not interested in a good faith discussion.

Attacking people for what they say is okay. Simply calling them names is not. Take the high road. Admittedly, I didn't always follow this rule, but I try.

Don't let the personal attacks bother you. The people calling you a monster reveal more about themselves than about you. Don't overreact or lose control, no matter how nasty or threatening the comments get. When in doubt, don't read them for a while.

Irony and humor work better than raw anger. Better to call someone a genius than an idiot.

Curse only in exceptional circumstances.

Back your arguments with raw data. If you are quoting from a source, screenshot or link to it so people can judge it for themselves.

As frustrating and upsetting as Twitter could be, it gave me the chance to reach an audience I otherwise could not have found. My audience grew day by day. In May, it surpassed one hundred thousand followers. That figure significantly understated its real reach. Many people told me they checked on my feed without officially following me, or posted screenshots of my tweets to Facebook for others to see.

Occasionally, my tweets hit a public nerve and became part of the news cycle. In May, a British newspaper discovered that Neil Ferguson had had an affair in late March. At the time, the entire United Kingdom had been locked down—*and Ferguson was personally supposed to be isolating himself because he had tested positive for the coronavirus.*

"Hey @Neil_Ferguson, fuck you: You shut down the world but ignored the lockdown to have an affair with a married woman," I wrote, and added a screenshot of the story. (A curse seemed appropriate under the circumstances.) More than 1.5 million people saw that tweet.[9]

More serious tweets could take off too, if they contained original reporting presented in a digestible way.

My tracking of Florida's hospital bed capacity was one example. Seeing that the state's hospitals were almost half empty in April 2020 helped people understand the state was far from disaster.

In late June 2020, as cases in Texas were rising and media panic swelling, I pushed an email from an executive at a chain of Texas emergency room clinics explaining why he believed the situation was under control. The tweet was arguably my most successful of the entire pandemic, because it was both substantive and very widely read. It was liked or retweeted more than thirty thousand times, and more than seven million people saw it on Twitter alone.[10]

I was grateful to the executive—J. B. Nieman, of a company called Complete Emergency Care—for having the guts to go on the record. And I was grateful that he was far from alone in reaching out to me over email.

If Twitter was an angry cesspool, my inbox was the opposite.

I received thousands of notes from people whose lives had been upended by the lockdowns. They were infuriating and heartbreaking and sometimes moving in their heroism. People shared personal stories and looked for reassurance that they weren't alone in seeing the media's hysteria as overblown.

A man in Manhattan reported that his neighbors hadn't left their apartment—or let their son and daughter leave—for almost two months. "They have groceries and packages left outside their door," he wrote. "Yes, this is child abuse."

A man with asthma explained his experience whenever he wore a mask: "I simply can't get enough oxygen in, and I can feel the carbon dioxide rushing back into my lungs. I can't do it." Because he didn't want to fight about mask mandates, he rarely left his home. "Having hardly any human interaction has left me depressed and isolated, like so many others." He went out of his way to reassure me that he was not suicidal.

But others were. One man wrote from Illinois: "The direction things have gone terrifies me and makes me want to commit suicide...there is no end in sight. The governor [J. B. Pritzker, heir to the Hyatt hotel fortune] is one of the richest men in America and he seems blind to any form of economic suffering. I can see no hope, no light from this. All Pritzker does is repeat we're all in this together, and other mindless PR-propaganda for children."

Pritzker's hypocrisy made him a target of particular scorn. He had sent his family to their estate in Florida while imposing a strict quarantine on his state's residents.[11]

In general, based on the emails I received, the anger and fear over lockdowns seemed worse in the Rust Belt, Pennsylvania through Illinois, than in coastal blue states with similar restrictions. My theory was that in California and New York, the real estate markets were relatively strong. People knew they could sell their homes and move to red states if they really wanted to do so. In places such as Illinois, people felt trapped.

"I don't really know why I'm writing you," the man from Illinois went on, "except your writing has been one of the only sources of hope I've had over the last month."

His suicidal intent seemed serious enough that I emailed back immediately: "Your email worries me—I hope you are getting the help you need. The lockdowns will end. Hang tough." I checked back with him a month later, and he said he was feeling better. As of mid-2021, he still was.

The frank pain of emails like his helped energize me against the blue-check negativity I faced. I didn't know if I was doing any good, but

I had to try. I was lucky enough to be able to say what so many others were thinking. As far as I was concerned, the people struggling to keep their jobs or lives together in the face of counterproductive lockdowns were the real heroes.

Physicians and scientists emailed too.

Most didn't want to be quoted publicly for fear of being ostracized. But they told me they believed I was on the right track and thanked me for speaking out. Sometimes they pointed me to papers I hadn't seen before.

In this way, my Twitter feed became almost crowdsourced. If someone passed along a paper that contained important new information, I would share it. On important issues, such as the fact that the virus was almost never transmitted outdoors, my feed could be weeks or even months ahead of the media and public health narrative.

One of the more fascinating examples came when a reader sent me a 1973 paper from what at the time was the *Journal of Hygiene* (now known as *Epidemiology and Infection*). The paper reported on an outbreak of respiratory illness in 1969 at a British research base in Antarctica—in the middle of the Antarctic winter, *after 17 weeks of complete isolation*. Out of nowhere, six of the twelve researchers at the base had developed colds. Despite intensive study, the researchers never figured out how the illness had started or what pathogen was behind it. I linked to the piece on Twitter as an example of the absurdity of hoping that lockdowns could ever completely contain a respiratory virus.[12]

■   ■   ■

When reporters at media outlets such as Vice and *Vanity Fair*[13] profiled me in April 2020, I tried to explain this dynamic to them. I even provided the *Vanity Fair* reporter with the names and emails of several former editors. I hoped he would see that even if I could be obnoxious on my Twitter feed, I was very serious about accuracy.

He didn't care. Almost none of the people writing about me did. They liked to call me a Covid "denier"—as if I had ever denied that Sars-Cov-2 was real and dangerous to some people—or a "truther."

Soon I stopped worrying about what they were writing. I knew they meant "truther" as an insult, but I didn't care. What could be wrong with reporting the truth about Covid's real risks? Or telling people hospitals were half empty *when in fact they were half empty*—because the media had scared away people who needed care? Why should I apologize for correctly reassuring parents that their kids were at almost no risk from the coronavirus?

I wasn't sure if I was developing a hero complex or just didn't want to be pushed around. But the harder the blue checks tried to shut me up and the nastier they were, the louder I became.

When they realized they couldn't shut me down, the elite media decided to ignore me. Fox News and conservative radio shows had me on regularly. The rest of the media refused, even outlets where I had previously appeared such as CNN, CNBC, and NPR. I said publicly I would happily appear live with no preconditions, and answer any question. Still, they wouldn't have me.

But they couldn't keep me from spreading the truth on Twitter. Day after day, my audience grew.

18

Masking, Unmasked

I n June 2020, for the first time since Joe Biden became the presumptive Democratic presidential nominee in February, Covid was briefly
not the most important story in the United States.

The video of Minneapolis police officer Derek Chauvin pressing a
knee into George Floyd's neck as Floyd pleaded, "I can't breathe,"
sparked massive protests. Police departments across the country were
under siege. Rioters burned a Minneapolis precinct and set up a
police-free "autonomous zone" in Seattle. Rising Democratic politicians
such as Alexandria Ocasio-Cortez called for "defunding the police."[1]

The height of anti–law enforcement fervor probably came on June
12, when the *New York Times* published an op-ed with the headline,
"Yes, We Mean Literally Abolish the Police" (which was *not* the piece
that led to James Bennet's firing).[2]

The same epidemiologists who had decried anti-lockdown protestors
a month before said the Floyd protestors had every right to be in the
streets. "We do not condemn these gatherings as risky for COVID-19

transmission," physicians and other public health experts wrote in an open letter. "We support them as vital to the national public health."[3]

I thought the Black Lives Matter protestors had every right to voice their grievances. Peaceful protest is a fundamental American right. But I disliked the hypocrisy of journalists and supposedly politically neutral scientists who decried lockdown protestors but had no problem with the George Floyd rallies, even when some turned into riots.

I was not alone. As a reader emailed to me,

> I took COVID seriously in early 2020. However after the George Floyd incident, and seeing the garbage proclamations from equally garbage woke healthcare "professionals" saying things like "racism is worse than COVID" and tolerating and encouraging very large groups to protest, twerk, and shout very closely to one another; and Mayor De Blasio of New York announcing that they told contact tracers not to ask people if they've been to a BLM protest, all while my mom's business collapsed due to the lockdowns....

This email was sent in June 2021, *more than a year* after the protests. People didn't forget.

As I mentioned earlier, at the time the first *Unreported Truths* booklet came out, I thought the media might use the protests as a way to pivot from the coronavirus. After all, the epidemic had turned out to be less catastrophic than initially predicted. Even blue states were slowly loosening restrictions in an effort to boost their economies—though the West Coast was notably behind.

I was wrong.

The media's obsession with the virus roared back by late June, as the protests faded and southern states saw cases rise. Outlets such as the *Times* turned out to be *committed* to the virus in a way I hadn't expected. A century before, the Spanish flu had rampaged worldwide, killing far more people than Sars-Cov-2 ever would, but the *Times* and other papers had published only a handful of front-page articles about it.

Many factors explained the difference. One was simply that reporters and other Americans had other massive issues to worry about in 1918 and 1919. Europe was remaking itself after the soul-crushing disaster of World War I. The United States was debating constitutional amendments to ban the sale of alcohol and let women vote. In Russia, Communists were battling to establish a state.

A flu, even one that killed millions of young people, simply didn't rate.

In 2020, the world was quieter. The media could devote its attention to the coronavirus. The coronavirus, Donald Trump, and the presidential election—three stories that could not be separated.

As the screaming over ventilators and testing faded, masks became the media's newest and most irritating obsession. Reporters spent endless time and energy arguing in favor of masks and mask mandates—and against anyone who did not want to wear them.

In truth, standard surgical masks do essentially nothing to control the spread of respiratory viruses such as Sars-Cov-2 or influenza. Cloth masks or bandannas are even more useless and may even be counterproductive.

Before March 2020, before the coronavirus hopelessly politicized epidemiology, this position was not even contentious. On February 6, 2020, scientists from Hong Kong published a meta-analysis—a study of studies—about masks in *Emerging Infectious Diseases*, a journal *published by the Centers for Disease Control*.

The analysis did not cover the coronavirus, of course. (In the appendix, the authors disclosed that they began working on the paper in 2018, more than a year before the first diagnosed Covid case.) Instead, it examined studies on whether masks slow the spread of the flu.[4]

A meta-analysis is not original research but an effort to sum up the overall state of scientific knowledge based on earlier published work. Scientists search the literature, looking for trials that touch on the question they're trying to answer. They then rank and weight those papers based on what are supposed to be objective criteria. A large study conducted by unbiased researchers will be more important to the overall meta-analysis than a small one that shows evidence of bias, for example.

In this case, the authors looked for randomized controlled trials that examined whether masks lowered the odds that people would be infected with the flu. Randomized trials are the gold standard for medical research. To perform them, researchers recruit people and split them at random into two groups balanced by age, sex, and other demographic factors. They then assign one group to take a drug or try an intervention such as a mask. The other group receives a placebo—a sugar pill—or no intervention.

Ideally, randomized trials are "double-blind" so that neither the researcher nor the subjects know who is receiving the real intervention and who the placebo. Sometimes companies will go so far as to conduct *sham surgeries* to hide the truth from patients.

Obviously this blinding can't work for a study of masks—people know whether they are wearing a mask or not. Still, the key is keeping the randomly assigned groups evenly balanced and prospectively registered. In other words, the groups are created *before* the trial begins and people aren't allowed to switch between them (except in certain rare and complicated trials designed in advance to account for such switching).

The authors of the February meta-analysis looked for research all the way back to 1946 (so they didn't include the 1919 paper from Dr. W. H. Kellogg of the California State Board of Health that found masks to be useless in stopping the Spanish flu). They found ten papers. Most showed no evidence that masks worked. A couple found a slightly positive effect. A couple were slightly negative. Overall, the studies found no benefit from masks.

The authors explained their findings clearly: "We did not find evidence that surgical-type face masks are effective in reducing laboratory-confirmed influenza transmission, either when worn by infected persons (source control) or by persons in the general community to reduce their susceptibility."

The meta-analysis did not include a 2015 randomized trial that examined cloth and surgical mask use by Vietnamese health care workers. That study had even more worrisome findings.[5] Researchers found health care workers wearing cloth masks—often handmade—actually had *more* flu-like infections than those wearing medical masks and than a control group, some of whom didn't wear masks at all.

Worse, the authors couldn't determine whether the higher infection levels resulted because surgical masks offered protection—or cloth masks actually *increased* infection rates. They noted that cloth masks blocked only 3 percent of airborne particles in laboratory tests. Health care workers "should not use cloth masks as protection against respiratory infection," the authors wrote.

■　　■　　■

Two arbitration cases in 2015 and 2018 made a similar point.

The decisions arose from efforts by hospitals in the Canadian province of Ontario to vaccinate nurses against influenza. The hospitals could not contractually make nurses get a flu shot, and some nurses refused. So the hospitals tried a quasi-mandate. Any nurse who refused a shot would be required to wear a surgical mask while working. Crucially, the hospitals were mainly concerned with using masks for "source control"—protecting *patients* from nurses who might spread the flu before they had symptoms.

In December 2013, the nurses' union filed a grievance against the policy. (Yes, the nurses did not want to have to wear masks.) A neutral arbitrator, James Hayes, heard testimony from 6 expert witnesses, consulted 249 exhibits, and read more than 100 scientific papers.

On September 10, 2015, Hayes issued a 136-page ruling saying that hospitals could not make nurses wear masks.[6]

The "scientific evidence said to support the [mask mandate] on patient safety grounds is insufficient," he wrote.

In addition, masks were uncomfortable, became moist, and could cause skin irritation, the nurses' experts said. One referred to a "grunge factor."[7]

The fight didn't end there. Some hospitals kept trying to make nurses wear masks. The nurses objected again—and won again.

In a September 6, 2018, decision, arbitrator William Kaplan agreed with Hayes's ruling. In fact, Kaplan went further than Hayes, calling the evidence for mask mandates "insufficient, inadequate, and completely unpersuasive." As he wrote in his ruling, "The preponderance of the masking evidence is compelling—surgical and procedural masks are extremely limited in terms of source control: they do not prevent the transmission of the influenza virus."[8]

These arbitrators were not anti-mask. They were chosen for their neutrality. But both reached the same conclusion after examining the evidence.

Of course, these decisions came in the context of the flu, not the coronavirus. But the viruses are roughly the same size. And they are transmitted in similar ways.

Further, the reason that standard cloth and surgical masks do not stop transmission of either the flu or the coronavirus is likely the same. Even when worn properly, they simply do not block enough of the very small particles that account for much viral transmission. They fail both ways—when people *inhale* particles that infect them and when they then *exhale* and spread the infection.

In 2009, four researchers examined how well surgical masks filtered small particles, those of one micron or less. A micron is a tiny unit of measurement, far too small to be seen. One thousand microns equal one millimeter. One *million* microns equal one meter, or about three feet. Yet a micron is actually about ten times the size of a Sars-Cov-2 viral particle.

The scientists tested five surgical mask brands. Even though they sealed their masks to the "faces" of their mannikins with silicone, four of the masks allowed at least 15 percent of 0.1 micron (virus-sized) to 1 micron-sized particles through. Two allowed more than half of those particles through.

The authors warned: "The wide variation in penetration levels for room air particles, which included particles in the same size range of viruses, confirms that **surgical masks should not be used for respiratory protection**" [emphasis added].[9]

The CDC used very similar language in a poster that remained available on its website as late as summer 2021. The poster explained that surgical masks do "NOT provide the wearer with a reliable level of protection from inhaling smaller airborne particles and [are] not considered respiratory protection."[10]

Even this discouraging language overstated the benefit of most masks. Many people don't even achieve whatever tiny protection masks might offer because they don't wear their masks properly. Wearing a loose mask, or a mask over a beard, is unequivocally useless. One infectious disease expert compared it to "fixing three of the five screen doors on your submarine."[11]

Further, that was the protection offered by disposable surgical masks, not the reusable cloth masks that many people wore. Those were even worse. They weren't manufactured to any consistent standard, and as the study of Vietnamese health care workers revealed, they seemed to perform *worse* than surgical masks.

Another alternative did exist.

Construction workers in dusty environments and nurses and doctors treating highly infectious patients typically depend on N95 respirators rather than surgical masks. N95s are certified to block at least 95 percent of small particles and often block up to 99 percent. And they are designed to be "fit-tested"—tightened to attach snugly to the wearer's face, leaving no gaps.

But N95s are more expensive than surgical masks and unpleasant to wear for long periods. And even they do not eliminate the risk of transmission, only reduce it somewhat. They are not a practical or reasonable option for widespread civilian use. The CDC never recommended them that way.

Of course, for people who are coughing or have other symptoms of infection, cloth or surgical masks may be useful. They capture larger droplets and respiratory phlegm. They also serve as a warning signal that their wearers are sick and other people should stay away. The World Health Organization and Centers for Disease Control have always encouraged sick people to wear masks.

But before the spring of 2020, they did not encourage people without symptoms to do so, even for "source control." As the WHO said in a January 29, 2020, bulletin, "[For] individuals without respiratory symptoms...a medical mask is not required, as no evidence is available on its usefulness to protect non-sick persons."[12]

Public health officials emphasized that same advice as the epidemic took off. Including the most important public health official of all. On March 8, Anthony Fauci told *60 Minutes*: "There's no reason to be walking around with a mask. When you're in the middle of an outbreak, wearing a mask might make people feel a little bit better and it might even block a droplet, but it's not providing the perfect protection that people think that it is. And, often, there are unintended consequences—people keep fiddling with the mask and they keep touching their face."[13]

As late as April 1, physicians writing in the *New England Journal of Medicine*—the most prestigious health care publication in the United States—explained, "We know that wearing a mask outside health care facilities offers little, if any, protection from infection....In many cases, the desire for widespread masking is a reflexive reaction to anxiety over the pandemic."[14]

But in a matter of days in early April, Fauci and other top public health officials reversed course. Masks were no longer useless for the general public. Quite the opposite.

By April 3, less than a month after telling people not to wear masks, Fauci had not just dropped his opposition. *He was promoting universal mask use even in people who did not have symptoms.* "If everybody does that, we're each protecting each other," he told PBS.[15]

This advice soon became summarized as, "My mask protects you. Your mask protects me."

Even now no one has explained convincingly why public health authorities changed their views in a matter of days, and in lockstep.

In the White House, Deputy National Security Adviser Matthew Pottinger had spoken to Asian public health authorities, who told Pottinger they believed masks had helped control the epidemic. On April 2, 2020, *Politico* reported that "Pottinger, in fact, has emerged as one of the biggest internal proponents of preventative mask usage."[16] Both Pottinger and his boss, National Security Adviser Robert O'Brien, regularly saw Trump and could make their case face to face.

But Trump's own public statements show he wasn't driving the new policy. On April 3, he grudgingly gave the new mask recommendation, while making clear he was unconvinced: "The CDC is advising the use of non-medical cloth face covering as an additional voluntary public health measure. So it's voluntary; you don't have to do it. They suggested for a period of time. But this is voluntary. I don't think I'm going to be doing it."[17]

"The science" wasn't driving the change. No one had conducted a convincing randomized controlled trial in March showing that masks protected their wearers—or anyone else.

In fact, when Danish researchers ran a trial on masks and the coronavirus later in the spring, they found that masks did *not* work. The trial was well designed and included more than six thousand people, a very large sample—larger than the samples in all the studies the researchers had reviewed for the CDC meta-analysis in February combined.[18] But the pressure to encourage mask-wearing was so heavy that the scientists couldn't find a journal to publish their findings for several months.

In the interim, journals repeatedly ran studies that purportedly showed benefits from mask wearing or mask requirements by comparing infection trends in states or workplaces that did require masks with those that didn't.

For example, one article looking at hospital workers in Massachusetts showed that infections had fallen among them after the hospital system required masks.[19] But the study *did not compare the workers' infection rates with those of the state's other residents*—who hadn't been under the mask requirement at the time. Those also declined, at about the same pace. So how could the hospital mask rules deserve the credit?

Other reports were even weaker, such as a CDC paper showing two hair salon workers with Covid had not infected any of the 139 customers whose hair they cut while wearing masks.[20] The results sounded impressive but were meaningless. The salon might have had very good ventilation. The salon workers might have been only lightly infected. Or some other unknown factor might have accounted for the lack of transmission.

Physicians and scientists depend on randomized controlled trials rather than anecdotes like these because randomized trials at least try to account for these potential "confounders"—hidden factors that might bias the results.

With no evidence that masks reduced infections in their wearers, health experts leaned heavily on the "source control" theory. They claimed masks reduced the amount of "droplet" particles a person with Covid released, reducing her risk of infecting others. Thus "My mask protects you; yours protects me."

Again, though, Fauci and other public health experts had essentially no real-world evidence to support the "source control" theory in early April, at the time they reversed their recommendation. Which only deepens the mystery behind the change.

Fauci and others would later claim that the new recommendation had been the right one all along—that they had only discouraged mask use in February because they feared people would panic and buy masks that health care workers needed. In June 2020, Fauci told TheStreet, "We were concerned—the public health community—and many people were saying this, were concerned that it was at a time when personal protective equipment, including the N95 masks and the surgical masks, were in very short supply."[21]

This explanation received very little pushback from reporters, but it was deeply troubling.

First, if true, it implied that top public health officials had *lied* and discouraged people from taking action to protect themselves as the pandemic took off.

Second, it did not account for the fact the CDC and federal authorities always knew N95 respirators were more valuable than ordinary masks and took action to hoard them. By early March, government agencies were buying all the N95s they could find from both manufacturers and distributors to ensure that civilians could not buy them.

By the second week of March, N95s were largely unavailable to civilians for any price. Stores had none in stock. Amazon, eBay, and other online retailers were blocking listings for them.[22] Surgical masks were also in short supply at the retail level.

So telling people not to wear masks *as a way to keep them from buying the N95 respirators or surgical masks that health care workers needed* was essentially useless advice by early March—and anyone giving such advice knew as much.

Third, it contradicted the fact that Fauci's pre-April public statements matched the guidance the CDC had always given. In other words, if public health experts had been lying about the value of masks for civilians in February, they had been lying for decades—long before anyone had worried about mask shortages. They had no reason to do so.

Finally, the mask guidance raised questions about a separate but closely related issue, the question of whether infected people could transmit Covid even if they had no symptoms. Again, the pre-March conventional wisdom on this issue had been very clear. As Fauci said at a January 28 press conference, "The driver of outbreaks is always a symptomatic person."[23]

The logic behind this theory was simple. People with higher viral loads were more likely to be sick—and also to exhale more virus with each breath. When researchers tried to find cases of people without symptoms transmitting the coronavirus to one another, they very rarely could. Cases of *presymptomatic* transmission were more common, but still rare.

"The extent of truly asymptomatic infection in the community remains unknown," the World Health Organization explained in a "scientific brief" on July 9, 2020. "Four individual studies from Brunei, Guangzhou China, Taiwan China and the Republic of Korea found that between 0% and 2.2% of people with asymptomatic infection infected anyone else." In contrast, studies showed that up to 15 percent of people with symptoms infected others.[24]

However, researchers found it difficult to reconcile models that predicted the rampant spread of the coronavirus with the number of actual symptomatic cases. To do so, they needed to posit a large number of cases spread through asymptomatic transmission. For example, in March 2021 researchers wrote:

> Using an epidemiological model that includes testing capacity, we show that many infections are nonsymptomatic but contribute substantially to community transmission in the aggregate. Their individual transmissibility remains uncertain. If they transmit as well as symptomatic infections, the epidemic may spread at faster rates than current models often assume. If they do not, then each symptomatic case generates, on average, a higher number of secondary infections than typically assumed.[25]

In other words, the debate about the risk of asymptomatic transmission again came down to modeled predictions against on-the-ground reality. And the stakes were enormous. If people without symptoms were unlikely to transmit the coronavirus, they had no reason to wear masks. After all, if my mask didn't protect me *or* you, why would I wear it?

Over time I grew to believe that a purely psychological explanation was the only answer that made sense. Masks were useless as protection, but the public health authorities needed them as a signifier. Seeing them on other people was frightening, a reminder of the danger of the coronavirus.

My mask scares you. Your mask scares me.

Fauci edged toward this explanation in May, telling CNN that he wore a mask even though "it's not 100 percent effective. I mean, it's sort of respect for another person, and have that other person respect you."[26]

And as talismans, masks proved incredibly effective. Just how effective became clear in May 2021, when the CDC dropped mask requirements for vaccinated people. The CDC obviously intended the change as a carrot to reverse falling vaccination rates. But the new guidance backfired. Within weeks, almost no one was wearing masks. Vaccination rates plunged further. For many people, the end of universal masking marked the end of pandemic.

■   ■   ■

But in the summer of 2020, mask-wearing was still on the rise. Reporters pushed it relentlessly. Not to wear a mask was to refuse to "follow the science"—no matter that almost no one knew what "the science" actually said. It was selfish, a sign that one cared more about one's own freedom than other people's lives.

Newspapers and magazines published insufferably arrogant pieces in which they told readers how to deal with the cretins who wouldn't wear masks. "It can be difficult to find common ground with someone who refuses to wear a mask for whatever reason," *Teen Vogue* said in July. "You might find the most resistance from people who are ideologically opposed to wearing masks because they believe doing so is a sign of weakness (it isn't)."[27]

The *Washington Post* went a step further, warning in September, "Some Covid-19 rule-breakers could be narcissists, experts say. Here's how to approach them"—as if people who'd decided to keep their faces uncovered were inherently dangerous. The article offered strategies to approach those awful people.

Craig Malkin, a psychologist, suggested telling them how important they were: "For example, [say,] 'You can make the difference between life and death because we're all in this together.'"

"The less significant they feel in all of this, the more they're going to have to pound their chests and push back," Malkin said.[28]

A study published in August would take this argument to the extreme. People who didn't wear masks were no longer just dumb or self-centered. They were sociopaths: "A new study by researchers from Brazil has found that people who are unconcerned with adhering to measures to mitigate the Covid-19 spread tend to manifest higher levels of traits tied to antisocial personality disorder, which is also known as sociopathy."[29]

In truth, I didn't want to fight about masks. I knew the propaganda had worked. Public opinion favored them, even among Republicans. In June 2020, about 65 percent of Americans said they wore masks in stores all or most of the time, according to Pew Research. By August the figure had risen to 85 percent.[30]

But I felt I had no choice. Pseudo-science and panic had driven every aspect of our response to the pandemic, including mask mandates. Encouraging people to wear masks was very different than requiring them.

If people wanted to try to protect themselves, even in a pointless way, so be it. If the government wanted to make people hide their faces from one another, it needed a good reason.

It didn't have one.

I also felt giving in on the issue would embolden politicians and public health authorities on even more important questions to come, such as reimposing lockdowns or requiring vaccines. I pressed back on masks, calling them face diapers, highlighting the research that showed they didn't work.

That position angered the media and public health experts more than any other, at least until vaccines came out. The left-leaning Media Matters site repeatedly tried to discourage Fox News from having me on. In September, Media Matters published an entire article devoted to refuting me, headlined "Masks Work. Fox Keeps Hosting Alex Berenson to Claim They Don't."[31] On Twitter, the attacks were more vicious and personal, of course.

By now, though, they bothered me less than they ever had.

The hate had turned into fuel.

19

Another Brick in the Wall

The debate over masks featured one kind of gaslighting, as mask advocates spun weak data and ignored generations of evidence on the uselessness of making healthy people wear masks.

But at least mask advocates had *some* evidence and theoretical justification. And even if masks were useless, they were unlikely to be (physically) harmful. Their danger came in their symbolism.

The debate over school openings was far worse, and the motives of Team Apocalypse far uglier.

Scientists knew that kids and schools played a major role in spreading influenza. Thus the 2007 CDC pandemic guidelines supported short-term school closings during flu outbreaks. They never anticipated permanent or semi-permanent closings. But they recommended considering shutting schools for up to four weeks for moderately severe epidemics, and twelve weeks for very severe epidemics—those likely to kill two million or more Americans.

As Sars-Cov-2 emerged from China, it seemed possible, even likely, that kids played a similar role in spreading the coronavirus. In March 2020, a limited pause to close schools appeared to be a reasonable choice.

Inside the federal government, no one advocated for school closures more loudly than Dr. Carter Mecher of the Department of Veterans Affairs. Yes, this was the self-same Dr. Mecher who in 2006 had fallen in love with a high school student's computer simulation "proving" lockdowns could reduce flu outbreaks by 90 percent. For much of February and March 2020, Mecher was busily sending emails to a group of similarly worried officials predicting doom and demanding school closures. As the *New York Times* reported on April 11,

> Dr. Mecher was urging the upper ranks of the nation's public health bureaucracy to wake up and prepare for the possibility of far more drastic action.
>
> "You guys made fun of me screaming to close the schools," he wrote to the group, which called itself "Red Dawn," an inside joke based on the 1984 movie about a band of Americans trying to save the country after a foreign invasion. "Now I'm screaming, close the colleges and universities."[1]

Still, scientists knew by early March that children and young adults were at low risk from Sars-Cov-2, as the March 16 Imperial College report showed. And some educational advocates worried about the collateral damage school closings might do to kids, especially poor kids. In the United States, almost thirty million children depend on schools for free or low-price lunches.[2]

For kids at high risk of abuse and neglect, school can be even more important. Teachers are among the main reporters of abuse to child welfare agencies. They may be the only adults who have the chance to check each day that children are not being hurt by their parents or caregivers.

Notably, New York City mayor Bill de Blasio pushed to keep open his system, the biggest in the country.[3] More than one hundred thousand of New York's million students were homeless and living in shelters. On Saturday, March 14, he said he would not close schools. "What are these kids going to do?" de Blasio asked. "Do we really believe these kids will hole up in their rooms for a month?"[4]

But pressure from the media and teachers' unions forced his hand. The next day, Sunday, March 15, he announced the schools would not reopen after the weekend—giving parents less than twenty-four hours' notice.[5]

New York was not alone. By the end of March, schools were closed almost everywhere worldwide—with the notable exception of Sweden. One and a half billion children and young adults, 20 percent of the world's population, were out of school.[6]

The near-overnight closures pushed many parents into a desperate scramble for childcare, as I saw first-hand. Even professional parents who were no longer going into offices and had resources had a hard time supervising their kids while trying to work. As weeks and months passed, the strain increased. As the *Baltimore Sun* reported in May in an article headlined "'We Feel Like We Are Drowning'":

> [P]arents are finding that teaching their children while juggling Zoom meetings and conference calls of their own is exhausting and unmanageable. While they are grateful teachers and school systems are cranking out lessons, some say their children can't keep up with the academic work by themselves. The formal education their children are getting is a fraction of what they would have learned in a classroom with teachers, they say.[7]

A poll in late April and early May 2020 found that adults with children reported significantly higher stress levels than those without—1.2

points higher on a 10-point scale. Almost half of parents reported their stress level was between 8 and 10. More than 70 percent specifically said that managing online learning was a source of stress.[8]

For hospital workers, grocery store clerks, and other essential employees who had to leave their homes, childcare became an even bigger crisis. The *Oregonian* newspaper told the story of a woman forced to leave her nine-year-old son and twelve-year-old daughter at home alone so she could work at a doctor's office:

> Jennifer, who asked that her last name not be used to protect the safety of her family, calls her children on her breaks to go over their schedules and spends every evening helping them with schoolwork....
>
> "I've been on the brink of a panic attack since this whole thing started," Jennifer said. "My daughter is in near tears every day."[9]

Even if they could find someone to watch their kids, some lower-middle-class single parents simply quit. They knew they would have more money if they stayed home and accepted enhanced unemployment benefits than paid for care while they worked. The burden fell primarily on women, who were more likely both to have low-paying jobs as essential workers and to be the main caregivers.[10]

Of course, the closures weighed most on kids.

Few schools had experience with remote learning. Even high-functioning suburban and private schools had to devise curricula and set up virtual classrooms on the fly. Many bigger urban districts—with slow-moving bureaucracies and powerful unions—barely tried at all during the spring. In cities where public schools barely functioned for many students in normal circumstances, closures effectively ended education.

Alec MacGillis captured the crisis in a devastating piece for ProPublica in September 2020, recounting the struggles of children in Baltimore, including Shemar, a twelve-year-old boy he knew personally:

Remote learning [for the Baltimore public schools] started in earnest on April 6. For Shemar, that meant just **four hours per week** of live online instruction—an hour for each of the four main subjects once a week, with nothing on Fridays....

The Remind app was another problem. Shemar downloaded it on his phone, which had no cellular service but could be used with Wi-Fi. But, when his mother lost or broke her phone, she borrowed Shemar's....

[But] the biggest challenge was not technological. No one made sure that Shemar logged on to his daily class or completed the assignments that were piling up. [emphasis added][11]

But even with engaged parents, even in schools with committed teachers who offered hours of live online instruction every day—such as the one our kids attended—virtual school simply didn't work very well.

The problems were obvious and unfixable. Smaller kids became bored and lost interest. Perhaps two hours of "school" each day was all they could handle. For older children, the extra screen time worsened galloping technology addictions. Everyone missed the chance to move and play with friends at recess.

Within months, the crisis was apparent. "Thousands of students in SC aren't doing their school work. Some have completely ghosted," a newspaper in South Carolina reported in May.[12] The longer the closures went, the larger the gaps became.

Instead of taking the problems seriously, the *New York Times* and *Washington Post* ran vacuous defenses of online school.

In May, the *Times* ran an op-ed by a thirteen-year-old New York City girl headlined "Why I'm Learning More with Distance Learning Than I Do in School: I'm Thirteen Years Old. I Don't Miss the Other Kids Who Talk Out of Turn, Disrespect Teachers and Hit One Another."[13] The piece should have been viewed as an indictment of New York's school system, not an endorsement of online learning. The *Post* offered

Jeb Bush telling parents, "It's time to embrace distance learning—and not just because of the coronavirus."[14]

Many other countries responded to the problems by reopening quickly, especially kindergartens and elementary schools. Liberal European countries with centralized educational systems were among the first to move. Denmark and Switzerland led the way, and Germany quickly followed.[15]

By May, Japan and other Asian countries had also partly reopened.[16] Most countries initially required masks and strict physical distancing restrictions, but over time the rules loosened.

The push to reopen increased as sophisticated contact tracing showed that children rarely spread the coronavirus to one another or adults. A French study published on April 11 was among the first to provide hard evidence.

A team of researchers tracked a group of cases in the Alps in early February 2020, a time when relatively few people were infected and scientists could devote close attention to small clusters. One of the infected was a nine-year-old, who went to three different schools and a ski class while showing symptoms. The child did not pass Covid to *any* other kids. "The fact that an infected child did not transmit the disease despite close interactions within schools suggests potential different transmission dynamics in children," the researchers wrote.[17]

In May, Chinese researchers reported that sixty-five out of sixty-eight children infected with Sars-Cov-2 "were household contacts of adults whose symptoms developed earlier."[18] The authors added, "There has been no evidence revealing the virus was transmitted from children to others." Data from the Netherlands, which had sophisticated contact tracing, showed the same.[19]

The most likely explanation was that younger kids beat the virus so fast and had such low viral loads that they were unlikely to spread it.

Further, as more children were exposed, hospital and death reports showed they were at even lower risk than scientists had first believed. Kids almost *never* died from the coronavirus. Not one of the nine million people under eighteen in California had died of Covid-19 as of mid-July.[20] The unfortunate children who did die often had severe underlying health problems.

A British report in 2021 would show that only twenty-five of the sixty-one British children and teens who were reported to have died of Covid before February 2021 actually had died of the virus. And of those twenty-five, thirteen had "complex neurodisabilities." Only six of them had not had what the researchers referred to as a "life-limiting" or other chronic condition.[21]

In other words, the odds that a healthy British child or teen would die of Covid during the first year of the epidemic were about one in two million.

On May 2, 2020, Dr. Nick Coatsworth, the Australian deputy chief medical officer, wrote, "I have examined all of the available evidence from Australia and around the world and, as it stands, it does not support avoiding classroom learning as a means to control Covid-19."[22]

Elite media outlets didn't report these reassuring findings.

Instead, they focused on a tiny handful of cases in which children—mostly with severe preexisting conditions, as the British study showed—had become seriously ill or died from Covid itself. On April 25, the *Washington Post* published an article headlined "New DC Hospital Numbers Suggest Kids Do Face Some Risk of Coronavirus Hospitalization."[23]

The word "some" was doing heavy lifting in that headline. As I explained in a Twitter thread, the story reported that 105 people under 25—not just kids, young adults too—had come to Children's National Hospital, the leading pediatric medical center in a region with millions of people. Of those, 28 had been hospitalized, fewer than one a day. Of them, 7 had needed intensive care. None had died. And most of the serious cases were in people over 15.

Even when they cast their nets widely, news organizations had a hard time finding cases in which healthy kids had died or even become seriously ill from Covid. The *Post* would later report about a Virginia teen who had required intubation after being infected—without disclosing that he was immunocompromised and had been hospitalized for the flu some years before.[24] (I learned the unreported details when angry readers who knew the truth about the case emailed me.)

So reporters went in a different direction.

Beginning in May, the *New York Times* published more than a dozen articles on the "post-Covid inflammatory syndrome" that was supposedly targeting kids. "Children Are Falling Ill with a Baffling Ailment Related to Covid-19," a front-page article on May 5 explained.[25] Article after article followed.

The inflammatory illness could supposedly affect even children who had suffered only mild Covid infections. It appeared similar to Kawasaki syndrome, a rare childhood illness that also followed infections. But the Covid syndrome often targeted the heart, with devastating results.

As usual, the rest of the media quickly followed the *Times*'s lead.

The real story was different. Severe cases of the syndrome—also called MIS-C, multisystem inflammatory syndrome-children—were rare. Other viruses, including the flu, were known to cause similar problems. And physicians had quickly figured out how to treat the syndrome with steroids. On June 3, a Texas television station reported that Dr. Coburn Allen, a pediatric infectious disease expert at the University of Texas, said "people do not need to worry too much about more people contracting MIS-C because many children have responded well to treatment. 'We've had enough experience now to know that, in general, most of these kids do fine,' Dr. Allen said."[26]

The British Kawasaki Disease Foundation went further. In a statement on May 15, it blasted "continuing sensationalist press pieces causing deep worry for families."[27]

On Twitter, I called the alarmist articles "kiddie panic porn," an ugly name for the ugly spectacle—an apparently deliberate effort to scare parents.

But the pushback came too late.

By the summer, many American parents believed, falsely, that the coronavirus was highly risky to their children. "Until we know more about risk of exposure, transmission, and multisystem inflammatory syndrome in children, I'll be keeping both my kids home infinitely [*sic*]," Kate Duchowny, a "social epidemiologist" at the University of California, San Francisco, told the *New York Times*.[28] On Twitter, parents bragged about having kept their children inside for months.

Teachers' unions took advantage of the fear and confusion to lead a drive against in-person school reopenings. At first they simply wanted to keep public schools closed through spring 2020. But by June, the unions were hinting they would try to keep schools closed at least through the fall.

They began to emphasize the risk to teachers, ignoring the reality that a study out of Sweden, where schools had remained open, had shown teachers were at no more risk than the average adult.[29] As the Swedish Public Health Agency reported on July 14, "Compared to other professions, the relative risk among teachers in day care, primary and secondary school were close to one, indicating no increased risk of exposure or infection."

Later studies showed that teachers were actually *safer* with schools open, because children were so unlikely to spread the virus.

The same paper also compared children in Sweden to those in Finland, where schools had remained closed, and found no difference in infection rates between the two countries. "Closure or not of schools had no measurable direct impact on the number of laboratory confirmed cases in school-aged children in Finland or Sweden," the report explained.

Yet the growing evidence base and international reopenings didn't matter in the United States. By late June, many cities and states, especially those run by Democratic mayors and governors, backed away from in-person schooling for the 2020–2021 school year. A few big school districts announced plans for classroom teaching. Others hesitated or suggested they would leave the decision to parents.

Then the president got involved, pressing for school reopenings.[30]

"The schools, hopefully, are going to be back in the fall," Trump said at a White House event on June 15. "They're going to be back in full blast. But the young people, they have very strong immune systems. I imagine that's the reason."

Trump's garbled language obscured the fact that he was correct. Children did have "very strong immune systems." He was on the right side on this issue. Unequivocally, absolutely, whatever adverb you prefer. Over the next several weeks, Trump and Secretary of Education Betsy DeVos repeatedly made the case for schools to reopen for in-person education in the fall.

I hoped having the White House push to reopen schools might make a difference.

It did.

For the worse.

Teachers' unions became even more opposed to reopenings. They called for massively expensive retrofitting of schools with new ventilation systems. They said publicly funded charter schools should be closed (on the theory that charter schools shared space with existing schools and worsened crowding). They called for randomized testing of students.

"There's no way that you're going to have full-time schools for all the kids and all the teachers the way we used to have it," Randi Weingarten, the president of the American Federation of Teachers, said on July 11.[31]

The Los Angeles teachers' union even insisted the police be partially defunded as a condition of reopening. "We must shift the astronomical amount of money devoted to policing to education and other essential needs," the union demanded.[32]

The unions' demands were utterly unrealistic. Even if the federal government had authorized the tens or hundreds of billions of dollars necessary for retrofitting schools, the work could not have been completed in a few weeks or months. In cities, even simple school construction projects routinely took years. Covid had further slowed construction.[33]

The impossibility of the demands was probably intentional. In essence, they were a way to ensure that schools could not reopen.

Rather than calling out the unions, journalists abetted them.

As the summer progressed, the media rarely reported that schools had opened all over the world without incident. They ignored researchers worldwide who had studied camps and schools and concluded children rarely transmitted the virus and were at little risk themselves.[34] As a Spanish newspaper reported in August, scientists in Spain had found that "children and adolescents who took part in 22 summer camps in the Barcelona area in recent months have been found to have a capacity to transmit the coronavirus that **is up to six times lower than that of the general population**" [emphasis added].[35]

Instead, reporters seized on a handful of incidents, such as an outbreak at a summer camp in Georgia, to play up the risks. Never mind that those outbreaks had led to few hospitalizations and no deaths. When a South Korean study purported to show children might spread the virus, the *New York Times* played up the danger: "Older Children Spread the Coronavirus Just as Much as Adults, Large Study Finds: The Study of Nearly 65,000 People in South Korea Suggests That School Reopenings Will Trigger More Outbreaks."[36] When other researchers pointed out deep flaws in the paper, the *Times* blandly called it "A New Wrinkle in the Debate."[37]

By the summer, many American parents had fears about schools and Covid's risks to their kids that verged on fictional. And the union pressure was unrelenting.

To maximize their leverage, local teachers' unions threatened strikes and encouraged teachers to seek disability leaves.[38] Some locals even encouraged members to write wills, as if being forced to teach in-person would be a death sentence. "Teachers are drafting wills along with lesson plans; one even wrote her own obituary," *USA Today* reported in August.[39]

"I Won't Return to the Classroom, and You Shouldn't Ask Me To," a teacher named Rebecca Martinson lectured in an opinion piece the *Times* published in July. "Please don't make me risk getting Covid-19 to teach your child."[40]

In the ultimate irony, Martinson explained that she taught nursing to high school students—training that almost by definition requires in-person instruction. "It amazes me how fast students adapted to remote learning," she wrote. "I've managed to teach them to ... suture wounds."

What could go wrong?

A handful of brave academics, led by Emily Oster, an economist at Brown University, tried to publicize the actual risks. Oster created a national database showing students and teachers were very unlikely to contract Covid. In an August 2020 interview with the *New Yorker*, she explained, "Kids tend to have very mild infections. They do not seem to get very sick in most cases. It's not that they can't get sick, but it's rare. The piece that is less certain is the degree to which they transmit the virus if they get it. And I think our best data suggests that younger kids probably do transmit it less efficiently than older adults."[41]

But even relatively restrained efforts such as Oster's to stand up to the unions generated blowback. As the *Times* would report in a June 2021 profile, Oster was called a "charlatan" and a "monster" on social media.[42]

I was not relatively restrained, of course.

"Please quit," I tweeted in response to Rebecca Martinson's op-ed. Those two words received almost twenty thousand likes or retweets—but plenty of vitriol, too. That tweet was the one that led Talia Lavin, a Brooklyn writer, to tell me to "eat shit death ghoul."

Of course, Talia did not have children[43]—a fact that didn't keep her from having a strong opinion on whether schools should open. From the beginning of Covid, people without kids had seemed more willing to tolerate school closures and lockdowns generally than those of us who did.

The rule had plenty of exceptions. Many parents kept their kids locked at home for months, and many childless people favored a return to normality. Still, from the admittedly unscientific sample I saw on social media, the correlation was real.

People without children didn't see first-hand just how damaging the lockdowns and school closures were to kids. But I couldn't help wondering if other factors played a role.

For all but the worst parents, raising children is a profound experience. Being responsible for another life means frequently putting your own needs second. *Don't want to get up at 3:00 a.m. to change a diaper? You'd rather sleep? Too bad.*

But having kids also helps feed optimism and a forward-looking attitude. Even on the worst days, children are hilarious and full of energy. And they remind us that life is bigger than all of us, and that it will continue after we are gone.

In the spring of 2021, I interviewed Valerie Kraimer, an Ohio woman whose teenage daughter Simone had died after being vaccinated against Covid. Valerie is a remarkable woman. She told the story of the horrific month her daughter had suffered carefully, cautiously, without drama or self-pity.

Only at the end did the depth of her despair become apparent, and for a reason I hadn't expected. Simone was her only child.

"I'm in my early fifties," she said. "I can't have any more kids. I've lost my opportunity to have grandchildren." Further, her brother and sister also had not had children. Simone's death meant that her family line would end with them.

We all have parents. But not all of us have children. And I couldn't help but wonder if balancing the needs of the young and the old comes more naturally to those who do.

■　　　■　　　■

Teachers' unions had simpler, baser motives.

Keeping schools closed would give their members a chance to work from home, convince the public the epidemic remained uncontrolled because of Trump's failures, and disrupt the economy. The only item not on their agenda was helping kids—particularly poor, inner-city children.

Yet the teachers *won*. Even more than law enforcement, American schools are funded and controlled at the city and state level. Property taxes fund them. Local school boards run them. Despite his bluster, Trump had no way to force schools to reopen.

By August, even school districts that had promised earlier in the summer that they would be reopening for full-time in-person instruction had changed their plans. Some big districts had given up even on "hybrid" instruction, the idiotic plan to split classes so kids would learn in school some days and at home on others. Full-time virtual learning was the norm from San Francisco to Chicago to Boston.

The absurdity of keeping schools closed became fully clear when districts nationwide told parents they would offer "supervised learning centers" where kids could learn online in groups.

And where would the "learning centers" be? Often *in schools*. As a Baltimore television station explained, "15 Schools, Rec Centers to Host City Students for in-Person Virtual Learning."[44]

Yes, "in-Person Virtual Learning," which would take place "in small groups led by a distance-learning proctor." In other words, children would go to school buildings and stare at computer screens while their teachers stayed home and instructed them over the internet.

The only major exceptions were in a few Republican states, including Florida, where Governor Ron DeSantis had ordered schools to open in-person despite objections from the state's teachers' union.[45]

In September 2020, only about one-quarter of schools nationally were open for in-person learning, according to Burbio, a private company that tracked school and local government announcements.[46] That number hardly budged during the fall. But after Joe Biden took office it rose sharply—even though the United States had far more Covid cases and deaths in January and February than in September and October.

For the entire 2020–2021 school year, fifteen states, including Virginia and New Jersey, offered in-person instruction for an average of less than half the year. Other big states, including Pennsylvania, New York, and Michigan, barely cracked 50 percent. California, home to about one in eight of all American children, was worst of all, offering barely 20 percent of its students in-person education.

Even those dismal figures overstated the number of students who were actually in school. Many parents who theoretically had the chance to send their kids to school kept them home either because they were afraid or because the in-person experience was so lousy. Kids were forced to wear masks and stay six feet apart, and in some cases were even taught virtually.

By the end of the 2021 school year, the extent of the damage from online schooling was clear. In Texas, most schools—especially in rural areas—stayed open. But enough had been closed for the state's standardized tests to capture a huge gap between in-person and virtual education.

The state reported in June 2021 that the number of students who met math benchmarks had *fallen* by 32 percentage points in districts that were more than three-quarters online. The decline was only 9 percent for districts that were less than one-quarter online. For reading benchmarks, the declines were 9 percent and 1 percent.[47] Black and Hispanic kids, who were more likely to live in troubled urban school districts, were especially hard-hit.

By then, virtual schooling had become so unpopular that the unions that had desperately tried to keep schools closed the year before claimed they had done nothing of the sort.

"Nothing should stand in the way of fully reopening our public schools this fall and keeping them open," Randi Weingarten of the American Federation of Teachers said in May 2021. In a tweet two months later, she went further, claiming her union had "tried to reopen schools safely since April 2020."[48]

Weingarten had a strange definition of "tried to reopen."

And tens of millions of American children had lost more than a year of school they'd never get back.

20

Another Brick in the Wall (College Remix)

T he educational insanity didn't stop at high school graduation.
Colleges and universities raced to implement the most draconian possible restrictions against their students, all in the name of protecting them. Online instruction was only the first step. Many colleges kept students from returning to campus at all.

The schools that did allow students on campus did everything possible to make them regret coming. They barred visitors. They forced students to wear masks—not just in group settings but alone in their rooms and outdoors. They banned gatherings of more than six people, effectively ending the extracurricular clubs and activities crucial to the college experience. Some required students to notify administrators or even ask permission to travel off campus.

At Bucknell University, for example, students who traveled more than thirty miles from campus had to quarantine off campus for eight days and provide a negative test upon returning. Otherwise they were required to leave campus for the semester.[1]

The University of California at Berkeley bizarrely banned students from *exercising outdoors*—a rule that seemed to have no purpose other than damaging students' mental health.[2] Worse, the school imposed the rule in February 2021, long after it was clear both that the coronavirus was almost never transmitted outdoors and that people of college age were at almost no risk.

Across the country, Northeastern University in Boston dismissed eleven students for having a party in a hotel room.[3] Adding insult to injury, the school refused to refund the students' $36,500 tuition, even though the party had happened at the beginning of the 2020 fall term.

"Cooperation and compliance with public health guidelines is [*sic*] absolutely essential," the school declared in a statement—proving that university authorities' understanding of grammar was as strong as their knowledge of the dangers of Covid to their students.

The ugly habit of snitching also spread on campus. As the *New York Times* reported at the start of the 2020–2021 school year, "Colgate University sent students a memo encouraging them to report classmates who violate social-distancing guidelines and to include names so action could be taken. Similar instructions were sent out at schools across the country."[4]

Some schools went further. The University of Miami paid students to walk around campus and report on people who refused to comply with mask-wearing and social-distancing rules.[5] Other schools promised more lenient punishments to students they had caught if those students informed on others. "As college kids have begun policing each other, campuses have become a place of paranoia, finger-pointing, and mistrust," *New York* magazine reported.[6]

In an indication of the success of the public health campaign to frighten young adults about Covid, many students happily accepted the rules, apparently believing that the coronavirus was a threat necessitating surveillance and punishment. "Save a life: be a snitch," a student at St. Louis University wrote. "Reporting students not obeying SLU's COVID-19 safety measure is in everyone's best interest."[7]

Others pushed back. Students and parents all over the country emailed me to complain about the rules—and the fact that the schools were charging full tuition for a distinctly second-rate college experience. The mother of a Michigan State University student explained,

> If students do not participate in contact tracing or break quarantine, they are suspended from the University. Our daughter lives on the street where most sororities are located, and she says the police drive up and down the street all day.
>
> Our daughter hasn't gotten Covid yet, but knows many people who have (all asymptomatic or just a slight cold). I've told her not to seek a test if she thinks she has it.
>
> I keep thinking the world is going to wake up and realize what damage is being caused by the overreaction to Covid, but I'm losing hope.

Gordon Gee, the president of West Virginia University, became the object of particular ire after he was caught in September shopping maskless in a drugstore.[8]

"This is after the university has suspended many students for going to parties w/o masks, refused to give refunds after going [switching] to mostly online classes, and him publicly scolding them," a reader wrote.

College athletics became a particularly thorny issue. For much of the summer of 2020, intercollegiate sports programs—including football, which generated fanatic interest and tens of millions of dollars in revenue for many big state universities—appeared likely to vanish.

The Ivy League, whose eight wealthy members did not need football revenue, canceled all its fall sports programs in early June. Bigger schools hemmed and hawed in the face of heavy media pressure to cancel their seasons.

On June 30, CBS Sports published an article predicting that up to seven college football players might die if colleges played.[9] The figure was based on an estimate that the coronavirus could kill as many as one in one thousand college-age people it infected—an estimate that over-stated the real risk to healthy young people by at least a hundred-fold.

The next month, German researchers published a study purporting to show that, of one hundred relatively young and healthy Covid patients, sixty showed signs of a heart inflammation called myocarditis.[10] The study was catastrophically flawed, as later research would demonstrate. (A May 2021 article written by three physicians, including two cardiologists, demolished the research in an article headlined "Setting the Record Straight: There Is No 'Covid Heart.'")[11]

But news outlets eagerly reported the German story, part of a pattern that persisted throughout 2020. Over and over again, studies that played up the risks of Covid received uncritical press attention. Those that showed the virus might be less dangerous were scoured for flaws—or simply ignored.

By August, the debate about intercollegiate athletics and particularly college football had, inevitably, become politicized. Each Saturday millions of Americans flocked to football stadiums far from major cities to eat, drink, and watch "student-athletes" tackle one another and generate billions of dollars for their schools. (While the players are not paid, some coaches are paid upwards of $5 million a year. The system was profoundly unfair, and it is now collapsing, but that's another story.)

Professional sports leagues had restarted their seasons in the summer of 2020. But they had done so without live fans and under severe restrictions. The reappearance of professional sports did not mark a return to normality. College football was symbolically crucial, particularly in political swing states such as Pennsylvania and Michigan. On August 10, Trump tweeted, "Play College Football!" Republican senators from Nebraska, Georgia, and Florida all pushed for the return of the sport.[12]

Naturally, the media almost universally took the opposite stance. "College Football during Covid-19 Teaches Wrong Lessons," the *New York Times* warned on August 29. "College Football Is Not Essential." *New York* magazine complained three days later that "college football is still recklessly barreling forward."

Confusingly, university athletic conferences in different parts of the country adopted different rules. The Southeastern Conference, the sport's most important, announced in late July that it would play. But the Big Ten, centered in the Midwest, canceled its season in August, then reinstated play in mid-September.[13] As the *Detroit Free Press* reported on September 16, "After more than a month of political wrangling, coach chirping, parent protests, player lawsuits, fan frustration and public outcry, the conference announced it plans to hold a season this fall after all."[14]

Notably absent from the lead of the story was any mention of health or the possible risks of Covid.

In the end, though a handful of games were postponed or canceled, the college football season went forward. Other sports did too. The predicted deaths did not occur. I have not found a single report of a college athlete dying from a Covid infection that followed competition or practice. (It is possible I have missed one, or a handful. But if any did occur, they were exceptionally rare. Reporters surely would have gone out of their way to publicize those incidents.)

Naturally, the media never acknowledged that Covid had proven far less dangerous to athletes than it had warned.

The fiasco over athletics was a microcosm of the way colleges and universities dealt with Covid. Whether from fear of lawsuits, a desire to appease left-leaning faculty members, pressure from their host towns, or a genuine misunderstanding of the tiny risks to their students, colleges engaged in "safetyism" at all costs.

In the 2018 book *The Coddling of the American Mind*, Jonathan Haidt and Greg Lukianoff defined safetyism as "a culture or belief system in which safety has become a sacred value, which means that people are unwilling to make trade-offs demanded by other practical and moral concerns."[15]

Driving provides a classic example of the trade-offs that a culture singularly fixated on safety cannot accept. A rigorously enforced speed limit of fifteen miles an hour might end *all* vehicle fatalities. But we have collectively decided that the risks of driving are low enough to permit much higher limits, even though a small risk across a large group of people can lead to eye-popping death totals. Vehicle accidents killed forty-two thousand Americans in 2020 (an increase of 24 percent from the previous year, possibly related to lockdown-related drug use or hidden suicides.)[16]

Safetyism is the broader cultural version of helicopter parenting, an effort at control that can produce children who are fearful and unable to make decisions for themselves.

As a psychologist and author of a parenting book told *Parents* magazine in 2018, "The main problem with helicopter parenting is that it backfires.... The underlying message [the] over-involvement sends to kids is 'My parent doesn't trust me to do this on my own.' This, in turn, leads to a lack of confidence."[17] Helicopter parenting is also associated with increased child anxiety and depression.

The obsession with minimizing Covid's risks seemed to produce similar effects on an entire generation of young people. Anxiety levels among teens and young adults skyrocketed. The CDC found that in February and March 2021, visits to emergency rooms for suicide attempts by adolescent girls rose 50 percent compared to the same period in 2019. For boys, attempts rose 3 percent.[18]

Inevitably, the bureaucratic pressure encountered some pushback. Off-campus parties continued, quietly. Roommates promised each other they would not get tested or report cases if they showed symptoms, in order to avoid having to quarantine.[19] "My roommates and I made a pact that none of us were going to get tested in Knoxville because it always gets reported back to the university," a University of Tennessee student told a local television station.[20]

Still, as the fall semester continued, universities only *tightened* their rules, despite the fact almost no students had been hospitalized or died after hundreds of thousands of positive tests. Schools such as the University of Missouri, which had begun the semester offering in-person teaching, switched to online learning.[21] And colleges continued to punish students caught violating rules.

Despite their anger, students and parents went along. Enrollment among first-year students fell 16 percent, as those who had a choice decided to take the year off. But the vast majority of students had little choice but to accept the rules. Overall enrollment fell only 4 percent, meaning almost all sophomores, juniors, or seniors returned.[22] Few wanted to jeopardize their educations or risk being expelled.

Once again, the bureaucrats and lawyers had won.

Viewed another way, universities had taught their students a vitally important lesson: established systems are incredibly powerful and nearly impossible to defeat without mass protest.

21

Deaths of Despair

I f life on campus was grim for young people in 2020, life off campus was worse.

Depression and suicidal ideation among teens and young adults rose, though American suicide rates actually fell slightly during 2020. Roughly 45,000 Americans killed themselves in 2020, a drop of 2,700 from 2019.[1]

The good news ended there. Other preventable deaths soared.

Most shocking were the deaths from drug overdoses. Those rose almost 30 percent, to about 93,000 Americans—an extraordinary increase after two years in which deaths had been roughly flat.[2]

Overdoses have been an American crisis since the 1990s, when a misguided (and drug company–funded) effort to increase prescription opioid painkiller use began. Last year's increase drove them to *five* times their level in 2000—and roughly ten times as many as the European Union suffered in 2018.[3]

Sloppy headline writers often blamed Covid for the increase. But lockdowns likely played a far larger role than the virus.

Strong evidence came from Canada, which has its own overdose crisis. Canada had significantly fewer Covid deaths than the United States, and almost no deaths under fifty, but a more severe lockdown. It also had an even faster rise in overdose deaths. The Canadian government reported in June 2021 that Canada had suffered 5,148 opioid overdose deaths from April to December 2020. That figure represented an 89 percent increase compared to the same period in 2019, and the equivalent of about 70,000 annual deaths in the United States. (Canada's figure did *not* include deaths from cocaine, methamphetamine, or other drugs.)[4]

Lockdowns drove overdose deaths in many ways.

Restaurant, bar, and retail store closings disproportionately cost young people their jobs and left them bored and stuck at home—even as unemployment payments provided them with steady income. Many twelve-step recovery groups became online-only, cutting off vital support for users trying to abstain. And people became even more likely to use drugs alone. If they overdosed, no one could call an ambulance or administer Naloxone to try to revive them.[5]

At the same time, Chinese-made fentanyl, a synthetic opioid far more potent than heroin, sometimes shipped directly from China, became even cheaper and easier to buy.[6] So the risks of accidental overdose rose alongside the odds people would use alone.

The Canadian government grimly summed up the situation in its June 2021 report: "A number of factors have likely contributed to a worsening of the overdose crisis, including the increasingly toxic drug supply, increased feelings of isolation, stress and anxiety and limited availability or accessibility of services for people who use drugs."[7]

Shocking as they were, the statistics could not capture the tragedy of young lives lost. The stories told by family members and friends had an ugly sameness.

From British Columbia:

> Butler and Dalton say COVID-19 caused Olivia's support group meetings to be cancelled. She relapsed and then lost her job. Soon, she was using alone in her apartment.

That's where Butler found her body on Oct. 22.

"My whole world just crushed at that moment," he said. "Ever since then...it's just been one bad day after another."[8]

And California:

Otto described his son as a charismatic and gifted high school athlete who made friends easily. But he said that during the pandemic he felt the teenager had too much time on his hands. He changed....

Otto said he and his wife got their son into a 30-day inpatient treatment program for addiction, but he relapsed a few days after completing the program. The parents tried to send their son back, but the treatment center lacked the space to take him right away, and due to COVID-19, local outpatient treatment options had an admission backlog....

When Otto went to check on his son a couple of hours later, he found him dead in his bedroom. Otto said the memory of that moment haunts him.[9]

And Massachusetts:

Susan Kinnane of Eastham lost [her] son Danny Vigliano to an overdose in August. The 35-year-old, whose struggle she said was made worse by the isolation, died alone on the floor of a Brockton MBTA [Boston regional train] station.[10]

And Pennsylvania:

Last month, Hinson [Michael Hinson, president of a non-profit housing group in Philadelphia] lost another friend to an overdose at age 42.

"He was in West Philadelphia for a whole week. They couldn't find him, and he was in the morgue for over a week," Hinson said. "He died of a drug overdose, alone."[11]

Overdoses were not the only crisis.

Homicides soared in 2020, rising more than 25 percent across the United States, as school closures left many young men with little to do. (Police inaction following the Floyd protests also appeared to play a role.)

Philadelphia, a racially divided city under Pennsylvania's harsh lockdown rules, was particularly hard-hit. Murders rose almost 40 percent in 2020. The city trailed only Chicago in the number of killings. With 1.5 million people, Philadelphia reported 1,214 overdose deaths and 499 murders for the year,[12] compared to about 2,400 deaths from Covid.[13]

The rise in murders, driving deaths, and overdoses cost tens of thousands of young Americans their lives. More than 155,000 people in the United States died of those causes in 2020, compared to about 120,000 in 2019.

Preliminary data suggested that deaths from alcohol abuse and alcoholism rose at a similar rate, adding at least another 20,000 preventable deaths to the grim total of what researchers frequently classify as "deaths of despair."[14] The United States was not alone; alcohol-related deaths in Britain soared 20 percent in 2020.[15]

In all, more than a quarter-million Americans died from drug overdoses, alcohol, traffic accidents, and homicides in 2020, a rise of over fifty thousand. Those deaths primarily occurred in younger people.[16] Even excluding traffic accidents, the rise in deaths of despair in people under fifty—not the total number, but the *increase* from 2019 to 2020—was *larger* than the *total* of seventeen thousand Covid deaths in people in the same age range in 2020.[17]

Yet practically no one was aware how bad the rise had become.

The same media outlets that lavished attention on Covid deaths showed almost no interest in these fatalities. The gap was especially galling and notable at CNN and MSNBC, with their up-to-the-second

Covid death tickers. Good luck finding anything similar for homicides or overdoses. As late as mid-2021, a complete and accurate national count of murders and overdose deaths in 2020 was not even available.

You manage what you measure, the business-school maxim goes. The corollary is that you measure what you care about.

The difference between our obsessive counting of Covid deaths and our lack of interest in these deaths of despair proved the point. On March 20, 2020, Governor Cuomo famously said, at a press conference announcing the New York lockdown, "When we look back at this situation ten years from now, I want to be able to say to the people of New York I did everything we could do. I did everything we could do. This is about saving lives and if everything we do saves just one life, I'll be happy."[18]

This is about saving lives and if everything we do saves just one life, I'll be happy.

In fact, the lockdowns in New York and everywhere else in the United States probably saved *no* lives. But even if they had, Cuomo's formulation was terribly flawed. It was single-entry bookkeeping, looking only at assets and not liabilities. It took into account only the lives quarantines might save and not those they might cost.

And all over the country, the price of that myopia was real.

22

Sunbelt Spike

The politicization of school and college reopenings disturbed me—and made me even more committed to fight for the truth. The strong sales and publicity the first *Unreported Truths* booklet attracted had cemented my role as a prominent lockdown critic.

My family tried to live as normally as possible over the summer, although doing so wasn't easy in a New York that remained mostly locked down. In June, after a mall over the state line in Connecticut opened, we drove to it, hoping to see life returning to normal.

Nope. Most stores were still closed, especially the ones you'd expect based on their Karen-heavy customer bases. Lululemon had a prissy little note explaining that the safety of shoppers and employees was all that mattered. Translation: *We've surveyed our customers and they're happy enough to buy online and let someone deliver their overpriced yoga pants.*

The stores that were open had clerks standing at the door, allowing shoppers in one at a time. Not that the capacity restrictions were necessary. The mall approached the post-apocalypse vibe of Manhattan back in April. It was nearly empty, a handful of people shuffling through its halls, their faces half-hidden behind masks. A picture taken at the time shows two cars in its enormous parking lot.[1]

By then I had realized masks were essentially useless. I wore mine pulled down over my chin. My Twitter avatar, with a bright pink mask around my chin, came from that time. If anyone challenged me, I covered my mouth. I didn't feel like arguing.

Our older daughter and I did take one longer trip at the end of June, to Denver. At the time Colorado appeared on track to have open and possibly unmasked schools in the fall of 2020. We were thinking about renting a house there for the school year.

Our Southwest flight had more passengers than I expected, probably because airlines had cut their flight schedules so sharply. No one seemed particularly worried about flying. That attitude was probably the result of selection bias—anyone who *was* concerned wouldn't be on the plane.

After we flew home, I tweeted:

> Flew today. Turns out that even when face diapers are required...they're not really required. I had a mask, of course, and if the flight attendants had wanted me to wear it I would have...but they didn't. Non-Karens are well aware they're viral theater.[2]

I didn't know it at the time, but this laissez-faire attitude would evaporate by the fall, as the theater around masks became more serious.

Colorado wasn't quite as pandemic-stunned as New York, but it wasn't great. Our hotel had just reopened, with the semi-logical rules that were popping up everywhere—one family to an elevator, masks at the gym, but enjoy the pool. Downtown Denver was mostly empty. But its heart, the 16th Street Mall, had more panhandlers, and they were more aggressive.

We didn't wind up renting a house in Colorado—a lucky break, because Colorado schools didn't open in the fall.

As the summer went on I appeared on Fox regularly, although other outlets would not have me. The media seemed to have decided that if it could not destroy me, it would ignore me. (This attitude persisted into 2021, when my questions about vaccines led to a second, angrier wave of attacks. More on those later.)

On Twitter, I found that blue checks I did not know had preemptively blocked me. Apparently, these people were terrified of reading what I was saying. Or maybe of letting *me* read what *they* were saying. In any case, they had decided the safest course was simply to cut me off. I found this attitude bizarre. Wasn't the whole idea of an open media platform to allow people with different points of view to debate?

I began to criticize the public health establishment, including Dr. Fauci, more directly. I knew I risked being dismissed as a conspiracy theorist. But I felt I had little choice.

Over time, Fauci's scaremongering and bias against reasonable reopening standards had become impossible to ignore. So had his thirst for media attention. In July he appeared on the cover of *InStyle* magazine wearing sunglasses, his legs crossed as he sat in a chair beside a pool. "THE GOOD DOCTOR," the cover headline read.[3]

A week later Fauci threw out the first pitch of the long-delayed baseball season in Washington as a national audience watched. (He missed the catcher badly, provoking jokes about "Fauci flattening the curve" and "socially distanced pitching.")

Then he headed into the empty stands of Nationals Park to watch the game. At some point, a photographer caught him with his mask pulled down to his chin, grinning as he sat next to his wife. I tweeted the picture the next day, along with the caption, "And there's Dr. Anthony Fauci showing us all he knows exactly how well masks work! Thanks for the lesson, doc."[4]

More than fifteen thousand people liked or retweeted the comment; given Fauci's loud post-March stance in favor of masks, the picture made him appear nearly as big a hypocrite as Neil Ferguson. Ultimately, he explained the photo away with the dubious claim, "I was totally dehydrated and I was drinking water trying to rehydrate myself."[5]

By then we had all learned that Sars-Cov-2 was not going to disappear anytime soon. A second major wave of the virus had struck. While the first wave had hit the Northeast and Midwest, the new epidemic was concentrated in the Sunbelt. The surge stretched from Miami to Los Angeles, from Houston to Nashville, a region encompassing almost 150 million people. The regional epidemic offered further evidence that the virus was highly seasonal—and that indoor transmission was its main driver. Summer humidity in the South and triple-digit temperatures in the Southwest had forced people indoors.

The usual media suspects predicted doom. On July 10, the investigative reporting website ProPublica published an article about Houston headlined "'All the Hospitals are Full.'"[6] But the headline had quotation marks around it. It was a comment by someone quoted in the article—the trick media organizations had learned to use when they wanted to offer frightening headlines that the data in their articles did not support.

"Houston hospitals have been forced to treat hundreds of COVID-19 patients in their emergency rooms—sometimes for several hours or multiple days," the writers went on, as if hospitals did not regularly board patients in emergency rooms on nights and weekends.

In fact, all the hospitals in Houston weren't full. They weren't *close* to full. They had thousands of empty beds throughout July. This information was no secret. The Texas Medical Center, a consortium of hospitals in downtown Houston, posted updated figures every day. They showed the system was strained but far from overrun.

As I tweeted ten days later:

Update from Houston: ALL THE HOSPITALS ARE (not) FULL! And they're not going to be, since new #Covid hospitalizations are down 30% in a week. Is there a word for panic porn as badly timed as that Mike Hixenbaugh/Charles Ornstein spectacular? They'll update it soon, I'm sure.[7]

They didn't, of course. They argued with me on Twitter a bit and then moved to their next story. I understood the impulse. Reporters generally hate admitting they were wrong. When I worked at the *New York Times*, I certainly did.

But these were not small mistakes, and they had real consequences. Spreading panic about Covid and pretending hospitals were full when they weren't could keep people from going to the emergency room for medical care. I had always thought one big difference between serious reporters and tabloid journalists was that serious reporters understood they had a responsibility to acknowledge when they were wrong. Apparently that distinction no longer existed.

A few days after the ProPublica story, on July 15, *The Atlantic* predicted that as many as 550,000 people in the Sunbelt might die before the spike burned out. "A Second Coronavirus Death Surge Is Coming," the magazine warned. Alexis Madrigal, the author, laid the panic porn on thick: "The testing delays, the emergency-room-nurse stories, the refrigerated morgue trucks—the first time as a tragedy, the second time as an even greater tragedy. One must ask, without really wanting to know the answer, *How bad could this round get?*" [emphasis in the original]

I had a hard time not seeing a certain hand-rubbing hope for disaster in these articles, their nose-in-the-air claims to the contrary.

I immediately attacked Madrigal's prediction on Twitter, offering a half-dozen reasons why it was wrong, starting with the most important:

> CASE MIX. The age of the infected is by far the most important factor in deaths, and reported infections have skewed much younger in the Sunbelt. Even The Atlantic admits this.[8]

Madrigal's estimates turned out to be about ten times too high. No matter. By the time the reality was clear, *The Atlantic* had moved on to new panic porn, mostly focused on kids and schools.

The *Atlantic* article also had elements of what became a subcategory of pandemic reporting in summer 2020, the Europe-handled-Covid-right-and-controlled-it-while-the-United-States-failed-because-of Donald-Trump article.

In these pieces, writers explained how sage European countries had imposed contact tracing and mask rules and ensured they had few new cases before reopening. Meanwhile, the United States had lurched forward without the necessary precautions. As Madrigal wrote, "No other country in the world has attempted what the U.S. appears to be stumbling into. Right now, many, many communities have huge numbers of infections. When other countries reached this kind of takeoff point for viral spread, they took drastic measures."[9]

Another *Atlantic* article, this one on July 2, was a first-person classic of the genre: "Do Americans Understand How Badly They're Doing? In France, Where I Live, the Virus Is under Control. I Can Hardly Believe the News Coming Out of the United States."[10] The author made sure to lay the blame on Trump: "As Donald Trump's America continues to shatter records for daily infections, France, like most other developed nations and even some undeveloped ones, seems to have beat back the virus."

The Atlantic wasn't alone. On July 20, *New York* magazine offered an article headlined "American Death Cult: Why Has the Republican Response to the Pandemic Been So Mind-Bogglingly Disastrous?" The author, Jonathan Chait, confidently averred, "Our former peer nations are now operating in a political context Americans would find unfathomable. Every other wealthy nation in the world has successfully beaten back the disease, at least significantly, and at least for now."[11]

On the same day, the *Wall Street Journal* explained "How Europe Kept Coronavirus Cases Low Even after Reopening":

> In the U.S., "we are pushing this idea that we have to live with the virus, that there's nothing we can do. That's not true: Europe shows you can turn the epidemic around," says

Jennifer Nuzzo, an epidemiologist and senior scholar at Johns Hopkins Center for Health Security.

While many European countries effectively used the lockdown to bring down case levels and build up the public-health capacity to track and trace new infections, in some U.S. states such efforts still lag behind.[12]

Anthony Fauci also made sure to laud Europe's response, telling Congress on July 31 that European countries had quelled their epidemics because they had locked down more strictly than the United States:

If you look at what happened in Europe, when they shut down or locked down or went to shelter in place, however you want to describe it, they really did it to the tune of about 95 percent-plus of the country did that....

We really functionally shut down only about 50% in the sense of the totality of the country.[13]

Weeks later, as the Sunbelt spike faded and France, Spain, and the rest of Europe headed into a second wave that dwarfed the first, these stories and Fauci's testimony would look unintentionally ironic.

Adding to the irony, in 2006 Nuzzo had co-authored the famous Donald Henderson paper arguing that "communities faced with epidemics or other adverse events respond best and with the least anxiety when the normal social functioning of the community is least disrupted."[14]

But reporters just didn't care. Over and over, they attacked Trump and the American response without comparing our death rates to those in Western Europe, the most obvious benchmark. (In fact, they ignored European nations except during those few weeks over the summer of 2020, when Spain, France, and Italy seemed to be doing better than the United States.)

CNN and the *New York Times* harped on the fact that the coronavirus death toll in the United States was far larger than America's share of the global population. "The U.S. accounts for 4 percent of the world's population, and for 22 percent of confirmed Covid-19 deaths," the *Times* reported on September 1, in a piece headlined "America's Death Gap."[15]

These figures were accurate. But—to use a charge often leveled unfairly against me—they were a form of misinformation. Wealthier countries accounted for a disproportionate share of Covid deaths. They had more older people at higher risk, and they counted deaths aggressively.

Month after month, deaths in four of the five biggest European countries roughly tracked those in the United States as a percentage of population (the fifth, Germany, was lower than the others, though over time its counts crept closer).

By summer 2021, the United States, with 4 percent of the world's population, had about 15 percent of reported Covid deaths. Britain, France, Italy, and Spain, similarly wealthy countries with under 3 percent of the world's population, had about 11 percent. And rates of obesity—something that would turn out to be a significant risk factor for severity of Covid cases[16]—are lower in Western European countries than in the United States.

If the comparisons of Covid deaths in the United States to those in the rest of the world were unfair and misleading, the comparisons between red and blue states were flat-out deceptive.

Through the summer, reporters and public health experts pointed to the low case and death counts in the Northeast as evidence that Democratic governors such as Cuomo and Phil Murphy were managing Covid better than Republicans. Naturally, strict lockdowns and slow reopenings received the glory.

"New York has been able to keep coronavirus at bay while other states see surges," ABC News said on July 16. "A professor of population health and medicine" at New York University "credited New York's strict social distancing orders for the turnaround and its extremely cautious reopening."[17]

Fauci added to the chorus the next day, saying on a PBS interview, "When you do it properly, you bring down these cases.... We have done it in New York....They did it correctly." It was not entirely clear what specifically Fauci thought New York had done correctly, although he mentioned closing bars and mask mandates.[18]

Meanwhile, Cuomo and Murphy were telling everyone who would listen about the amazing job they had done. "We have crushed the curve of new cases," Murphy said on June 24. "We've gotten to where we are through shared sacrifice."[19]

Cuomo bragged in a not-exactly-challenging interview with ABC on June 17, "We went from the worst infection rate to the best infection rate." He added that he had survived the crisis by imagining what his father would do. "My father's spirit lives in me. I know what he would say. I know his advice."[20] Cuomo added, "New Yorkers who died did not die because we failed them."

Less than a month later, Cuomo felt bold enough to attack Trump directly. At a press conference, he said:

> The President is attacking science. What a surprise. No surprise. He's been attacking science from day one. The denial of reality was to deny science and he's done that from day one....
>
> Trump was wrong from day one and New Yorkers have been right from day one. There's no argument. There's nothing to tweet about. The facts are in. The numbers are in. Look at the number of bodies.[21]

Look at the number of bodies?

At the time New York, with about 6 percent of the United States population, accounted for more than 20 percent of American coronavirus deaths. Of course, the spring 2020 wave had struck New York hardest. (That fact was probably the primary reason cases and deaths stayed relatively low in New York through the fall of 2020 and winter of 2021. The city and state had more people who were recovered and immune than almost anywhere else in the United States.)

But a *full year* after Cuomo's comments, following three separate coronavirus waves that had touched essentially every state and evened out the burden nationally, New York still had more deaths than any other state except California, which had twice as many people. It had 40 percent more deaths than Florida, which had more residents and far more elderly residents.

By July 2021, New York had recorded more than fifty-four thousand deaths, almost three per one thousand residents, the second-most deaths per capita. Only New Jersey had more deaths per resident. No obvious demographic factors explained the vast difference between New York and many other states—highlighting Cuomo's decision to send Covid patients to nursing homes as a key potential factor.

Yet in the summer of 2020, most journalists seemed reluctant to challenge Cuomo on his claims, perhaps because doing so might have meant taking Trump's side. Only later—only after Trump had lost the election, in fact—would outlets such as the *New York Times* and *Washington Post* begin seriously to challenge Cuomo.

23

The Forever Lockdowners

The Sunbelt spike led some public health experts to call for a second lockdown, this one even harsher than the spring version.

On July 26, 2020, Andy Slavitt, who had run Medicare and Medicaid under President Obama and throughout 2020, made a habit of near-endless Twitter threads predicting doom, promising his hundreds of thousands of followers that "we can virtually eliminate the virus any time we decide to."[1]

Easy, right?

All we'd have to do was "keep the bars & restaurants & churches & transit closed." Oh, and "prohibit interstate travel."[2] Slavitt didn't say so out loud, but taking *that* step would probably have meant declaring martial law and suspending the Constitution.

Slavitt wasn't done yet. He also wanted to suspend most food production and medical services and retail supply chains. He called it a "90% lockdown": "Meaning most of the Americans who couldn't stay home in April because they were picking crops or driving trucks or working in health care would stay home with us."[3]

Slavitt made shutting down the entire country sound like a summer vacation. *We'll all hang out and watch TV...and when the power goes out we can tell ghost stories from the olden times when we had a Constitution!*

Slavitt was not alone. On August 7, Michael Osterholm, director of the Center for Infectious Disease Research and Policy at the University of Minnesota, co-wrote an opinion piece for the *New York Times* demanding: "A more restrictive lockdown, state by state, to crush the spread of the virus....People must stay at home and leave only for essential reasons: food shopping and visits to doctors and pharmacies....The lockdown has to be as comprehensive and strict as possible."[4]

Osterholm's plan, nearly as bizarre as Slavitt's, would have resulted in among the most restrictive lockdowns anywhere in the world. If followed strictly, it would have banned not just shopping and working in offices—*but all outdoor activity, including going outside for exercise, in the middle of August.*

Yet the *Times* offered it as a serious option.

Again, strangely, Osterholm had offered less panicked advice early in the epidemic. On March 21 another opinion piece by him, this one co-written with Mark Olshaker, published in the *Washington Post*, and headlined "Facing Covid-19 Reality: A National Lockdown Is No Cure," had explained:

> As a country, with momentum building for a possible national shutdown directive, we are on the verge of ringing a giant bell that we don't know how to un-ring.
>
> [We] don't, for example, have good data on the real impact of closing public and private K–12 schools on the spread of covid-19....The second-order effect of shutting schools is that hardest hit will be those least able to afford to miss work to care for homebound children.[5]

The events of the ensuing months had entirely vindicated that fear.

Osterholm and Olshaker had concluded, "The best alternative will probably entail letting those at low risk for serious disease continue to work…while at the same time advising higher-risk individuals to protect themselves through physical distancing and ramping up our health-care capacity as aggressively as possible. With this battle plan, we could gradually build up immunity without destroying the financial structure on which our lives are based."

The March article offered a sane and sober perspective. And in the five months between Osterholm's two pieces, we had learned Covid was *less* dangerous than it had appeared in March.

Yet Osterholm and the entire public health establishment had gone the other way. I could find no explanation for the change that didn't center on Donald Trump. When I publicly asked Osterholm and others to explain, they ignored me.

As Osterholm's summer piece mentioned in passing, the Sunbelt spike was already fading by early August. (This phenomenon was nearly as common as the Covid hysteria itself: peaks in media panic were almost always a sign that a regional epidemic was topping out.)

Hospitalizations for Covid declined in Arizona after mid-July, and in Florida and Texas later in the month. Nationwide, reported Covid cases peaked at about seventy-five thousand a day, higher than their spring levels, in part because testing was so much more widespread. But hospitalizations and deaths remained lower than their April peaks.

Several factors accounted for the lower death rates. The rise in testing meant many newly reported infections came in low-risk young adults. Southern states generally avoided the Cuomo mistake of sending patients with Covid back to nursing homes. Dexamethasone, following its clinical trial success, had become a standard treatment regimen, reducing mortality. And doctors now knew they should use ventilators only as a last resort.

The pattern in the Sunbelt matched that of every other major coronavirus wave in 2020 *everywhere in the world*. The virus turned out to be both unpredictable and deeply predictable. Scientists might not know when a wave would begin, but once one did, it followed a steady pattern.

But—on those rare occasions when they even reported on the end of the Sunbelt spike—the media generally gave lockdown and mask restrictions the credit.

In fact, lockdowns clearly did *not* deserve credit for the rapid turn. No Sunbelt state imposed harsh restrictions on work or shopping during the summer, though some did close bars and mandate mask-wearing. As the BBC reported in mid-July, Florida governor DeSantis had "joined President Donald Trump in emphasizing the importance of keeping the economy open."[6]

The BBC almost surely meant the words as an insult, but DeSantis's focus on keeping businesses going paid off. Economies across the South recovered quickly even as the epidemic spread over the summer. By September some southern states had nearly reached pre-March employment levels.

That good news contradicted the claims of health experts that economies could not recover as long as Covid remained a threat. In fact, lockdowns were far more damaging to the economy than the virus itself. In states that had more restrictions, such as New York and California, unemployment remained higher than in more open states such as Florida where the virus was more common over the summer. In August, New York's unemployment rate was 12.5 percent, while Florida's was 7.4 percent. Before the lockdowns, differences in state unemployment rates had been smaller, usually no more than 2 percent.

Other signs of lockdown fatigue appeared by late summer. Mobility data compiled by Apple showed that after plunging in March and April, requests for directions across the United States had surpassed pre-Covid levels by June.

As work and travel patterns moved toward normal, cooperation with government bureaucracies fell. All over the country, state health departments complained that people wouldn't cooperate with their efforts to "contact trace."

Tracers ask anyone who has had a positive coronavirus test to give up the names of people he or she has been around. Those contacts, in turn, are encouraged to be tested. They are also asked or sometimes forced to submit to a quarantine of up to fourteen days, whether or not they are sick.

Throughout 2020, public health experts aggressively pushed contract tracing as an essential tool to slow the spread of the virus.[7] "To suppress their epidemics to manageable levels, countries around the world have turned to contact tracing," Stat News reported in May, in an article headlined "Contract Tracing Could Help Avoid Another Lockdown."[8]

States rapidly added to their armies of contact tracers. New York alone announced in April it would hire up to seventeen thousand tracers, nearly one for every one thousand people in the state.[9] Cities, countries, and schools also had their own forces.

The public health authoritarians wanted more. A group of them, including Scott Gottlieb and Slavitt, demanded the federal government help states hire *another* 180,000 tracers at a cost of $12 billion.[10] They also asked for $4.5 billion to rent hotels for people forced to quarantine and $30 billion in daily $50 stipends for people who couldn't work because of quarantines—a total of $46.5 billion in all.

At $700 for a 14-day quarantine, the proposal implied that more than 40 *million Americans* would be caught in quarantines over the next 18 months.

But the contract tracers immediately ran into trouble. Many people had no interest in talking to them. "We still struggle with the fact that most people aren't answering the phone when we call," the assistant city manager of San Antonio told the *San Antonio Express-News*. "Right now, we really need the public's help."[11]

The unwillingness to cooperate was not confined to Republican states. New Jersey governor Phil Murphy reported in December that 74 percent of his state's residents refused to cooperate. "Quite frankly, this is unacceptable, and we need to turn it around," he said.[12]

But despite the bluster, neither Murphy nor any other governor had real leverage. Even Americans who no longer supported lockdowns might be willing to tolerate them sullenly. But efforts to use state power to support or enforce quarantines against individuals caused instant backlash, as health officials in Kentucky found out in July 2020, when they put a husband and wife on "house arrest" after they refused to sign an isolation order.[13]

One reason people may have been disinclined to help was that contact tracing was essentially useless to control any disease that had spread as widely as the coronavirus. Tracing was labor-intensive and depended on following plausible transmission chains both to and from an infected person. But in cases where the virus was everywhere, chasing its spread was the respiratory equivalent of trying to track chlamydia at an orgy.

"If new cases of COVID-19 accrue too quickly for tracers to keep up, the system fails," an infectious disease epidemiologist explained to the Live Science website for an article headlined "Why Hasn't Contact Tracing Managed to Slow the Massive Surge of Coronavirus in the US?"[14]

The fact that coronavirus test results could take up to a week to come back only worsened the problem. By the time tracers contacted an infected person, he might well be recovering—after having passed the virus to other people in the days following his test. A *Lancet* paper in July suggested that a delay of more than three days in returning test results made contact tracing essentially useless.[15] But three days was faster than many commercial sites could return results.

The most important factor behind the tracing failure, though, was not practical but philosophical.

In August, a reader who lived in New York State walked me first-hand through the tracing and isolation process. He and his wife had been ordered to isolate after returning from a trip to the West Coast. (As a way to bask in New York's low summer infection rate, Cuomo had declared other states hot spots and told people who were visiting or traveling from them they needed to isolate for two weeks when they arrived in New York.)

We started our quarantine today. My wife and I have different last names so we have 2 different folks working our adventures. I got my first call at 10 am and the gentleman was pretty nice overall. He even joked that Cuomo was an idiot, that might have been defensive as I was still low on coffee and a bit surly to start.

Overall the call was quick and they answered my questions reasonably. I am not to ride my motor bikes, even though I wear a full face helmet and look essentially like a lost spaceman, Covid is dangerous. Got it. I asked about groceries and he said someone would call us if we didn't have Instacart options in our area. I explained we live on a mountain...don't think he's heard that one before....

I got a follow up text message asking if I had any symptoms. I misread it and entered the wrong thing (yay dyslexia) and discovered that there is no way to correct an error, or someone to contact to correct the error....

Generally I don't give a shit about the government, I think that for the most part they don't care enough about me or are too incompetent to find me. I don't like being on their radar, especially for something as silly as Covid-19. My wife had a bit of a cry because of it all and it really made her anxious (which is not something she has an existing issue with)....

This is all a bit too 1984 for me.

And this couple was not even being asked to give up information about anyone else, just to stay home for two weeks. The unenthusiastic national response suggested that though some Americans might participate in the quarantine, most had little interest in doing so, and even fewer intended to set health officials on the people around them.

"They're not willing to share their friends, who they saw, the stores they went to," a California public health official complained in August to NPR. "And that's been a huge problem."[16]

Problem was one word for it.

Anecdotal evidence that many people were tired of lectures about the virus was also visible.

In early August, almost a half-million motorcycle riders gathered for the annual Sturgis, South Dakota, rally. The usual media doomsayers predicted widespread infections and deaths among attendees. "Crowds seen at motorcycle rally raise fears of super spreader event," CNN claimed.[17] In fact, six weeks after the rally, health authorities had traced 414 Covid cases and one death to the rally.[18] (Five people died riding motorcycles at the rally, and at least 56 others were injured.)[19]

Stores and restaurants were also filling up. As the chief executive officer of Darden Restaurants, which operates Olive Garden and other chains, told investors in September, his restaurants were as full as state rules allowed: "We have seen no change in demand based on Covid levels in a market unless capacity restrictions change.... We see a pretty resilient consumer out there."

So the United States muddled along.

In Europe, though, anger over the lockdowns picked up in the fall, as the second wave took off and countries such as Britain,[20] France,[21] and Germany[22] imposed new restrictions. In London, Paris, and Berlin, thousands and in some cases tens of thousands of protestors turned out. But the protests did not stop governments from imposing new lockdown rules.

In poorer countries, especially South American and African nations that endured harsh lockdowns and economic hardship from the global recession, the anger was more visceral.

One of the world's strictest and longest quarantines was in Colombia, where the government imposed a near-total quarantine and closed borders and airports through the summer of 2020. "Colombia's long virus lockdown fuels anxiety and depression," the Associated Press reported in August.

Many Colombians like Nilva Rodriguez, 50, in Barranquilla, have scarcely left their homes. Only twice in four months has she been outside the house she shares with her elderly parents, brother, his pregnant wife and a teenage child.

When she talks to relatives in Miami, she says they are stunned to learn that she cannot even go to a nearby beach because it remains closed.[23]

Unemployment skyrocketed to 25 percent in Colombia's cities, including Bogota, the capital, where millions of people had lived in severe poverty even before the crisis.[24] Then, on September 9, police in Bogota killed Javier Ordoñez, a taxi driver and part-time law student whom they caught drinking after the lockdown curfew. As a reader—an American expatriate with a home in Colombia—emailed me, Ordonez "was killed by police after they confronted him for violating social distancing laws (that is the only 'crime' anyone is accusing him of)."

Video showed Ordoñez pleading for his life, and his killing set off riots across Colombia.[25] Police reported that demonstrators had damaged 56 station houses and injured 147 officers.

But when they wrote about the riots, major English-language outlets largely ignored the role lockdowns and economic shutdown had played in stirring them. Instead they focused on Colombians' anger at police brutality, which was real, but not the primary driver.

"The reality is that the population is incensed…and on top of that you have crime levels and economic misery pouring fuel on the fire," the expatriate explained—and other readers offered similar analyses.

Colombia was not alone in seeing lockdown-related violence and protests.

"Police say people's pent-up frustration over being confined to their homes without income for months together saw them vent their fury," the *Times of India* reported about an August 2020 riot in the southern city of Bangalore.[26] A month earlier, thousands of protestors in Bangkok had rallied against lockdown laws that they said the Thai government was using to punish political opponents.[27] And in August, tens of thousands of Argentinian protestors marched in Buenos Aires and other cities to demand loosened lockdown rules. "A significant part of the population in Argentina is saying 'We've been at home for five months, we need to start living again,'" one analyst told CNN.[28]

Yet throughout 2020, the protests never quite took off. The media covered them grudgingly, when it covered them at all, and often focused on the fact that some protests had nationalist or right-wing elements.[29]

In addition, the difficulty of organizing protests on social media—Facebook in particular frequently censored anti-lockdown groups—meant that the rallies never disrupted cities or had millions of participants. They waxed and waned but never reached a volume or intensity that meant politicians had to heed them.

In poor countries and rich, anti-lockdown anger simmered, but it did not boil over.

24

This Is Only a Test

Meanwhile, late summer 2020 brought evidence that a crucial and poorly understood technical decision early in the year had caused cases and deaths to be overstated, perhaps substantially.

The issue involved PCR testing—which was the way nearly all coronavirus infections were diagnosed. Ironically, the *New York Times* brought the story to light, in an August 29 article headlined "Your Coronavirus Test Is Positive. Maybe It Shouldn't Be."[1]

PCR stands for polymerase chain reaction. PCR tests were not specifically designed to find the coronavirus. They can be used to search for any type of genetic material. They are an important part of the DNA-matching that police laboratories use, for example.[2]

The details of PCR tests are complex. For Sars-Cov-2 tests, a nurse or medical technician takes a swab of cells from a patient who may be infected with the virus. At first, the swabs were generally taken from high in the nose with Q-tips that had especially long handles.

The original "nasopharyngeal" swabs were uncomfortable, at best. They regularly brought tears to the eyes of people undergoing them. A reporter for the San Jose *Mercury* News described "an incomparable sensation like someone itching the back of my eye socket, deeper than one would even think the nasal canal goes."[3] A WebMD article even more bluntly asked, "Brain Scraper: Why Do Some COVID Tests Hurt So Much?"

Now less intrusive swabs taken lower in the nose are more common. Either way, the swab is bagged and sent to a laboratory for a PCR test. There a technician adds chemicals to the sample to extract potential coronavirus RNA, or ribonucleic acid.[4] (You may recall from chapter 7 that RNA is the virus's genetic material, the stored information that determines its structure and how it interacts with and attacks our cells.)

An enzyme is then added to transform the RNA into double-stranded DNA, deoxyribonucleic acid, because the PCR amplification process only works on DNA. The newly created DNA is heated in what is called a thermal cycler to break apart its strands. More chemicals and enzymes are added to the newly torn-open DNA.

The crucial moment comes when the newly added material fuses with the broken halves of the DNA strand, creating *two* identical strands where only one existed before.

The process is then repeated over and over. If the original sample contained coronavirus RNA, each thermal cycle doubles the amount of DNA. Meanwhile, the technician adds a florescent chemical tag. If the target DNA is present, the florescent tag will attach to it, proving the viral RNA was present in the original sample taken from the patient.

As the Mayo Clinic explained,

> The copies accumulate, round by round, exponentially, so that millions and millions of copies are generated....
>
> If SARS-CoV-2 complementary DNA is present in the sample, the primers can copy the targeted regions. As they copy these regions, probes stuck to these new fragments release a visual signal that can be read by the instrument used in this process.[5]

In other words, a glowing vial equals a positive test.

Even this explanation, complicated as it is, understates the intricacy of the PCR test—and its risks.

From the beginning, public health authorities framed the tests as yes-or-no questions. The results were positive or negative. People were infected with Sars-Cov-2, or they weren't. What only experts understood was that *the number of PCR cycles the machines ran was crucial to whether the test would return a positive result or not.*

PCR tests are exponential growth at its purest. After 10 cycles, a single piece of DNA becomes 1,024. After 20, more than 1 million. After 30, over 1 billion. And after 40, more than 1 trillion. One trillion is an unimaginably large number: one million million: 1,000,000,000,000.

One viral RNA particle multiplied to one trillion pieces of DNA. The feat boggles the imagination.

And the more cycles the machine runs, the greater the odds of false positive tests coming from laboratory contamination. Among other potential problems, trace amounts of genetic material remaining on the lab equipment from an earlier test can be multiplied and detected in the testing process.

Worse, the endless doubling can cause an even bigger problem—positive results that are true but meaningless.

Any PCR test that takes more than 30 cycles to become positive shows that the original sample contained minimal amounts of coronavirus RNA. In fact, Sars-Cov-2 may not have existed at all in its complete form in those samples, since the PCR process is not designed to amplify the virus's entire RNA strand, just a piece of it.

In contrast, samples that turn positive at lower cycle thresholds—below 25 and especially below 20—indicate that patients have high viral loads and are at much increased risk of dying of Covid. A June 2020 paper showed that half the patients at New York–Presbyterian Hospital whose admission samples were positive at fewer than 20 cycles died. Only about 1 in 20 people whose samples required more than 32 cycles to be positive died.

Even after adjusting for age and other factors, the gap remained large. Those whose samples had a cycle threshold below 25 were six times as likely to die as those whose sample had a threshold over 30.[6]

In other words, viral load was a crucial predictor of how sick someone was. A positive finding at 30 cycles or more, and certainly 33 or more, was a weak positive.

For people who did not need hospitalization—and most people with weak positives did not—a high-cycle positive indicated that the patient was past the peak of his infection, had beaten back the virus, and was at little risk. It could also mean the sample came from someone whose infection had never been more than trivial. In rare cases, it could indicate that the test had caught the infection very early, when viral loads were still increasing.

Positive tests that occurred at thresholds over 35 were even less significant. They generally did not indicate the presence of transmissible virus at all, just fragments left over from old infections. They were not exactly false positives—they were past positives.

"I'm shocked that people would think that 40 could represent a positive," Juliet Morrison, a California virologist, told the *Times*.[7]

High-cycle positives were especially likely to be meaningless in patients who had no Covid symptoms. A paper published in September 2020 by the government of the Canadian province of Ontario reported that only 5 of 32 asymptomatic people who had CT-positives above 35 had *any* virus in their bodies.[8]

In other words, testing people without symptoms for surveillance purposes was especially likely to produce useless positives. This led cynics to say that high-cycle PCR testing was producing a "testdemic" or a "casedemic."

Just as important, people who tested positive with high cycle thresholds appeared to be much less infectious than those with lower thresholds. In a sample of 324 patients, English researchers found infectious virus in almost 90 percent of patients who had positive CT thresholds in the low 20s, but in fewer than 10 percent of those whose thresholds were in the mid-30s.[9]

This finding made sense. People with positive tests only at high CT-positive thresholds had less virus in their bodies to excrete. The smaller amount of virus they were carrying was less dangerous, both to themselves and to others.

The problem with the PCR tests was that high-threshold and low-threshold results, which really meant two very different things, were treated the same by health authorities. As the BBC explained in September 2020, "A person shedding a large amount of active virus, and a person with leftover fragments from an infection that's already been cleared, would receive the same—positive—test result."[10]

Anthony Fauci was well aware of the issue. He said as much in a June 2020 interview with the *Journal of the American Medical Association*. "If it's 35 or more, even though it's technically positive, the chances of that being replication competent are extremely low," he said. "In other words, you could have a PCR-positive test and yet still not be contagious."[11] He repeated the point in nearly the same language the next month on *This Week in Virology*, a podcast produced by the American Society for Microbiology.[12]

"Replication competent" essentially means "live." Even virologists and infectious disease experts use the terms interchangeably. Viruses cannot reproduce on their own, so they are not *alive* in the way that other organisms are. Instead they take over a cell's machinery to make copies of themselves.

A virus that is not replication competent lacks that ability. It is harmless.

The broader question and answer on the virology podcast with Fauci highlights the issue. The podcast's hosts worried that overly sensitive PCR tests were catching patients who were no longer infectious. They hoped Fauci would agree those people could be discharged from hospitals.

One host asked, "A number of reports of patients who shed viral RNA for weeks, as determined by PCR, doesn't seem to be infectious virus, it doesn't seem to be a threat for transmission, and I'm wondering if you think we could use a cutoff of viral loads as determined by PCR to say this patient can go home."

Fauci's answer made clear he understood the problem: "If you get a cycle threshold of 35 or more, the chances of it being replication competent are miniscule.... You almost never can culture [grow] virus from a 37-threshold cycle, so I think if someone does come in with 37, 38, even 36, it's just dead nucleotides, period."

Fauci was not alone in this realization. Scientists worldwide were aware of these potential problems by late spring.

By July, the European Centre for Disease Prevention and Control was publicly encouraging physicians to examine high-cycle positive results skeptically. The European CDC warned that any result over 35 cycles could be due to laboratory contamination and should be confirmed with a second test "in countries where the epidemic is not yet widespread."[13]

So PCR tests were not the yes-or-no indicator that patients had been told. The cycle threshold mattered enormously.

■   ■   ■

But many—perhaps a majority—of positive tests had thresholds above 30. Exactly how many is impossible to know. If public national data on the distribution of cycle thresholds in positive tests exists, I have not been able to find it.

One fragmentary piece of data came out in December 2020, when Rhode Island reported, in response to a public information request, that more than half of its positive PCR tests from February through June were at cycle thresholds over 30.[14]

The *Times* reported even higher percentages of thresholds over 30 in its August 2020 article, including 63 percent in New York State and almost 90 percent in Massachusetts in July. As the *Times* explained in a moment of surprising clarity, "up to 90 percent of people testing positive carried barely any virus."[15]

It is worth noting that the first wave of the epidemic in Massachusetts had passed in July 2020, and the rate of low-virus, high-cycle positives tends to rise as an epidemic is ending. Thus 90 percent may be an artificially high percentage. Still, if even half the positive tests were real but meaningless, the implications were enormous.

First, calling those tests "positive" unnecessarily frightened many people. People with positive results over 30 cycles, and certainly above 33, should have been told that if they had minor or no symptoms their results probably put them at little risk.

Instead, when people were given their test results, they were only told the test was positive or negative, not the threshold. (Some states did refer to very high-threshold results, in the 37 to 42 range, as indeterminate.)

But scaring people was only one problem.

As Fauci had acknowledged, high-cycle positives kept patients in hospitals after they could be safely discharged. They also forced some people at no risk of transmitting Covid into contact tracing protocols. Their positive tests required them to isolate from families, friends, and their jobs for weeks. Meanwhile, their close contacts were supposed to quarantine.

Tightening the rules for positives would have meant that fewer people would be subject to those rules. Public health efforts could have focused on people with higher viral loads, who were at higher risk of infecting others.

Those civil liberties and practical concerns were the main reason the *Times* had published its article. As it explained, "On Thursday, the United States recorded 45,604 new coronavirus cases....If the rates of contagiousness in Massachusetts and New York were to apply nationwide, then perhaps only 4,500 of those people may actually need to isolate and submit to contact tracing."[16]

But the problems went still further.

For CNN and other media outlets, counting positive tests—which they always called "cases"—was a focus second only to the death count. Including high-cycle PCR tests in the case numbers painted a picture of an exploding epidemic with hundreds of thousands of new patients becoming ill each day—a picture that did not match reality. Most infected people had no or mild symptoms even if they had positive tests—Italian data showed about half of infected people had no symptoms and another one-quarter had only very mild symptoms.[17]

CNN and the other purveyors of panic porn never reported that fact.

The last problem caused by ultra-sensitive PCR testing received even less attention.

Including marginally positive tests pushed up death counts. Why? Because of the death matching process that states used. Most of the "with" Covid deaths—that is, people who died from Alzheimer's or cancer or other terminal illnesses but were counted as Covid deaths—are likely high-cycle positives which states matched after their dates of death, sometimes significantly after.

Indeed, as the epidemic dragged on, a strange phenomenon occurred. Many deaths were reported as Covid-caused not weeks but *months* after they had taken place, often as the result of certificate matching.

Even deaths that legitimately appeared to be from Covid might not be. An asymptomatic person might have a positive test and then two months later die from a heart attack. Under the matching rules, that death would forever be listed as Covid-linked. And since Covid can cause cardiac problems, a heart attack would not stand out as an obviously wrongly coded death, as overdoses or hospice cancer deaths did.

Knowing how many high-cycle-positive deaths might have been miscategorized—how many were "with" as opposed to "from" Covid—is nearly impossible. The existence of these deaths dubiously ascribed to the virus did not mean that Covid had not killed hundreds of thousands of Americans. But a more rational PCR standard would have led to somewhat lower death counts.

Why didn't the Centers for Disease Control and state health departments set such a standard? And why didn't they encourage Americans to use faster, cheaper tests called "rapid lateral flow tests" once those were developed?

Lateral flow tests are more like pregnancy tests. They could be performed at home in a matter of minutes and would come back positive or negative. They were somewhat less accurate than PCR tests, but they still caught the vast majority of cases. One at-home test approved in December 2020 was 96 percent accurate, for example.[18]

Those questions remain among the big unanswered mysteries of the pandemic—along with the government's unwillingness to conduct national randomized antibody sampling and aggressively test inexpensive, low-risk treatments such as ivermectin. (I distinguish these questions from those that are obviously politically influenced, such as the unwillingness to open schools despite massive scientific evidence.)

Health officials clearly worried they might miss cases if they set the PCR threshold too low. Technicians did not always push the swabs as high into the nose as they were supposed to. Running 40 cycles reduced the risk of false negatives. Anyone who had *any* coronavirus at all would be caught. So, as it was conducted, the PCR test had very high "sensitivity," meaning that it found practically everyone who had the coronavirus. (This assumption could not always be made about children, who could be so resistant they were nearly impossible to swab. I watched my five-year-old son wriggle his way through several tests without ever giving a meaningful sample.)

Running the test with fewer cycles also risked missing a tiny number of people who had *just* been infected and whose viral loads were increasing but still low. Those people were about to approach peak infectivity and had few symptoms. Catching them quickly was crucial to containing the coronavirus through contact tracing.

As it turned out, though, authorities had no hope of containing the virus—not just in the United States but everywhere else. By May 2020 at the latest, authorities should have realized that contact tracing was a false hope, because not enough people were cooperating and because the virus had spread too widely for it too work.

Worse, even very accurate tests could lead to many false positives if they were used too widely. Imagine a situation where the test is 99 percent accurate.

That figure is very high. Even so, at times when only a few people have the coronavirus, widespread testing with a 99 percent accurate test will lead to a huge number of false positive results.

Here's how the math works. Suppose only 0.1 percent of people are actually infected. That figure translates into 10 infections out of 10,000 people. In other words, 9,990 people out of every 10,000 *don't* actually have the virus.

If the test is 99 percent accurate at identifying people who are not infected, it will find 99 percent of those 9,990 people negative. In other words, of the 9,990 tested people who don't have the virus it will find 9,890 true negatives—and 100 false positives to go with the 10 *real* positives it correctly finds.

Even though the test is very accurate, 100 out of the 110 positives it returns are wrong.

This statistical example may seem complicated. But the takeaway is simple.

Widespread random population testing, as public health experts have demanded since the spring of 2020, may cause as many problems as it solves.

Ironically, this reality is *especially* true of PCR tests, despite their accuracy, because they are both expensive and slow to return results when they are used on large numbers of people.

As the government of Wales explained in July 2020, "The performance of the existing [PCR test] is at its best when its use is targeted, for example, when used to support diagnosis in symptomatic individuals. It is unsuited to the non-targeted screening of asymptomatic individuals, especially in populations with a low prevalence of infection."[19]

But the United States went the other way, engaging in a desperate and futile hunt for asymptomatic and barely symptomatic positive cases.

By mid-July, American labs were running 800,000 tests a day—about 20 million a month.[20] At an average cost of $150 or more, the United States was spending $3 billion monthly on Covid tests alone.

And still the public health mandarins were not satisfied. The more tests the United States conducted, the more they said were needed. A report in September 2020—when the United States was reporting about 40,000 new cases a day—suggested the nation might need 193 million tests a month.[21]

As with the insistence on contact tracing, the testing fervor seemed driven mainly by the desire of public health officials to *do something*, whether or not it made sense.

All these questions remained essentially out of the public view until the *Times* ran its August piece. Yet the piece did *not* lead to a widespread reconsideration of testing policies, including the high PCR thresholds.

When it ran panicked stories about hospital overrun or children getting Covid, the *Times* set the agenda. But on those rare occasions when it offered a more sober perspective, the rest of the media was less likely to follow.

So the casedemic continued unabated.

25

Long, Long Covid

As the summer wave in the Sunbelt faded, reporters focused on yet another supposed coronavirus crisis—"long Covid," also called "long-haul Covid."

Unsurprisingly, *The Atlantic* magazine and its science writer Ed Yong led this trend. It may be worth noting that Covid was good to both *The Atlantic* and Yong. The magazine's subscriptions soared in 2020, and Yong won a Pulitzer Prize for his articles. As the panic faded in 2021, subscriptions fell, and the magazine's web traffic crashed.[1]

In an August 19, 2020, article headlined "Long-Haulers Are Redefining Covid-19," Yong laid out the terror of long Covid:

Lauren Nichols has been sick with COVID-19 since March 10....She has lived through one month of hand tremors, three of fever, and four of night sweats.

When we spoke on day 150, she was on her fifth month of gastrointestinal problems and severe morning nausea. She still has extreme fatigue, bulging veins, excessive bruising, an erratic heartbeat, short-term memory loss, gynecological problems, sensitivity to light and sounds, and brain fog. Even writing an email can be hard, she told me.[2]

This laundry list of symptoms was telling, though not for the reasons Young realized. "Hand tremors," "sensitivity to light and sounds," "bulging veins," undefined "gynecological problems," and the inevitable "brain fog"—all these were symptoms of something.

How they fit with a respiratory illness that did its most serious damage to the old and morbidly obese was another question.

I will admit to a cynicism about long Covid even greater than my skepticism about masks, the value of lockdowns, or almost anything else coronavirus-related.

In 2008, I wrote a piece for the *New York Times* headlined "Drug Approved. Is Disease Real?" about fibromyalgia, a difficult-to-define chronic pain disorder that afflicts millions of Americans, mostly middle-aged women. The article began,

> Fibromyalgia is a real disease. Or so says Pfizer in a new television advertising campaign for Lyrica, the first medicine approved to treat the pain condition....
>
> [But some doctors,] including the one who wrote the 1990 paper that defined fibromyalgia but who has since changed his mind, say that the disease does not exist....
>
> The diagnosis of fibromyalgia itself worsens the condition by encouraging people to think of themselves as sick and catalog their pain, said Dr. Nortin Hadler, a rheumatologist and professor of medicine at the University of North Carolina who has written extensively about fibromyalgia.
>
> "These people live under a cloud," he said. "And the more they seem to be around the medical establishment, the sicker they get."

I talked to Hadler long enough to see he had real sympathy for fibromyalgia sufferers. He just didn't think they had an illness that could be treated with pain medicine.

Efforts to define fibromyalgia either clinically or biologically have largely failed. For years, the diagnostic criteria included "tender points." If people felt pain in at least eleven of eighteen separate spots, they were said to have fibromyalgia. Even that incredibly vague rule proved too restrictive. Now the diagnosis of fibromyalgia is based simply on having widespread pain for months.

Pain is fibromyalgia. Fibromyalgia is pain. What was a symptom has become an illness.

In late 2005, I threw out my back so badly I could not walk for weeks. When I tried to, I suffered sciatic nerve pain that made me feel like my left leg was on fire. At one point I found myself sitting on the ground on a sidewalk in Times Square, with the traffic rushing by me, thinking, *I can't stand up, if I can't get myself into a cab I'm going to have to call an ambulance.*

I got myself into a cab.

Back pain is notoriously hard to diagnose or treat. Some people whose radiological scans look terrible have little pain. Others with mostly normal scans are miserable. Surgery helps some people, not others. Even the best surgeons do not know in advance who will benefit.

I opted for conservative management and physical therapy. After a few weeks the pain faded. But over the next fifteen years it came and went—and came back, sometimes for months. I viewed the problem as mostly my own fault. (My wife agreed.) I hadn't taken proper care of myself. Though I exercised moderately and even ran a marathon in 2013, I didn't do the right core strengthening or stretching. I sat at desks and in coffee shops for too long. I spent too much time bending my neck staring at screens.

I treated my body badly. It returned the favor.

All of which is to say that I understand the intersection of modern life and pain first-hand. Sometimes I had to take lots of ibuprofen—lots as in 16 pills, 3200 milligrams, the maximum allowed daily dose—for months. But I always avoided opiates and drugs such as Valium (which was a muscle relaxant before it was an anti-anxiety drug). I wasn't morally opposed. I simply feared those pills would take as much they gave. Or more.

Maybe most important, I avoided medicalizing the condition, even though I could have. I never thought of myself as sick or disabled, just as an idiot with a bad back.

In a 1978 essay called "Illness as Metaphor," Susan Sontag famously wrote, "Everyone who is born holds dual citizenship, in the kingdom of the well and in the kingdom of the sick. Although we all prefer to use only the good passport, sooner or later each of us is obliged, at least for a spell, to identify ourselves as citizens of that other place."

Published just before the crisis of AIDS—another illness that stood out as a social signifier—Sontag's essay was especially timely.

Yet today her vision seems almost backwards. *We all prefer to use only the good passport.* Really?

The number of novel poorly defined illnesses, diseases, and syndromes has swollen enormously since Sontag's essay. An incomplete list would include irritable bowel syndrome, reactive airway disease (coughing), restless leg syndrome, chronic Lyme disease, and of course the granddaddy of 'em all, chronic fatigue syndrome, which also goes by the far more frightening name myalgic encephalomyelitis.

Some of these grew up adjacent to actual diseases. Chronic fatigue emerged after AIDS, for example. Irritable bowel is a cousin of celiac disease and ulcerative colitis, two sometimes disabling illnesses. Drug companies appear to have invented others more or less out of whole cloth, such as restless leg syndrome.

In general, these syndromes lack defined biological underpinnings, unlike more traditional diseases. Cancer can be defined as the growth of abnormal cells that if unchecked will destroy normal tissue. Coronary artery disease occurs when blood vessels feeding the heart are blocked. AIDS comes when HIV destroys the body's T-cells.

These and many other traditional illnesses have standard and reproducible biological markers as well as clinical signs. T-cell counts are a standard measure to determine the progress of HIV infection. Cancer cells come in different types that pathologists can easily distinguish. Cancer is typically "staged," with ranges from a single tumor location (stage 1) to widespread disease that has spread to multiple organs (stage 4).

The new diseases generally lack those biological indicators—or even basic causes. Despite decades of diligent and expensively funded research, no one has ever found a cause for chronic fatigue syndrome, for example. Contrast that with AIDS, whose root viral cause was found barely two years after physicians first saw patients with the illness.

The new diseases have other commonalities, though.

Their symptoms are generally self-reported, such as pain. Thus they are impossible to prove true or false in an objective way. Their incidence waxes and wanes with broader societal trends. They come with high rates of disability. They have generated vocal support groups of sufferers insisting they are real. And they have physician advocates, many of whom treat them "off-label"—with medicines that have never been shown to work in clinical trials against these diseases.

For example, physicians who have made a business treating chronic Lyme disease regularly prescribe long-term courses of antibiotics, despite a lack of evidence.[3] As the Centers for Disease Control explains, federal studies have shown that "long-term outcomes are no better for patients who received additional prolonged antibiotic treatment than for patients who received placebo. Long-term antibiotic treatment for Lyme disease has been associated with serious, sometimes deadly complications."[4]

At a time when we can model the structure of an individual viral particle, have mapped the entire human genome, and even unlocked many of cancer's secrets, these new diseases are stubbornly unknowable. They exist without cause, course, or cure. They are nothing more or less than their self-reported symptoms. They are metaphor as illness. From the first, long Covid fit perfectly among them.

While men were more likely to become severely ill from the coronavirus than women, and older people were far more likely than the young, long Covid had exactly the reverse profile. Its sufferers were disproportionately young to middle-aged women, often with pre-existing diagnoses of depression or anxiety.

Not surprisingly, the constellation of symptoms for long Covid is both diffuse and heavy on psychiatric or quasi-psychiatric conditions. In September 2020, a British group of lawmakers identified sixteen:

1. Exhaustion
2. Vomiting
3. Diarrhoea
4. High temperature
5. Hair loss
6. Chest pain
7. Hallucinations
8. Lasting breathing problems
9. Purple toes
10. Chills
11. Disorientation
12. Muscle/body ache
13. Insomnia
14. Arrhythmia (a problem with the rate of rhythm of the heartbeat)
15. Tachycardia (where the heart beats more than 100 times per minute)
16. Cognitive problems—memory loss, confusion[5]

It was not entirely clear why the coronavirus might cause "hallucinations" or "hair loss." But the lack of biological plausibility didn't seem to matter to Ed Yong or the other reporters writing story after story about long Covid.

Similarly, a March 2021 study of patients in California found: "Women were more likely to become long haulers....Presenting symptoms included palpitations, chronic rhinitis [stuffy nose], dysgeusia [loss of taste], chills, insomnia, hyperhidrosis [sweating], anxiety, sore throat, and headache among others."[6]

In response, I tweeted:

Today on World's Greatest Medical Mysteries:
    Is it the meat sweats...or long Covid?
    Your coworker's cologne...or long Covid?
    An old mattress...or long Covid?
    Your husband's unwillingness to take out the garbage when you tell him...or long Covid?
    Tune in tonight!

Tweets like these were the reason people hated me (and liked me). But I couldn't help myself. I found the claim that sweating might be a long-term symptom of a serious respiratory illness to be idiotic.

To be clear, Covid patients who require intensive care or ventilators often need months to recover. People who need mechanical breathing devices to survive rarely return to normal overnight. That's true whether they were ventilated because of Covid or influenza or even car accidents.

But the severity of self-reported long Covid symptoms has little to do with the severity of the initial illness. Most sufferers have never been hospitalized.

Many had never tested positive for Covid at all.

"People who fell ill in March are still suffering with life-limiting symptoms," *Wired* magazine reported in September 2020. "Many never received positive Covid-19 tests...."[7]

Saying that many long Covid patients had "never received positive Covid-19 tests" wasn't quite accurate. It implied some patients simply hadn't been tested.

In reality, many patients had tested *negative*.

In a May 2020 survey of self-reported long Covid patients, only 23 percent had ever had a positive Covid test. Forty-nine percent had not been tested, and the remaining 28 percent had had a negative test.

Yes, even when long Covid was only months old, its sufferers were insisting on personal experience over biological credibility. They knew better than anyone what kind of disease they had.

Still more oddly, some long-haulers reported problems that had begun before they could plausibly have gotten Covid. In September 2020, a Yahoo News editor offered his tale of woe:

> How did this "Dante's-Inferno"-like journey start? . . .
>
> After returning home to the U.K. from a long weekend in Reykjavik, I ended up in the emergency room for lung and heart pain....I asked if it could be the coronavirus; the doctor didn't even know what I was talking about. After several hours, I was sent home. My diagnosis? A viral chest infection and pericarditis—inflammation of the lining around the heart.

The doctor "didn't even know" about the coronavirus because this emergency room visit came in *January 2020*—at a time when Sars-Cov-2 was rare outside China. Two months later, when the editor had "fever, nausea, vomiting, dehydration and chills so bad that I was shaking," he was given a coronavirus test.

It was negative.

Finally, in April, he tested positive.[8]

If you're having a problem following this timeline, no wonder. It is incomprehensible. If anything, it suggests the opposite of "long Covid." The symptoms began months before his coronavirus diagnosis.

Naturally, the most common self-reported symptom of long Covid is fatigue.[9] Which affects approximately all Americans approximately all the time.

I am barely exaggerating. A 2017 survey from the National Safety Council found that 97 percent of American workers reported at least one risk factor for fatigue, such as working more than 50 hours a week. Forty-three percent said they did not get enough sleep.[10]

With symptoms this vague and common—and no requirement for a positive test—*anyone* can self-define as a long-hauler. That's no exaggeration.

The Yahoo editor is just one person, but similar examples of shoddy reasoning pervaded long Covid coronavirus research—and the reporting on it.

In October 2020, for example, British researchers examined brain function in eighty-four thousand people and found a decrease in IQ in those who had had Covid. "COVID-19 infection likely has consequences for cognitive function that persist," the researchers wrote.[11]

In reporting the study, media outlets offered panicked takes. "Coronavirus could age the brain by 10 years or cause IQ to fall," the *Times* of London warned.[12]

Those headlines didn't explain that the researchers had divided the patients into five groups, ranging from those who had shown no symptoms to those who required ventilator support. Not surprisingly, the ventilated patients showed a sharp mental decline, losing the equivalent of 8.5 IQ points.

But only *sixty* of the eighty-four thousand respondents had been on ventilators.

In contrast, the 9,000 people who said they were ill without respiratory symptoms showed a decrease of less than one point—change that is nearly impossible to measure even with sophisticated testing and for all practical purposes makes no difference. The 3,600 people who said they had respiratory symptoms showed a decrease of less than two points, whether or not they received medical assistance.

If anything, the overall findings should have *reassured* people who feared that Covid might damage their intellectual abilities long-term. Its message was not: Covid is bad for your brain. It was: being put on a ventilator is bad for your brain.

But an honest portrayal of that finding would have been far less likely to drive clicks.

■   ■   ■

Now we have reached the next stage of long Covid, its full medicalization. Clinics are springing up to treat long haulers, the federal government is pouring money into research, and interest groups are demanding even more.

In February 2021, the National Institutes of Health announced a $1.15 billion grant program to examine long Covid—now given the name of "post-acute sequelae of SARS-CoV-2 infection, or PASC."[13] (A Latin-flavored disease name is a crucial first step in the medicalization process. An acronym helps too.)

Within months, the American Medical Association called for still more spending. "More resources needed to help millions living with 'long COVID,'" the AMA's website proclaimed.

The AMA also demanded "an ICD-10 code or family of codes to recognize Post-Acute Sequelae of SARS-CoV-2 infection"[14]—codes that would make billing insurance companies easier.

Long-hauler groups multiplied too.

Among them was "Survivor Corps," which as of summer 2021 claimed more than a hundred thousand members. Its goal: "mobilizing COVID-19 Survivors to support all medical, scientific and academic research to help stem the tide of this pandemic."[15]

Its founder, Diana Berrent, advocated for increased funding for long Covid research, treatment, and disability payments. In July 2021, Berrent told a Florida television station, "Our members are getting denied disability every day and this is a recognition of the wrap-around services that we are going to need to provide to **all survivors** of COVID. . ." [emphasis added].[16]

What Berrent didn't disclose was that she was a longtime Democratic operative tied to the Clintons.

"I spent my entire adult life working for Bill Clinton," she had told the *New York Times* in 2004.[17] She spent 2016 campaigning for Hillary Clinton, working as a member of Hillary's "National Advance Staff," according to her LinkedIn page.

Further, Survivor Corps received money from a San Francisco non-profit group called "Multiplier." Formerly called the Trust for Conservation Innovation, Multiplier is focused on sustainable development initiatives such as "low environmental impact infrastructure systems."[18]

Multiplier's interest in long Covid might have seemed odd at first.

But it fit perfectly with the left's desire to use Covid to remake society, with more government intervention in the economy and medical care. Even if Covid itself vanished, long Covid could last forever. It offered an opportunity to open disability payments to millions of new recipients.

Fauci himself had lifted the veil on this sort of thinking in an August 2020 paper. He and a co-author wrote in the journal *Cell* that international travel and other "living improvements achieved over recent centuries come at a high cost that we pay in deadly disease emergencies." (Despite the "deadly disease emergencies," those "living improvements" had nearly doubled human lifespans and helped nearly eradicate many infectious diseases, a fact Fauci somehow omitted.)

The paper ended with an exhortation:

> Our human activities represent aggressive, damaging, and unbalanced interactions with nature [and] we will increasingly provoke new disease emergencies....
>
> [Covid] should force us to begin thinking in earnest and collectively about living in more thoughtful and creative harmony with nature.[19]

Fauci left vague exactly what he had in mind. Presumably it didn't include *more* economic growth.

Treating long Covid was a growth industry, though.

A physician in Maryland told the *New Republic* magazine he had a waiting list of up to nine months. But then his screening process was not exactly strict: "He does not require patients to present a positive Covid test.... He will see anyone who continues to experience chronic fatigue, elevated heart rate, or 'disabling symptoms' more than three months after a Covid infection."

The *New Republic* fully supported this nonexistent standard, complaining that other clinics "said they continue to require a positive Covid test to receive care for long-haul symptoms."[20]

These new clinics spared no expense to care for their patients. *Scientific American* reported that a University of North Carolina clinic offered first-time patients "an exhaustive medical workup by a variety of specialists [and] a rehabilitation physician, an internist, a psychiatrist, a neuropsychologist, a physical therapist and an occupational therapist cycled through each patient's exam room to assess their condition."

This level of care was equivalent to an expensive concierge medicine service. *Scientific American* left the question of who might be paying for it delicately unanswered. (The North Carolina clinic required a positive test, at least.)

The article noted that "physicians are feeling their way through treatment protocols," before noting that "neurological stimulants such as Adderall, Dexedrine and Ritalin have proved effective at improving energy and focus."[21]

Neurological stimulants? Adderall and Dexedrine are amphetamines, plain and simple. Ritalin is a close chemical cousin. Amphetamine, a.k.a. speed, has "proved effective at improving energy and focus" at least since soldiers on all sides received it in World War II. (Which is presumably where it got the nickname.)

Of course, amphetamines are also addictive and can cause extreme weight loss and psychosis after long-term use.[22] They have also been shown to damage immune responses in animals. In one study, influenza-infected mice were more likely to die if they received amphetamines.[23]

Which might make amphetamines an odd treatment option for people who supposedly have a chronic post-respiratory illness—like, say, long Covid.

But for physicians who want to make patients who are feeling vaguely lousy feel better fast, amphetamines work great. As *The Onion* said in 1998, "Report: Aspirin Taken Daily with Bottle of Bourbon Reduces Awareness of Heart Attacks."[24]

The Onion, of course, is satire. *Scientific American* doesn't mean to be.

26

Herd Immunity

Day after day, week after week, the emails flooded in.

During summer 2020, many centered on schools. Would they open in the fall for in-person learning? Could parents do anything?

Masks were another big topic, especially after I pointed out in August the delay in publishing the Danish study on whether masks protected their wearers. (You may recall that the study's authors had a hard time finding a journal to publish it, because it showed masks didn't work.) People wanted evidence to help them fight mask mandates.

Others lamented lost jobs, or being unable to see their elderly parents, or the welter of strange rules that made interstate travel difficult.

Whatever their nominal topic, the emails had something deeper in common: a feeling of profound dislocation. Many, if not most, of my readers were conservatives. But others were self-described independents or Democrats. These were not conspiracy theorists. Many were professionals with advanced degrees. A surprising number were physicians.

They wrote of their sorrow and anger at realizing for the first time that they could not trust the *New York Times* and other elite media outlets to report the truth—a feeling I understood all too well. Some went further, expressing their fears that the United States would not recover easily from the hysteria. In September one doctor emailed:

> I wish I could say that my physician and scientist friends and colleagues are seeing through covid—but they are not. They have literally lost their minds....
>
> As an example, physician friends with whom we vacation want to cancel vacation because of covid fears. Specifically, they are concerned about their teenage children, one of whom...tested positive and recovered promptly. When I pointed out that, in that case, there was truly no concern as the teenager had already had covid and therefore was immune—they replied that there was now documentation of second infections....
>
> My colleagues and friends are not outliers—this is a real mass hysteria.

Like so many people who wrote me, this physician simply could not understand the media's insistence on portraying the pandemic as a modern plague.

My Twitter feed became a community of sorts for skeptics, reminding them they were not alone or insane. It was an island of cool-headed—maybe sometimes *too* cool-headed, maybe sometimes cold-blooded—reality in an ocean of hysteria.

I wish I could say that Twitter had a similar effect on my marriage. My wife's frustration grew as I became a more public figure, my appearances on Fox rising to multiple times a week.

Her feelings had nothing to do with any fear of Covid. She also believed we had overreacted. She had gotten Covid in the spring while running her hospital's Covid unit for psychiatric patients. She had a positive PCR test to prove it. She had recovered within two days. She said she might not have even known she was infected if she had not briefly lost her senses of smell and taste.

So she understood first-hand that Covid presented few risks to most healthy people. But she felt my tone on Twitter was counterproductive. I wasn't a physician or scientist. I should debate humbly and with an understanding of what I didn't know, she said. Instead, I acted arrogantly and alienated potential allies.

I tried to explain I felt I needed to be aggressive to be heard. She didn't understand how superheated the politics around Covid had become, I said. Even basic facts had taken a backseat to the anger at Donald Trump.

She told me I was just making excuses, that I preferred fighting and snark to civil discussions that might change minds.

The flak she received from her hospital colleagues didn't help. Many despised me, even in those pre-vaccine days. They claimed my stance on masks was a public health threat. Even if masks helped only a little, why not encourage people to use them?

The administration at her hospital had made clear they viewed me as a liability to her and her career. Right or wrong, I had taken a controversial stance on a public health issue. And people knew we were married. She shared my last name. Early on, I retweeted something she had written, a major mistake.

Worst of all, even when I was right, the tweeting was a constant distraction, she said.

I told her Twitter had amplified my reporting in a way nothing else could have. Almost by itself, it had turned me into one of the leading voices against lockdowns and masks. People around the world followed my feed. And I knew how to use it. I avoided wasting time on long individual arguments with random people.

Jackie was unconvinced. She pointed out that I tweeted dozens of times a day, several hundred times a month. How long did each tweet take? Anywhere from a few seconds to a few minutes. Three to five minutes on average? The math was stark. I spent a minimum of one to two hours tweeting every day, and more reading other people's threads and responses to my tweets.

When she married me, I'd been a journalist, a reporter for the *New York Times*. I still *was* a journalist, as far as I was concerned. Jackie said I had become something more and less at the same time. People knew my name, but that didn't mean they liked me. I overestimated my influence and my ability to change policies.

This critique would have stung me more, except that *no one*—not even the president of the United States—seemed able to turn us off the course we had set in March.

For a few weeks in late summer and early fall, we seemed to be moving toward more rational policies, despite the complaints of lockdown advocates such as Andy Slavitt. In August, Dr. Scott Atlas, a Stanford University radiologist, had joined Trump's coronavirus task force. Overnight, Atlas became Trump's closest Covid medical adviser.

Atlas came from outside the public health and infectious disease establishment. He was skeptical about the value of lockdowns and other aggressive measures. He also had a deep understanding of the science and data around Covid, and his medical credentials made him difficult to dismiss. He argued aggressively, both inside the administration and in public appearances, for reducing restrictions.

"The impact of prolonging the lockdown is worse than the impact of the disease," Atlas said in an interview with the BBC Radio Newshour on September 4. "What I'm advocating is using logic and rational reasoning to understand the harms of locking down."[1]

Atlas faced immediate pushback from Fauci and other public health grandees, who weren't used to facing challenges from physicians inside the government. "New Trump Pandemic Adviser Pushes Controversial 'Herd Immunity' Strategy, Worrying Public Health Officials," the *Washington Post* reported on August 30, just weeks after he started.[2]

As the *Post* headline explained, Atlas's rise became inextricably linked to the debate over "herd immunity."

Herd immunity is the point at which so many people become immune to Sars-Cov-2 (or any pathogen) that although the germ or virus can continue to infect individuals, it cannot cause widespread outbreaks. The pool of vulnerable people is just too small. Even if individual cases or minor clusters of infection occur, they will fade away on their own.

The exact percentage of people who must be immune before herd immunity is reached depends on how contagious a pathogen is. The more contagious, the more people must be immune. For an easily spreadable illness such as measles, more than 90 percent of people must be protected before herd immunity can exist.

People can gain immunity in one of two ways—either natural recovery from an infection, or inoculation with an effective vaccine.

As the World Health Organization explains: "'Herd immunity,' also known as 'population immunity,' is the indirect protection from an infectious disease that happens when a population is immune either through vaccination or immunity developed through previous infection."[3]

But no vaccines were available for the coronavirus in the summer of 2020. In their absence, the only way to generate herd immunity would be to allow enough people to be infected with the virus and recover.

In its purest form, herd immunity is a strategy both simple and radical.

I tended to critique lockdowns, masks, and other mitigation efforts because they did not reduce infections. But for true believers in pursuing herd immunity, mitigation efforts were largely pointless *even if they worked*.

In fact, they could be worse than pointless: the better they protected people, the more counterproductive they might actually be in the long run.

Why? Without an effective vaccine, the coronavirus—or any virus—will infect people until it runs out of people to infect. If our mitigation measures slow the rate of infection, we simply drag out the process.

Thus we should try to slow the spread of the virus only to the extent that we allow our health care system to handle the burden of sick people when infections peak. (In other words, we should try to "flatten the curve," nothing more.)

Of course, whether such a strategy is societally acceptable depends on the objective fact of how dangerous a virus is—*and* on our subjective tolerance for those deaths. To take an obvious example, the United States would never tolerate allowing the unchecked spread of a virus like smallpox, which could kill up to 100 million Americans before it burned out.

What about a virus that killed two to three out of every thousand people it infected, or up to one million Americans? The answer might depend on whether the dead were children or the extremely elderly—as well as how the media presented those deaths.

In a rational world, a serious debate about herd immunity would have been worth having. But in the United States in 2020, reporters and the public health establishment would not tolerate one.

"Coronavirus 'Herd Immunity' Is Just Another Way to Say 'Let People Die,'" the *Los Angeles Times* opined in September, above a picture of Scott Atlas. "There's so much we don't know about the new coronavirus that a laissez faire approach is unacceptably reckless."[4] The liberal website Vox would later call herd immunity "the worst idea of 2020."[5]

The blowback was so intense that on September 4 Atlas denied to NPR ever having suggested to Trump that herd immunity might be a viable strategy—though he had clearly danced around the idea before joining Trump's team.[6]

By late September, the public health establishment had sharpened its knives.

On September 28, Robert Redfield, the head of the Centers for Disease Control, was overheard on a phone call on a flight to Washington saying about Atlas, "Everything he says is false." He complained Atlas was misleading Trump about herd immunity.

After the flight, Redfield confirmed that he had been talking about Atlas[7]—something he obviously did not have to do, raising the question of whether he had made the call expecting to be overheard, so that he could bash Atlas without criticizing him officially.

On the same day, Fauci attacked Atlas on CNN. Most public health experts "are working together," he said. "I think you know who the outlier is.... You know my differences with Dr. Atlas, I'm always willing to sit down and talk with him and see if we could resolve those differences."[8]

Fauci complained Atlas was giving Trump information that was "really taken either out of context or actually incorrect."[9]

Yet with coronavirus cases and deaths falling nearly in half in the United States from late July to late September, Trump and Atlas seemed to have a window to reset the narrative and argue that the coronavirus was a manageable health problem rather than a singular national crisis.

On September 25, Florida governor Ron DeSantis removed all restrictions on businesses in his state, allowing bars and restaurants to operate at full capacity. His order also banned Florida cities or counties from enforcing mask mandates against individuals.[10]

Two months before, DeSantis had ordered Florida's schools to open for full-time instruction in the fall even if local school boards did not want to do so.[11] The September order cemented DeSantis's stance as the leader of the red-state governors pressing for a return to normal, an increasingly popular stance among Republicans.

On the same day he criticized Atlas, Fauci complained about Florida's reopening. "That is very concerning to me," he told *Good Morning America*. "You're really asking for trouble."[12]

DeSantis shrugged off the complaints and moved ahead.

A week later, the publication of an anti-lockdown manifesto called the Great Barrington Declaration grabbed attention.[13] Co-authored by epidemiologists from Stanford, Harvard, and Oxford, it declared, "Coming from both the left and right, and around the world, we have devoted our careers to protecting people. Current lockdown policies are producing devastating effects."

The declaration did not *quite* call for a full-bore herd immunity strategy, although it did argue (correctly) that sooner or later the world would reach herd immunity in any case: "We know that all populations will eventually reach herd immunity—i.e. the point at which the rate of new infections is stable—and that this can be assisted by (but is not dependent upon) a vaccine. Our goal should therefore be to minimize mortality and social harm until we reach herd immunity."

Instead of a completely unfettered reopening, the declaration called for "Focused Protection," reopening schools and universities and allowing societies to return to normal while trying to save those most at risk. The declaration didn't have many specific details on how to accomplish this goal, as critics noted. It was more a statement of goals than a bureaucratic memo.

The declaration drew immediate attention. "Epidemiologists Stray from the Covid Herd," the *Wall Street Journal* headlined an interview with two of the authors later in October.[14]

The public health establishment counterattacked, calling the declaration simply an effort to rebrand herd immunity. "The official medical term for the herd immunity approach is 'let 'em sicken and die.' I believe they teach it in Evil Doctor School," Dr. Esther Choo, a CNN regular, tweeted.

Gregg Gonsalves, the same Yale epidemiologist who seven months before had called Covid a chance to remake society, complained, "This fucking Great Barrington Declaration is like a bad rash that won't go away."[15]

On October 15, Fauci took direct aim at the declaration, saying its essential plan was, "'Let everybody get infected that's going to be able to get infected and then we'll have herd immunity.' Quite frankly that is nonsense and anybody who knows anything about epidemiology will tell you that is nonsense and very dangerous."[16]

Quite frankly that is nonsense.

The refusal even to discuss herd immunity captured Fauci's arrogance in a nutshell. Though he could act friendly to interviewers who were properly submissive, he grew haughty and dismissive when challenged. "Quite frankly" became his go-to phrase. "Quite frankly, the attacks on me are attacks on science," he would say in June 2021.[17] Weeks later he would tell Senator Rand Paul, "Senator Paul, you do not know what you are talking about, quite frankly."[18]

Defenders of the lockdowns also complained that the declaration had been written at the American Institute for Economic Research, a conservative think tank, as if that fact meant its points should be ignored. But the authors took no money from the institute, whose involvement was largely limited to hosting the meeting and the gbdeclaration.org website.

"The AIER kindly provided the location for the meeting," Dr. Jay Bhattacharya explained in an email to me in August 2021. "They did not pay me anything to write it. They offered me a small honorarium for coming to the meeting that I turned down. I have taken no personal money for any of my COVID-related activities during the epidemic, and I believe the same is true for [the other authors]."

Almost a million people signed the Great Barrington Declaration after it was released. The number might have been even higher, but technology companies appeared initially to censor the declaration. In much of the world, searching for the declaration on Google returned results denouncing it, while burying links to it.[19] Moderators on the biggest Reddit message boards about the coronavirus refused to allow users to post it.[20]

Still, the declaration helped open the debate around herd immunity by providing some academic cover to lockdown skeptics.

It might have done even more.

But two days before it was released, President Trump had become the world's most famous Covid patient.

27

Trump

Perhaps it was inevitable that President Trump would be infected with Sars-Cov-2, despite the protections the Secret Service tried to provide him.

Those protections were never as airtight as they seemed from the outside, as I knew first-hand.

I had visited the White House in September 2020 to talk to National Security Adviser Robert O'Brien—one of the Trump administration's unquestioned grown-ups. It was the first time I had been inside since I'd taken a tour as a kid in 1981, before the assassination attempt on Ronald Reagan started the process of turning the people's house into an armed fortress.

I came to Washington to see O'Brien because I was fishing for information about the origins of the virus. He was polite and cordial and didn't give me anything classified.

Still, I was somewhat surprised I wasn't required to take a coronavirus test to enter the grounds. I also didn't have to wear a mask once I was inside the White House itself. I knew O'Brien had already recovered from Sars-Cov-2 and was immune. But what about his aides?

People who met Trump personally were required to be tested. But even very reliable tests couldn't catch every infection as soon as it happened. Had I been infected at the time, I could have passed the virus on to someone who could have given it Trump.

In any case, as the presidential campaign heated up, Trump clearly became less worried about contracting Covid. Whatever his history as a germophobe,[1] he knew that large rallies energized his base and provided a contrast with the man he called "Sleepy Joe" Biden, who spent most of his time sequestered at home.

At one early Trump rally, in Tulsa, Oklahoma, Herman Cain apparently contracted Sars-Cov-2. Cain died of Covid on July 30 in Atlanta, at age seventy-four.[2] Almost two years after the epidemic began, Cain remains probably the most prominent public figure to die of Covid—a striking fact, given that he was hardly a household name outside of Republican political circles.

Cain's death prompted a wave of articles about Trump's callousness. "Will Herman Cain's Death Change Republican Views on the Virus and Masks?" the *New York Times* asked solemnly.[3] A writer for an Illinois newspaper owned by the national chain Gannett went further, claiming that "in a just world, Donald Trump would be tried and convicted of involuntary manslaughter in connection with the death of Herman Cain."[4]

Not surprisingly, the criticism did not change Trump's plans. He held large rallies in the South and Southwest in August and September.[5]

But Trump was almost certainly infected at a smaller event. On Sunday, September 27, he announced at the White House that he would nominate Amy Coney Barrett for the Supreme Court. The event was held outside, but more than a hundred people were present. Several attendees, including Chris Christie and Kellyanne Conway, soon tested positive for the coronavirus.[6]

Rumors that Trump might be infected began on Thursday, October 1, after his aide Hope Hicks tested positive.[7] Just after midnight on Friday, Trump announced he and his wife Melania had been infected—in a tweet, inevitably:

> Tonight, FLOTUS and I tested positive for COVID-19. We will begin our quarantine and recovery process immediately. We will get through this TOGETHER![8]

Trump's infection immediately became the world's top story.

The only other major national leader known to have had a serious case of Covid was Boris Johnson, the British prime minister. In early April 2020, Johnson was hospitalized. He needed three nights of intensive care and supplemental oxygen. He said afterwards that his physicians had seriously considered putting him on a ventilator, a move he had resisted.[9]

Johnson was fifty-five at the time of his infection. Trump was seventy-four and significantly overweight. Trump's age and obesity placed him at a real risk of dying from Covid, perhaps as high as 3 percent. The fact that his symptoms had developed so quickly was another worrisome sign.

Friday afternoon, October 2, not even eighteen hours after the initial announcement, Trump shuffled across the White House lawn to a waiting helicopter, which carried him to Walter Reed National Military Medical Center.

At this point, many major media outlets could barely contain their excitement—an ugly word, but it accurately describes the tenor of the coverage. Discussions of the Twenty-Fifth Amendment, which governs succession if a president is incapacitated, began almost immediately.

"Here's what happens if Trump gets too sick to govern," a CNN commentator wrote.[10] The *Washington Post* and other outlets ran similar pieces.

The frenzy peaked on Saturday, when Trump's physicians acknowledged he had received supplemental oxygen on Friday after his oxygen levels fell below 95 percent. Dr. Sean Conley, Trump's personal physician, said he had not had a fever since Friday morning and had only a mild cough and fatigue.[11]

"The president this morning is not on oxygen, not having difficulty breathing or walking around," said Dr. Sean Dooley, a pulmonologist who was also treating Trump. "He's in exceptionally good spirits."

But Mark Meadows, Trump's chief of staff, undercut these optimistic assessments. In a separate briefing, Meadows told reporters that Trump's vital signs "over the last 24 hours were very concerning and the next 48 hours will be critical in terms of his care."[12]

Further, despite their optimism, Trump's physicians acknowledged that he was receiving aggressive care. His treatments included remdesivir, the drug that Fauci had lauded months earlier. He also had been given monoclonal antibodies, which regulators had not yet approved, from the drug company Regeneron.[13] The fact that Trump's doctors were using those treatments led reporters and some physicians to speculate his illness was more severe than the White House would admit.

"Doctors say giving Trump the antiviral drug remdesivir is a sign his infection may be serious," Business Insider reported on Saturday afternoon.

■   ■   ■

Barely forty-eight hours later, Trump was back in the White House. The president and his physicians had been right. The naysayers, including Meadows, had been wrong. As National Public Radio reported,

President Trump walked out of Walter Reed National Military Medical Center on Monday evening, planning on receiving the remainder of his treatment for COVID-19 at the White House.

He was seen pumping his fist in the air on the way out of the building.... Upon arriving back at the White House, Trump walked up the staircase of the South Portico entrance, removed his mask, gave reporters standing below a thumbs-up and saluted Marine One.[14]

Trump's critics tried to give the credit for his rapid turnaround to his aggressive care.

"Most Patients' Covid-19 Care Looks Nothing Like Trump's," the *New York Times* huffed the day after Trump returned to the White House.[15] "Ethicists say Trump special treatment raises fairness issues," the Associated Press complained,[16] as if anyone would not expect the president of the United States to receive the best possible care. The monoclonal antibodies received particular scrutiny, though regulators authorized their use for everyone about six weeks later.

In reality, even with minimal care, Trump would probably have recovered fairly easily. Even at Trump's age, most people infected with Sars-Cov-2 did not require hospitalization. People in their eighties and nineties were at much higher risk.

And though Trump was overweight, he had always been physically robust, an avid golfer capable of long stretches of campaigning. If we had learned anything during the first months of the epidemic, it was that Sars-Cov-2 played favorites, ravaging people who were already unhealthy.

Trump returned to health even faster than most patients. By October 12, a week after leaving Walter Reed, he had repeatedly tested negative for Sars-Cov-2, meaning he no longer needed to isolate and could resume campaigning.[17]

No matter. By then the media and public health experts had already found a new narrative around Trump's illness.

Naturally, it was negative. Trump and his political allies had been irresponsible by not wearing masks at the Amy Coney Barrett event. Trump had risked his own life and the lives of White House staff. He had not treated Sars-Cov-2 with the proper respect.

"We had a super-spreader event in the White House and it was in a situation where people were crowded together and were not wearing masks," Fauci told CBS News on Friday, October 9. "So the data speak for themselves."[18]

Indeed, they did.

Trump didn't die of Covid. Melania didn't die. His son Barron didn't die. As far as I can tell, of people who became infected from the Barrett event, only Trump himself and former New Jersey governor Chris Christie were hospitalized.

Christie, who was morbidly obese and asthmatic, also recovered completely, though his hospitalization lasted a week.

■   ■   ■

But even the absence of severe illness in the highest-profile Covid outbreak imaginable did not change the media coverage or public perception of the pandemic.

On October 2, the day Trump was hospitalized, Dr. Mike Ryan of the World Health Organization said he believed 750 million people worldwide had been infected with Sars-Cov-2. Ryan, the executive director of the WHO's Covid response program, made the comment at an internet seminar hosted by the Royal Irish Academy, Ireland's premier scientific organization.[19]

His estimate was stunning. It represented 10 percent of the entire world's population. It was far higher than previous estimates and far higher than the number of positive PCR tests for active infections.

Then again, when antibody tests were conducted, not just in the United States but everywhere, they showed much higher rates of infection and recovery than PCR tests did. The difference was even larger in poor countries, which could not afford to conduct pointless PCR tests of asymptomatic or barely symptomatic people.

For example, a study from late July 2020 found that about 3 million Kenyans, more than 5 percent of the country's population, had antibodies.

At the time, Kenya had reported barely 2,000 Covid cases and 71 deaths.[20] In other words, the PCR tests were catching only 1 out of 1,500 Covid infections.

If Ryan's estimate was correct, it suggested that the virus's infection fatality rate was even lower than had previously been reported. By late October (to allow for a lag between infection and death) governments had reported that about 1.3 million people worldwide had died of Covid, suggesting that the overall death rate worldwide was in the range of 0.15 percent to 0.2 percent.

That rate was still three to four times higher than an average flu strain—but it was only one-twentieth as high as the first estimates out of China, and less than one-fifth as high as the 1 percent figure reporters commonly used.

Put another way, Ryan's estimate suggested that at least 998 out of 1,000 people worldwide who were infected with Covid would survive.

Yet until I tweeted about it, the estimate received no attention at all outside Ireland.

On October 5, as Trump prepared to leave Walter Reed and return to the White House, he tweeted, "Don't be afraid of Covid. Don't let it dominate your life." I found this simple call to action inspiring, especially considering that it came out of Trump's personal experience facing the virus.

"Maybe the smartest comment [Trump] has ever made," I tweeted in response. "For too long we have let this virus—and the media's hysteria around it—dominate us. We need to take back our lives, our schools, and our whole world."

Yet most of the media felt exactly the opposite. The backlash was immediate. "'Don't Be Afraid of Covid,' Trump Says, Undermining Public Health Messages," the *Times* headlined an article about Trump's tweet. "Experts Were Outraged by the President's Comments."

The *Times*'s article began:

> Public health experts had hoped that President Trump, chastened by his own infection with the coronavirus and the cases

that have erupted among his staff, would act decisively to persuade his supporters that wearing masks and social distancing were essential to protecting themselves and their loved ones.

[Instead,] the president yet again downplayed the deadly threat of the virus.[21]

The experts—so quick to be outraged at *any* suggestion that we should try to return our lives to normal, put the virus's death toll in context, or acknowledge that many people infected with Covid might never even know they had it.

Journalists even claimed that Trump's call to be unafraid was hurtful to Americans who had died of Covid—as if calls to beat cancer insulted people who had died of that disease. Apparently the only acceptable way to face Covid was on bended knee, hoping that the dread plague wouldn't take you.

Don't be afraid of Covid. Don't let it dominate your life.

But, after eight months of obsessive death counting and panic pornography, far too many of us were. And it did.

28

A House Divided

I n November 2020, Donald Trump lost unfair and square.

I don't mean Joe Biden or the Illuminati or anyone else stole the election. But the media, Hollywood, academia, and much of corporate America did not want Trump to win re-election and openly worked to defeat him.

The best comparison may be to the 1996 election in post-Communist Russia. Boris Yeltsin, who five years before had helped to overthrow the Soviet regime but was now clearly ailing, faced a strong challenge from Gennady Zyuganov, a Communist.

Fearing Zyuganov might win, the Russian establishment lined up behind Yeltsin and did everything short of actually rigging votes to help him. Michael McFaul, who would later serve as the American ambassador to Russia, wrote in 1997: "Yeltsin grossly violated the campaign finance limits, the media openly propagated Yeltsin's cause, and counting irregularities again appeared in Chechnya and some other national republics...."[1]

And Yeltsin won, ensuring that Russia would not return to Communism. McFaul added, "The historic events of the 1996 presidential election appear to point to true progress in making a Russian democracy."

That assessment proved optimistic. At best.

Yeltsin's worsening alcoholism,[2] along with the *democracy-is-fine-as-long-as-our-guy-wins* attitude of the Russian elite, worsened the raging cynicism of ordinary Russians and paved the way for Vladimir Putin's power grab in 1999. Of course, maybe the situation in Russia would be even worse now if Zyuganov had won in 1996—though it's hard to imagine how.

America's democracy is more firmly rooted than Russia's.

But anyone looking at the last several years must feel alarmed at the trend line. Both Trump and his Democratic opponents violated long-standing democratic norms, although the media focused only on Trump's transgressions—both real and imaginary. The notion that "Russian interference" played a major role in Trump's election in 2016, for example, is absurd. Despite a massive fundraising edge and overtly friendly media, Hillary Clinton simply could not convince enough independent voters to choose her.

And if not for the coronavirus and its economic impact, Trump could have squeaked through again in 2020, repeating his 2016 win by taking a minority of the popular vote but a majority of the Electoral College. That outcome might not have been great for democracy either, but it would have been constitutionally sound. Besides, the rules are the rules, and both parties know them.

Instead, Trump's personal vulgarity and the establishment's thumb on the scale gave Biden the victory. Trump alienated too many suburban women to carry Rust Belt states such as Pennsylvania that had given him the win in 2016.

I didn't vote for either man.

For the first time in my life, I left my ballot blank. Trump had proven himself feckless and unfit for the job, in my view. The Democrats had pressed coronavirus policies that were fundamentally dangerous to personal freedoms. I hated not voting, but after months of deliberating, I couldn't.

Of course, I lived in New York State, so I knew my vote wouldn't matter much anyway. Biden's victory there was a foregone conclusion.

Elsewhere the outcome was not so clear. For much of the 2020 election night, we seemed to be replaying 2016. Trump won Florida, which was supposed to be leaning towards Biden. He won easily in Ohio, a supposed toss-up. Nationally, he ran substantially ahead of the polls, which had shown him nearly ten points behind Biden on the eve of the election.[3] And as the night progressed, he surged ahead in Pennsylvania and Michigan and Wisconsin, the three historically Democratic states that had delivered him the win four years before.

When I went to sleep at 3:00 a.m.—very late, but not quite late enough—Trump appeared to be on his way to an electoral surprise even bigger than his 2016 win.

Within hours, the picture changed dramatically. Heavily Democratic cities such as Milwaukee and Philadelphia began to report results that ran hugely in Biden's favor. Pennsylvania and other states began counting mail-in ballots, also favoring Biden. On Wednesday and Thursday, Biden erased Trump's lead, then pulled ahead. By Friday morning his victory was all but assured. And just before noon on Saturday, November 7, four days after the election, CNN and other networks called the election for him.[4] "Victory for Joe Biden, at Last," read the *New York Times* headline.[5]

It is possible some mail-in ballot fraud occurred. Fraud and mass ballot harvesting are theoretically easier when people are voting at home instead of at centralized polling stations where neutral observers can watch them. In fact, France and many other European countries ban mail-in voting for this reason.[6]

But since Biden defeated Trump, Republicans have not shown widespread election fraud occurred—and not for lack of trying. Further, Trump's loss was *not* due to Biden's posting unusually high margins in heavily Democratic cities. Trump lost badly in Philadelphia and other Democratic bastions, but Republicans always do. The numbers are clear.

Biden won because swing voters in the suburbs, especially women, turned against Trump.[7] No one has suggested those suburbs are particularly vulnerable to vote fraud.

For a couple of days after the election, I tried to investigate the possibility of vote fraud. I interviewed young men in Georgia who had had a strange experience with a volunteer who was apparently trying to cure a spoiled ballot after Election Day. But I rapidly backed off. I simply couldn't see any realistic possibility that fraud had led to Trump's loss.

Worse, I quickly realized that in chasing the phantom of widespread fraud, Republicans were doing massive damage to the anti-lockdown cause.

On Tuesday, November 10, one week after the election, I told Tucker Carlson:

> So as Biden takes office, and I think we all expect he is going to take office in 10 weeks, Republicans are going to really have to raise their voices...if we're not going to have national mask mandates, which is something else that Biden has indicated he wants very aggressively.
>
> And in the weeks between now and January 20th, Republicans are going to have to decide what to do. Are they going to, you know, fight what looks like a losing battle on behalf of Donald Trump? Or are they going to fight for COVID restrictions that are reasonable and that get us moving forward? I guess, I should just say, fight against COVID restrictions, because a lot of us on what I like to call Team Reality are going to be depending on, you know, Republicans at the national and the state level to push back.[8]

My comments reflected the fact that the partisan divide over how to respond to the virus—tiny in the spring—had become a Grand Canyon-sized chasm.

A Gallup poll in September 2020 showed that almost 80 percent of Democrats worried personally about getting the coronavirus. Only about

25 percent of Republicans felt the same. The differences extended to behavior. Fifty-five percent of Democrats but only 24 percent of Republicans said they always socially distanced. Perhaps most shocking, only 4 percent—one in twenty-five—of Democrats said they were "ready to return to normal activities right now." More than half of Republicans were.[9]

The differences were mirrored in policies at the state level. Florida and other Republican-led states were mostly back to normal by fall 2020. But blue states such as New York and Oregon lurched forward and back. They ended broad lockdowns but retained rules that made traveling to other states difficult, along with restrictions on bars, restaurants, theaters, worship services, and other indoor events. Some targeted team sports. Others restricted retailers.

Worse, they routinely changed their opening benchmarks to justify new restrictions. Hospitalizations were the standard that made the most sense, the *only* metric that truly mattered. But as hospitals emptied out, health departments insisted that the number of new "cases"—that is, positive tests—had to fall almost to zero before the restrictions could be lifted.

California went further, telling counties they had to make progress on "health equity" before they could reopen. As NPR explained on October 6, "In order to advance to the next phase of economic reopening, counties like Los Angeles will need to reduce the levels of the virus in their most vulnerable communities."[10]

In other words, a county's businesses and schools might have to stay closed if too many black or Hispanic people had positive tests compared to the number of white residents.

Biden's reluctance to campaign live suggested that his personal fears mirrored the feelings of his strongest supporters, including the teachers' unions fighting to keep schools closed. Now he would be dictating national coronavirus policy. Republicans needed to stand against government overreach, not give Democrats and the media an excuse to tag them as conspiracy theorists who wouldn't accept an election that Trump had lost by millions of votes.

So I believed.

Of course, I could afford to tell the truth.

I was a journalist who prided himself on being politically independent, not a Republican officeholder who would face a primary challenge if he even breathed Trump hadn't won. In the summer of 2021, long after the election fight was lost, I spoke to a group of Republicans in Congress about Covid. *You're not going to get anywhere until you admit Trump lost*, I said. But they mostly wouldn't.

This counterproductive—to say the least—attitude reached its zenith on January 6. My forty-eighth birthday! Yay! I was at the local Honda dealership getting my SUV serviced and lamenting the fact they no longer offered cookies (since Covid, they had eliminated snacks) when the news of the Capitol riot hit.

For a few minutes I assumed the media was hyping the story, looking for another excuse to trash Trump.

No. The riot was real, the tear gas was real, and Trump was disgustingly slow to condemn what was happening. An insurrection? It wasn't an *insurrection*, exactly. I'd seen those first-hand in Iraq when I worked for the *Times*. Insurrections came with mortars and car bombs. It wasn't a coup, either. Did you see any tanks in the streets preventing a peaceful transfer of power? Me neither.

But it was a giant ugly mess, and an awful day for the United States of America, and Trump was responsible. *What did he think was going to happen?* Did he think Congress wasn't going to certify the Electoral College votes? Did he think he wouldn't have to leave the White House in two weeks? Probably not. He's not stupid. He just reveled in causing trouble, as he had so often before—and in giving the 20 or 25 percent of the country that loved him one last show.

But the consequences of Trump's theater of the absurd were devastating.

The riot gave the media and the left the cudgel they had wanted for years. Sure, leftist groups in Portland, Oregon, had aggressively targeted the federal courthouse and other government buildings for months, in riots the media famously wrote off as "mostly peaceful protests."

No matter. The Capitol was uniquely symbolic, and a peaceful national transfer of power uniquely important. Thus its attackers were not merely rioters or criminals, but rebels, even terrorists. *Insurrection* became the word that MSNBC and CNN used to describe the riot.

The shift in language justified social media giants to throttle political dissent. And all dissent is ultimately political. To oppose Covid lockdowns or mask or vaccine mandates—not just masks or vaccines themselves, mask or vaccine *mandates*—was to endanger the public health. It was to blaspheme and risk banishment from the public sphere.

This effort had begun as soon as Covid arrived in the United States, but it accelerated dramatically after January 6. Two days later, Twitter banned Trump's account, which had nearly ninety million followers.[11] The service explained:

> After close review of recent Tweets from the @realDonaldTrump account and the context around them—specifically **how they are being received and interpreted on and off Twitter**—we have permanently suspended the account due to the risk of further incitement of violence. [emphasis added][12]

In other words, Trump was to blame for the way people read his tweets—an interesting take on freedom of speech. But Twitter did not back down, and much of the media cheered its action. "Twitter's Trump Ban Deemed Necessary, Derided as Long Overdue," a Bloomberg headline proclaimed, adding that the suspension "may be too little, too late."[13]

And the ban had an immediate impact—both by preventing Trump from using what had become his favored form of communication and because of its symbolism. A social media application that *had not even existed* fifteen years before had muzzled the most powerful person in the world. He seemed to have no recourse.

Soon enough, I would discover Twitter's power to censor for myself.

29

Here We Go Again

B ut Trump's defeat was not the only big development in the pandemic in November 2020.

A fresh wave of cases accelerated in the United States and worldwide, leading to new lockdowns in Europe and some states. Covid deaths globally, which had ranged from thirty-five to forty thousand a week since the spring (more than one million human beings die each week of all causes), began a steady climb that lasted through January.

As had been the case all year, the epidemic was highly regionalized and seasonalized. In the United States, California, which had escaped the first wave and outperformed the rest of the Sunbelt during the summer spike, was especially hard-hit.

Reporters wrote the usual puzzled stories trying to explain why the state was doing so badly: California had reopened too soon. Its citizens hadn't listened to public health experts and properly masked or socially distanced. They were suffering from "lockdown fatigue."

The stories rarely noted that the state had begun to reimpose stay-at-home rules as early as November 16, when Governor Gavin Newsom said he was "pulling an 'emergency brake,'" with cases rising.[1]

More restrictions followed in December. "California Will Impose Its Strongest Virus Measures since the Spring," the *New York Times* reported on December 3.[2] "Millions of people across Southern and Central California are likely to see outdoor dining shuttered, playgrounds roped off and hair salons closed within days."

Of course. Close restaurant patios and playgrounds, where transmission was non-existent. The public health mandarins—in California and everywhere—were proving beyond a doubt that they had learned nothing from their spring escapades. Sure enough, California's cases and hospitalizations and deaths continued to soar.

The state's experience provided yet more real-world evidence that lockdowns could be imposed in only two possible ways—too early, or too late. Too early, and locking down caused economic carnage, while leaving nearly the entire population vulnerable to viral spread when the restrictions were lifted. Too late, and forcing infected people to stay home with their families risked *accelerating* transmission.

Yet even a year into the epidemic, public health experts and journalists refused to see reality, much less admit it. "California Has Lost Control," *The Atlantic* said on December 21, before offering this brilliant non-explanation for what was happening: "Why California—a state that had been an example of a reasonably effective response—and why now? Some officials have pointed to lockdown fatigue. Thanksgiving alone is not the culprit, as cases were clearly rising in early November. The state's reversal of fortunes is so sharp and sudden that the reasons remain unclear, but its time as a big and relatively bright spot in a dark winter has definitively come to an end."[3]

If the media covered the winter surges in blue states with befuddlement, it treated those in red states far more censoriously.

On December 3, weeks before its report on California, *The Atlantic* (I realize I seem to be picking on *The Atlantic*, but its coronavirus coverage really was this bad, month after miserable month), ran an article headlined "Iowa Is What Happens When Government Does Nothing." It warned, "Public-health experts predict that the state's lax political leadership will result in a 'super peak' over the holidays, and thousands of preventable deaths in the weeks to come. 'We know the storm's coming,' Perencevich [Dr. Eli Perencevich, an Iowa epidemiologist] said. 'You can see it on the horizon.'"

The magazine knew just whom to blame—Kim Reynolds, the state's Republican governor—and just what to do:

> The crisis in Iowa's hospitals could be improved in a matter of weeks if Iowans started wearing a mask whenever they leave the house and stopped spending time indoors with people outside their households....
>
> Reynolds needs to order bars closed and restaurants to move to takeout only, at least until the surge is over, public-health experts told me. Reynolds and other state leaders could frame mask wearing and self-isolation as a matter of patriotic duty.[4]

Otherwise Iowa faced the bleakest of futures.

Or not.

The Atlantic's panic porn was impeccably timed. It came out almost three weeks after coronavirus cases peaked in Iowa and *the very day* that deaths began to drop—based on a weekly average in both cases. Two months later, in February 2020, Iowa Covid deaths had fallen about three-quarters, from 62 a day to 16. Over the same period, deaths in California rose more than 6-fold, from 80 to 510.

Even accounting for California's much larger population, its death rate was three times as high as Iowa's by February. Yet Iowa supposedly had done everything wrong through the winter, California everything right. (In a follow-up article in February 2021, *The Atlantic* would claim, laughably, that "one key reason" its promised apocalypse in Iowa had not come to pass "could be that Iowans drastically changed their behavior just in the nick of time." Sure.)[5]

In reality, the changes probably had nothing to do with the policies either state had followed and everything to do with the fact that the fall wave had started in the Upper Midwest and Plains states before coming to California.

Or, as I sometimes wrote, *Virus gonna virus.*

As positive tests—"cases"—nationwide soared past 100,000 and then 200,000 a day and deaths surpassed the spring daily high of about 2,250 (again, based on the 7-day average), the coverage took on its usual cast.

Coronavirus patients were overrunning hospitals. Well, they weren't *quite* overrunning them, but they were close. "California hospitals at 'brink of catastrophe' as many run out of ICU beds," the Associated Press reported on December 31.[6]

Entire medical systems were desperately short of oxygen. Well, they weren't *exactly* desperately short, but they might be soon. "Oxygen supply issues forced five Los Angeles–area hospitals to declare an 'internal disaster,'" a CNN article warned on December 29—before acknowledging that "generally the problem is not an absolute shortage of oxygen."[7]

States around the country were spending hundreds of millions of dollars on field hospitals to deal with the overrun. Only those temporary centers remained basically deserted week after week. As a Los Angeles television station reported in July 2021, "California spent nearly $200 million to set up, operate and staff alternate care sites that ultimately provided little help. . . . It was a costly way to learn California's hospital system is far more elastic than was thought at the start of the pandemic."[8]

The stories were the same everywhere, in every wave. Hospitals were always *about* to collapse. But they never did. And the field hospitals, which should have provided the most tangible evidence that Covid patients were too great a strain for the system, instead showed the opposite.

Yet neither journalists nor epidemiologists ever learned to adjust their predictions or expectations. Through the fall, they had insistently predicted the horrors of a "twindemic"—a combined Covid and flu season that would devastate hospitals.[9]

The twindemic didn't happen either. Influenza simply disappeared in the 2020–2021 winter. Once again, no one quite knew why.

Pro-maskers claimed that the answer lay in the magic of masks—a bizarre explanation given that Sars-Cov-2 and influenza were transmitted exactly the same way and Covid was still rampant. Conspiracy theorists said the flu was being misdiagnosed as Covid. But that idea didn't hold up either, as the two viruses were easily distinguishable. (In the most conspiratorial version of this theory, Covid didn't exist at all—it had *never even been cultured in a lab*, or some such nonsense. These were the emails I tried not to read.)

A more likely answer seemed to be that Sars-Cov-2 was simply better at infecting people than standard flu strains. As the CDC had said as early as September 2020, "Viral interference might help explain the lack of influenza during a pandemic caused by another respiratory virus that might outcompete influenza in the respiratory tract."[10]

Again, though, when bad-news predictions proved wrong, they were simply forgotten. Some conservatives believed that after Biden's victory, and certainly after his inauguration, the media would pivot quickly to focusing on good news stories about the epidemic. I had my doubts. Nearly a year in, reporters still seemed committed to the narrative—and fixated on death counts.

The governmental response to the fall and winter wave was even harsher—and more confused—in Europe.

France imposed a new national lockdown on October 29, then replaced it with a curfew on December 15. On December 10, the BBC reported, "France will delay the reopening of cultural venues and introduce a night-time curfew as it struggles to curb the spread of Covid-19. [French] Prime Minister Jean Castex said the infection rates **were not** falling as fast as the government had hoped after a lockdown was imposed in late October" [emphasis added].[11]

Surprise, surprise.

Across the channel, England imposed a new national lockdown on November 5, ended it December 2, and then reversed course again weeks later.[12]

Smaller island nations such as Ireland and New Zealand seemed especially desperate to prove they could keep the virus out, whatever the cost to their economies and societies. New Zealand largely barred foreign visitors[13] and shut down repeatedly[14] in so-called "snap lockdowns" when it found even a handful of Covid cases.[15] Ireland prevented its own citizens from traveling more than three miles from their homes after a rise in cases in the fall.

Despite scattered protests, most people in Europe and other advanced democracies still appeared willing to tolerate Covid restrictions as 2020 ended. Perhaps the clearest sign came in New Zealand, where Prime Minister Jacinda Ardern swept to re-election on October 17, her Labour Party winning 49 percent of votes—its biggest share in fifty years.[16]

Ardern's commitment to keeping New Zealand free of Covid, even if doing so meant cutting the nation off from the rest of the world, drove her victory. "Ardern Wins 'Historic' Re-Election for Crushing COVID-19," Reuters reported.[17]

Meanwhile, for reasons that remained unclear, East Asian nations dodged the pandemic throughout 2020. After its initial wave subsided, China reported almost no new cases or deaths. Even with the near lockout of Western media, the country's post-February figures appeared trustworthy. China's seeming success appeared to show the value of tough early lockdowns.

Vietnam used a similarly harsh strategy, putting millions of its citizens into quarantine as the year progressed. It finished 2020 with only thirty-five coronavirus deaths out of almost one hundred million people.[18]

Yet Japan found similar success with *no* lockdowns. The country's constitution didn't permit them.[19] Mask-wearing, although common, was not universal. Japan tested almost none of its people, so the "test-trace-isolate" plan couldn't possibly be the answer.[20] And demography wasn't the explanation. Japan had one of the world's densest cities and oldest populations.

So why hadn't the virus overrun Tokyo and the rest of Japan? No one had a good answer. Japan had very little obesity[21] and relatively low rates of lung cancer despite lots of smoking.[22] Perhaps genetic or environmental factors had simply made the Japanese less vulnerable. But no hard evidence supported that explanation. The fragmentary evidence from antibody tests released in September that showed Sars-Cov-2 had spread widely in Tokyo only added to the mystery.[23]

I watched the world's struggles with Covid as closely as anyone, trying to understand governmental responses that appeared increasingly out-of-tune with our knowledge about the risks of the virus. Why had we not changed our attitude after those first panicked days in March?

Like a lot of other Team Reality members in blue states, I found myself frustrated as the fall progressed. The rules made no sense. My kids were in school—but the school was being conducted *outside*, under canopies. (They weren't even tents. Tents have sides. Canopies don't.) So why did the kids have to wear masks?

For that matter, why did I have to wear a mask when I was walking into a restaurant, but not after I sat down? Why were coffee shops closed but malls open?

I had always liked working at coffee places—a way to counter the loneliness of writing. With that option foreclosed, I spent much of the fall of 2020 driving to a fancy mall forty-five minutes from our house. I camped in the food court there hour after hour, working on an *Unreported Truths* booklet on the uselessness of masks. My own mask sat on the table in front of me, a devotional symbol that I was a good camper who knew the rules. I had a cup of coffee with me, which meant I was drinking, which meant Covid couldn't get me, and I didn't have to wear my mask.

In the event, no one cared. No one said anything. Of course, the mall was nearly empty. People in New York were still scared, or didn't know it was open, or preferred to buy online.

Only a couple of times during the fall and winter did I meet open animosity for going maskless.

"You've forgotten your mask," a man at a local pizza place said to me.

"No," I said.

"Oh, you're one of *those* assholes." He had an English accent.

My temper rose, but I didn't argue. My order was ready. I took it and went to the car. My masked friend followed me out, phone in hand, taking a picture of me and my license plate, thrilled at the chance to tattle on me. I could only laugh—if he decided to post the picture, my followers would be thrilled! An on-brand moment.

And yet, despite the nonstop fearmongering about "twindemics" and "dark winters" and "pandemic fatigue," November brought one very real reason to hope we might be near the end of Covid.

The vaccines had arrived.

30

Free at Last

On the morning of Monday, November 9, 2020, the joyous headlines poured in, following Pfizer's all-caps press release: "PFIZER AND BIONTECH ANNOUNCE VACCINE CANDIDATE AGAINST COVID-19 ACHIEVED SUCCESS IN FIRST INTERIM ANALYSIS FROM PHASE 3 STUDY."[1]

"Pfizer says early analysis shows its Covid-19 vaccine is more than 90 percent effective," CNN reported. "Dow futures soaring to record territory, up more than 1,500."[2]

Three days later, Dr. Anthony Fauci offered an even more optimistic take at an event sponsored by a British think tank: "Certainly it's not going to be a pandemic for a lot longer, because I believe the vaccines are going to turn that around."[3]

On November 16, the news got even better, as Moderna announced its mRNA vaccine was 94 percent effective.[4] Then Pfizer, which was partners with the German company BioNTech, posted more complete results showing its shot offered 95 percent protection.[5]

Further, both companies said their products looked safe. "No serious safety concerns have been observed," Pfizer reported. Moderna said its vaccine "was generally well tolerated." Considering that more than twenty thousand people had received the Pfizer shot during the trial and another thirteen thousand the Moderna, the apparent lack of serious side effects was very reassuring.

After nine grim Covid-filled months, the vaccine findings looked like a giant victory for science and medicine. They offered a path back to normal life. And they had come much faster than expected. When Covid emerged from China in early 2020, vaccine experts had predicted shots against Sars-Cov-2 would not be ready until late 2021 at the earliest.

The experts had also warned the vaccines might offer only modest protection. In Senate testimony in September 2020, Dr. Robert Redfield, the head of the Centers for Disease Control, even said vaccines might not work as well as masks.[6]

But scientists had come together in a government-academic-private partnership to offer protection to a desperate planet. Debates about which lucky people should be vaccinated first began immediately. The stocks of Moderna and BioNTech, which had jumped during 2020 alongside rising hopes for the vaccines, soared even further.

Company executives and scientists basked in praise. A November 10 article in *The Guardian*, a British newspaper, explained how a husband and wife in Germany—Dr. Uğur Şahin and Dr. Özlem Türeci, both physicians, both the children of Turkish migrants—had founded BioNTech.

"They are the 'dream team' scientist couple who came up with a big idea that could protect humanity from a virus that has killed more than a million people," *The Guardian* reported.[7]

About the only person who was not thrilled was Donald Trump. He went back and forth between demanding credit for the vaccines and grumbling that Pfizer had withheld its early results until after Election Day in order to hurt his chances of victory.[8]

By December, even he had come around. Both he[9] and Vice President Mike Pence[10] would refer to the vaccines as a "miracle."

I was briefly impressed, too. On November 10, I tweeted:

> Been thinking a lot about the vaccine announcement yesterday. Assuming it holds up, a true example of science and scientists at their best—a small group of people working together to produce an advance that is almost magical both in its complexity and its impact.…[11]

Assuming it holds up.

What neither I nor almost anyone else outside the companies understood at the time was what Pfizer and Moderna *weren't* saying.

But within days my natural skepticism had taken over. My skepticism—and the years I had spent covering the pharmaceutical industry for the *New York Times*. I had seen first-hand that its top companies could not be trusted to disclose side effects or other problems with their medicines.

Drug companies know far more about their products than anyone outside, including regulators. But they don't always use that knowledge for the public good. They have a history of hiding negative clinical trial results, marketing their drugs for unapproved uses, and paying physicians incentives (bribe is such an ugly word) to write prescriptions.

I had seen all those practices up close. After years of reading internal emails, listening to trial testimony, and examining research data, I probably understood the games the companies played as well as anyone who didn't work for them.

And I understood the crucial role clinical trial design played in the approval of new medicines.

Vaccines and pharmaceuticals are not like other consumer products. Patients can't buy them for themselves. Physicians have to prescribe them. And before they can do so, regulators have to approve them as safe and effective.

In the United States, the Food and Drug Administration has that job. But the FDA does not pay for or design clinical trials or run "preclinical" work—research on animals and in laboratories. It has to rely on the data from the "sponsors," the drug companies. Companies structure their trials so that they maximize the benefits the drugs provide, or seem to provide, while minimizing side effects. Everyone in the industry knew the game.

So I looked hard at the clinical trials that Pfizer and Moderna had conducted, along with the other data and research on mRNA vaccines. The harder I looked, the more flaws I found.

I wound up writing my fourth *Unreported Truths* booklet about the vaccines. I worked on it for almost four months before publishing it on March 23, 2021. It totaled about fourteen thousand words, making it the longest of the four, and the most intensely reported and forward-looking.

I wish I could print it in its entirety here, but Regnery says *Pandemia* is too long already. (Besides, I have to save some material for the book I am going to have to write about the vaccines, right?)

Still, the booklet shows that potential problems with the vaccines were obvious long before regulators and the White House acknowledged them. In the next chapter I reproduce four passages from it, about four crucial problems with the vaccines: 1) the fact that the vaccines were hardly tested on the elderly people at high risk of death from Covid, 2) the pressure on regulators for approval, 3) the lack of preclinical work to ensure safety, and 4) the concerning side effects, which cropped up almost immediately.

I offer them as they appeared in the booklet—with a handful of minor copyediting fixes and some additions to the notes. I have also added a subhead describing each excerpt.

31

The Excerpts:

Basic Facts You Need to Know about Potential Problems with the Vaccines

EXCERPT 1

The vaccines were hardly tested on the elderly people at high risk of death from Covid.

The Covid vaccines—like most vaccines—may work much better in younger people, who are at lower risk from Covid anyway.

Until recently, this risk could only be classified as theoretical. But on March 5 a team of German researchers published their findings from a study that tested how well people over eighty responded to Pfizer's vaccine compared to those under sixty.

Unfortunately, the researchers found that vaccines produced a markedly weaker immune response in older people than those under sixty. Seventeen days after receiving their second dose, about one in three people over eighty had *no* detectable "neutralizing antibodies" to the coronavirus in their blood—a crucial measure of immunity. Only 1 percent of younger people had no neutralizing antibodies.[1]

Other studies show that the protection the vaccines offer probably peaks between one to four weeks after the second dose and then slowly declines.[2] Thus the researchers were measuring people at what should have been the peak of their vaccine-generated immunity. Yet many people over eighty were still apparently vulnerable to the coronavirus at that point.

Our real-world experience with flu vaccines raises similar concerns. The evidence that influenza vaccines reduce deaths in people over 65 is weak. In fact, a 2020 study that looked at 170 million flu vaccinations in Britain found they appeared to be linked to slightly *higher* rates of deaths and hospitalizations.[3]

The Covid vaccines have been given for fewer than four months, so scientists are only beginning to accumulate data on how well they work in the real world. What we can say for sure at this point is that the clinical trials did not answer the most important question about the mRNA and all Covid vaccines—whether they actually save lives....

Pfizer and Moderna ultimately reported 366 Covid infections in their big trials (counting from one to two weeks after the second shot, when the vaccines become fully effective).

Nineteen infections occurred in people who received the vaccines. The other 347 occurred in those who got placebo shots.[4]

Nineteen versus 347. Those were the numbers the companies highlighted in November, the numbers that excited the world.

But what no one seemed to understand, then or now, was that those were not hospitalized patients, much less people who needed intensive care or died. They were almost all mild or moderate cases—meaning a positive Covid test along with symptoms such as a cough or low-grade fever.

Serious illness from Covid in the trials was vanishingly rare—not just among people who received the vaccine, but those who got the *placebo*. Out of the more than thirteen thousand people in the Moderna trial who received the placebo, only nine required hospitalization for Covid.

For Pfizer, only nine placebo patients out of twenty thousand became what the company defined as "severely" ill, compared to one vaccine recipient. Hospitalizations were rarer still.

The trials also had almost exactly the same number of *deaths* in people who received the placebo or vaccine. No one died of Covid in the Pfizer trial. One Moderna placebo recipient died of Covid, the only patient to die of Covid of all seventy thousand people in the two trials. Counting every death that occurred for any reason, or "all-cause mortality," eight people who received the vaccine died, compared to eleven who received the placebo.[5]

Given the size of the trials, that tiny difference offers no evidence to suggest the vaccines either save or cost lives.

Why did so few people die in the trials if Covid has really killed more than 500,000 Americans—1 out of every 600 people?[6] Because both companies tested their vaccines mostly on healthy people and those under 65. **They included only a few elderly people with serious medical conditions, who are the people far more likely to die from Covid than anyone else** [emphasis added]....[7]

EXCERPT 2
The regulators who approved the vaccines did so under pressure.

Pfizer and Moderna knew they wouldn't need to answer the question of whether their vaccines reduced deaths. As long as the top-line data looked impressive, the pressure for approval would be huge. No one would look too hard at what the trials had actually proven—that the vaccines reduced moderate illnesses in people who were at low risk from Covid anyway.

And Pfizer and Moderna were right. The lack of data did not stop regulators from rushing the vaccines ahead. Internal documents from the European Medicines Agency, which is Europe's equivalent of the U.S. Food and Drug Administration, show the pressure that the EMA and FDA faced to approve the vaccines quickly.

The documents are mostly emails that were hacked from the EMA sometime in late November or early December.[8] (On January 25, after previously refusing to do so, the agency confirmed that they were real, saying in a press release that "individual emails are authentic.")[9]

The pressure began almost as soon as Pfizer announced its initial results on November 9. It only increased in the days that followed. On November 16, Marco Cavaleri, the EMA's Head of Health Threats and Vaccines Strategy, told his colleagues the FDA was being "pushed hard by Azar and US GOV." Azar refers to Alex Azar, the Secretary of Health and Human Services, the FDA's parent agency.

Initially, the FDA had told the EMA it did not expect to authorize either vaccine before year-end, giving it a bit more than a month to review the data, the emails show. But the FDA and EMA believed the British government intended to move faster, putting pressure on them to do the same.

"They [the British] are going to rush," Cavaleri wrote....[10]

EXCERPT 3
The preclinical work to ensure safety was inadequate.

In early 2020, as epidemiologists warned of tens of millions of coronavirus deaths worldwide, the risks of rushing a vaccine seemed small compared to those of the virus. The United States government called its multi-billion-dollar effort to jump-start vaccine development "Warp Speed"—a reference to *Star Trek*'s fantasy that spaceships could travel faster than the speed of light.[11] (The Merriam-Webster dictionary now defines "warp speed" as "the highest possible speed.")

Unfortunately, even after we realized the coronavirus was far less dangerous than we'd initially feared, governments rushed vaccines ahead. Normally, drug companies spend years on "preclinical" development, testing potential medicines in laboratories and on animals. Their goal is to choose the best possible candidate before trying it on a few healthy volunteers.

Then they spend months or years more reviewing those early human trials and making sure they know everything about possible side effects.

Only then do they begin the large "pivotal" clinicals necessary to approve their drugs.

But Pfizer/BioNTech and Moderna compressed that five- to ten-year timeline into months. Moderna started testing its vaccine, called m1273, in humans on March 16, 2020—barely ten *weeks* after the first reports of the coronavirus emerged from China.[12]

BioNTech began its human testing about a month later, in April.[13]

Moderna was in such a hurry it did not even finish a proper pre-clinical study for its vaccine, as European regulators disclosed in their vaccine review. They called the company's work "inadequate for evaluating the repeated dose toxicity of mRNA-1273." They gave the company a pass on the dubious grounds that it had submitted similar preclinical data from other vaccines it was developing....[14]

EXCERPT 4
Significant side effects cropped up almost immediately.

In the excitement, nearly everyone appeared to ignore deeply sobering figures on side effects. The trials made clear neither Pfizer nor Moderna had fully put to rest the concerns that had slowed development of mRNA vaccines for a decade. Their vaccines cause serious side effects in many people, especially after the second shot.

In vaccine trials, drug makers record two kinds of side effects, called solicited and unsolicited events. Solicited events are those that occur shortly after the vaccination itself and are presumed directly related to it, like arm pain or a fever or nausea the day after the shot. Solicited events are generally temporary—unpleasant effects that fade as the immune system finishes reacting to the vaccine....

The rates of solicited adverse events were far higher in vaccinated people [in the clinical trials]. Pfizer reported almost 80 percent of people who received the vaccine had pain or swelling where they were injected. Only about 10 percent of placebo patients reported similar problems. The gap worsened as the pain levels increased. About 30 percent of vaccinated people said they had moderate or severe pain, compared to 1 percent of people who received the placebo.[15]

Of course, a sore arm is not life-threatening. And for most people the pain faded within a couple of days. But rates of "systemic" solicited adverse events—like fever, nausea, or diarrhea—were also far higher in people who received the vaccine....

Even a lot of serious short-term side effects do not necessarily mean the mRNA vaccines are deadly. And no deaths in the clinical trials were definitively linked to the vaccines. But the fact that people in the trials had so many severe adverse events shows they can cause a strong immune reaction—whether because of the lipid nanoparticles, the mRNA itself, or some other reason.

Data from both animal and early human studies contained other warning signs, **especially about potential blood and cardiovascular problems** [emphasis added]. European regulators noted that in animals, Moderna's mRNA vaccines reduced lymphocytes—which help fight infection—and increased inflammation. They even caused some precancerous bone marrow changes. The regulators said the changes "were generally reversing" after two weeks.[16] But they did not say the animals had actually returned to normal.

Meanwhile, Pfizer and BioNTech reported their drug caused lymphocytes to drop temporarily in volunteers in an early clinical trial—a sign the vaccine might leave people more open to infection in the days after it was given.[17]

None of these reports by themselves provided reason to reject the vaccines. They did provide hints of potential problems that should have been investigated further, or at a minimum tracked once the vaccines were made publicly available. Yet regulators didn't press the companies to run more studies on how the vaccines might damage blood or bone marrow cells....

Both the United States and Europe have systems allowing health care workers to file reports if they see someone have a medical problem after receiving a vaccine. Patients can also file reports directly. The United

States system, called VAERS—the Vaccine Adverse Event Reporting System—includes details from the reports themselves, though not the identity of patients. The European system, EUDRA, offers only a broad overview of reports.

Both systems have received far more reports of side effects after Covid vaccine shots than other vaccines. By mid-March, VAERS had received more than thirty thousand reports of side effects from Covid vaccines—as many as all other vaccines combined during the last year.

The gap is even larger for reports of serious side effects or deaths. With about 110 million doses of mRNA vaccines given in the United States, the VAERS system had received more than 1,800 death reports, the CDC reported on March 16. In comparison, it received about 20 reports of deaths out of 180 million flu vaccinations in the last two flu seasons.[18]

■ ■ ■

I finished the *Unreported Truths about Covid-19 and Lockdowns, Part 4: Vaccines* booklet on what I hoped was a balanced note:

In many ways, the Covid vaccines—especially the mRNAs—have become a real-world Rorschach test.

Vaccine advocates see a scientific leap forward that may work not just against the coronavirus but influenza, other viruses, and even cancer. Just as the terrible injuries of wartime led to advances in surgery, the pressure of the Covid epidemic led companies and governments to work together. They introduced these new vaccines far faster than would have otherwise been possible. Even if some kinks need to be worked out, the mRNA hypothesis has now been shown to work in the most dramatic possible way.

But to vaccine skeptics—anti-vaxxers—the mRNA vaccines are just another in a long line of overhyped vaccines. They are far more dangerous than the scientific community admits and have potentially catastrophic long-term risks. The speed of their development is cause for alarm, not celebration. In the long run, they may cause infertility, devastating brain diseases, or the emergence of devastating new variants of the coronavirus. By the time we know the truth, it will be too late.

As is usually the case in these dogmatic battles, the truth is likely somewhere in the middle. Both sides are so focused on their own gospel that they have failed to see the vaccines for what they really are—a new technology that carries both promise and risk....

Make no mistake, regulators failed at every point in the development of these vaccines—the preclinical work, the major clinical trials, and the approval process. Then again, they had little choice. Dr. Moncef Slaoui, who oversaw Operation Warp Speed, told the *New York Times* that the United States government had realized that "what was very important was to be a full, active partner in the development and the manufacturing of the vaccine. And to do so very early."[19]

How could the FDA or EMA possibly have stood up to that pressure? A few extra weeks of preclinical development might have given us more information about the vaccines' pregnancy risks and other rare but serious side effects. A few thousand extra older people in the trials would have answered once and for all the question of whether the vaccines save lives.

But those questions were never answered. Now they may never be....

In the coming months, the pressure to be vaccinated is only going to increase. Even raising the basic data-driven issues I have discussed in this booklet causes massive backlash, as I have learned since January.

But that doesn't make them any less real.

32

Bad News

B y the time I wrote those words in March, I knew I was on lonely ground.

Not shaky. Lonely.

Of course, the Team Apocalypse blue checks would brook no questions about the vaccines. Their inability to think critically came as no surprise. From the beginning they had done everything they'd been told without question. They had stayed inside and masked and bleached their groceries and tried to shame their neighbors and everyone else into doing the same. Then they'd begged for more.

As late as January 2021, many *still* seemed to believe Covid was an automatic death sentence, even for healthy young and middle-aged adults. They had been hiding at home for a year. They were desperate for a solution, any solution.

They found it in the vaccines.

As always, Molly Jong-Fast—the Brooklyn writer who in March 2020 had predicted that as many as twenty-three million Americans might die from Covid, and had spent months locked in her apartment[1]—

summed up the view of the terrified left. In a December 2020 piece for *Vogue*, she wrote:

> "Yes, the vaccine is coming," I told myself as I spent my first Thanksgiving without any of my 70-something parents in the hope of keeping them safe. Yes, the vaccine is coming, I tell myself as I look ahead to what will be an even lonelier Christmas. Yes, the vaccine is coming, I tell my father, who hasn't seen his grandchildren in months. Yes, the vaccine is coming, I silently mouth as I look into my children's bedrooms as they stare into the blue lights of their computer screens, deprived of school, friends, family, and what used to be called normal life.[2]

The vaccine was coming. One magic prick at a time.

Through the winter and spring, lefty blue checks offered their grateful thanks for the blessing of mRNA. Vaccination centers were our new houses of worship, the shots our modern sacraments. You didn't even need to kneel to receive them. (Though you did have to wait fifteen minutes to make sure you didn't go into anaphylactic shock.)[3] And like all true believers, the vaccine fanatics couldn't wait to spread the good word.

I'm not exaggerating.

"The #COVID19 vaccine is the miracle so many have waited and worked for, and will end the pandemic," New York mayor Bill de Blasio tweeted on December 22. "Get this shot of hope and help set our city free."[4]

"Take whatever COVID vaccine you can get," six members of Biden's Covid advisory board—all doctors or scientists—wrote on February 12. "The best thing you can do is get vaccinated as soon as you're able."[5]

Martina Navratilova, the tennis great and liberal activist—her Twitter avatar was a campaign poster for Joe Biden and Kamala Harris—tweeted proudly on February 28, "Just got my first shot—Pfizer—and I am so excited and relieved and happy etc—if there are any antivaxxers out here—if you can—please get the vaccine."[6]

■   ■   ■

Ironically, many people on the left had spent decades criticizing the pharmaceutical industry for its corruption of science and the prices of prescription drugs. In the months before Biden was elected, journalists and Democratic politicians had specifically warned against the risks of a rushed vaccine. As early as May 2020, when Trump suggested a vaccine could be ready by year-end, NBC told viewers only a "miracle" would allow Trump to meet that promise.[7]

On September 5, 2020, Democratic vice presidential nominee Kamala Harris told CNN that approval or authorization of a vaccine before the election is "going to be an issue for all of us."[8]

Just weeks later, Andrew Cuomo went further. "I'm not going to trust the federal government's opinion," Cuomo said at a press conference. "New York state will have its own review when the federal government has finished with their review."[9]

But when Biden won, the left reversed course.

Long before he was inaugurated in January, the media and public health establishment had begun a full-court press on the vaccines. "Trump Is Right: Andrew Cuomo Should Accept F.D.A. Approval of a Coronavirus Vaccine," the *New Yorker* opined on November 16—*after* the election, but *before* the agency had even held its first public advisory meeting in December to discuss the trials.[10]

Two *Vanity Fair* headlines on stories written by the same author summed up the woke media's incoherence.

On October 7, "Trump's Rush to Release a COVID Vaccine Has Americans Worried."[11]

On December 18, "The White House's Incompetence Is Apparently Holding Up 'Millions' of COVID Vaccines."[12]

The handful of investigative reporters who specialized in chasing complex pharmaceutical stories simply refused to look at the vaccine clinical trials or rush to authorize their use. Aside from me and Serena Tinari and Catherine Riva, who wrote for the *British Medical Journal*, almost no one asked even basic questions.

Meanwhile, many conservatives who had supported me throughout 2020 grew increasingly frustrated with me.

Their desire to see the vaccines move ahead quickly came from a somewhat different place than the left's vaccine enthusiasm. Covid didn't necessarily terrify them. But they hated lockdowns and mask mandates and school closures. They figured getting jabbed with sixty (or two hundred) micrograms of mRNA was a small price to end the pandemic.

And they simply couldn't seem to imagine the vaccines might actually be dangerous or ineffective. After all, the shots had gone through huge clinical trials. The Food and Drug Administration and Centers for Disease Control had signed off on them. The entire medical and scientific establishment couldn't be wrong, could it?

These conservatives showed a strange naiveté. They had either forgotten or never known about drugs such as Vioxx, a painkiller from Merck approved by the FDA in May 1999. Merck withdrew Vioxx from the market in September 2004 after a clinical trial showed it nearly doubled the risk of heart attacks compared to a placebo.[13]

In the five years Vioxx was on the market, Merck had advertised it aggressively to the public. In 2000 alone, Merck spent $161 million advertising Vioxx, the most on any prescription drug, more money than was spent to advertise Pepsi or Budweiser.[14] The advertising worked. Tens of millions of people took Vioxx before it was recalled.

With so many people using Vioxx, even a relatively small increased risk of heart attacks translated into a huge death toll. In early 2005, *The Lancet* published a study from FDA scientists showing Vioxx might have caused as many as 140,000 cases of heart disease and 55,000 deaths.[15] Internal Merck documents revealed researchers at the company—including Dr. Edward Scolnick, Merck's chief scientist—had been concerned about Vioxx's heart risks long before Merck withdrew it.[16] Merck wound up spending billions of dollars to compensate victims.

Vioxx is just one of many examples of Big Pharma's malfeasance. It stood out mainly because it had harmed so many people. But mainstream conservatives tended to believe in corporate America (at least when it wasn't censoring them or annoying them with woke behavior).

Thus Republicans happily endorsed the vaccines. A few days before Christmas, South Carolina senator Lindsay Graham posted a photo of himself receiving his first dose and tweeted in apparent sincerity:

> Thank God for nurses who help people in need and know how to use a needle. Thank God for those who produced these vaccines. If enough of us take it, we will get back to normal lives. Help is on the way.[17]

Younger, slicker Republicans expressed similar sentiments, if not as humbly. In January, Robby Soave of *Reason* magazine, a self-described libertarian and proponent of reopening schools,[18] tweeted:

> People who say "well, the vaccine doesn't actually prevent infection" are wrong. The vaccine almost certainly prevents infection. It is akin to a cure. If you got it, you don't have to wear a mask. You will neither contract nor spread the disease.[19]

Such confidence!

Such mistaken confidence.

Other conservatives liked to remind the world that the *Trump* White House had conceived and funded Operation Warp Speed. Trump had promised Americans the vaccines by the end of 2020, and he'd delivered. Questioning the vaccines meant denying him his only (apparent) Covid victory.

"Operation Warp Speed's Triumph: Trump's Vaccine Bet Was Government's Best Pandemic Decision," the *Wall Street Journal*'s conservative editorial page crowed prematurely, on March 2. "American governments, federal and state, have made many mistakes in the Covid-19 pandemic. But the great success—the saving grace—was making a financial bet in collaboration with private American industry on the development of vaccines. That effort is now letting the country see the possibility of a return to relatively normal life as early as the spring."[20]

A month later, right-wing provocateur Ben Shapiro complained to his more than three million Twitter followers about the CDC's cautious guidance telling vaccinated people to continue to wear masks in many situations. "Once you are fully vaccinated, take off the mask and go live your life because the vaccines are a scientific miracle," Shapiro wrote.[21]

■   ■   ■

What conservatives didn't seem to understand when they criticized me for pushing back on the vaccines was that I agreed the CDC's insistence that vaccinated people needed to wear masks was absurd.

But not because they were vaccinated. Because the CDC's guidance on masks was absurd, whether or not people were vaccinated.[22]

The choice of vaccines or pandemic was a false dichotomy. We didn't need vaccines—whether they worked well, poorly, or not at all—to stop wearing masks. Or end lockdowns. Or reopen schools. We just needed to put the dangers of the coronavirus in reasonable perspective. We needed to treat it as a medical problem, not a societal crisis.

We needed to change our perspective, not look for yet another miracle answer that would likely fall short. Vaccines would help protect those at high risk from Covid—the old, frail, and morbidly obese. (Maybe.) The rest of us could take our time in deciding whether we wanted them, given their nasty side effect profile and broader questions about mRNA technology.

But I learned quickly how unpopular a position I had taken.

The November clinical trial results had seduced everyone: leftists, rightists, and even Covid centrists—the rarest of breeds, sometimes seeming to consist of only one person, Dr. Monica Gandhi.

The consensus among the edumucated loudmouths who dominated Twitter went something like this: Ninety-five percent protection! If not better! It's all over but the shouting. Just get shots in arms double-quick. The proles can go back to drinkin' and fightin' and screamin' at NASCAR races while those of us with college degrees return to our thoughtfully curated lives: hot yoga, buying CBD-infused iced tea at Whole Foods, and travel soccer for the kids.

"Please be assured that YOU ARE SAFE after vaccine from what matters—disease and spreading. Two vaccinated people can be as close as 2 spoons in a drawer!" Gandhi tweeted on January 9.[23]

On February 17, Martin Varsavsky, a blue check tech entrepreneur with a hundred thousand Twitter followers, went further. "We should explain that after millions of vaccinations there is NOT ONE fully vaccinated person who got severe Covid and died of Covid."[24] (This statement was false even at the time. Fully vaccinated Israelis had already died.)[25]

A wildly misleading chart also became popular on and off Twitter. It showed that no one who had received the vaccine had died of Covid during the clinical trials for the mRNA (or other) vaccines.[26] What the chart failed to note was that only *one* person who had received the *placebo* in the mRNA trials had died of Covid.

On February 19, David Leonhardt of the *New York Times* said, "The evidence so far suggests that a full dose of the vaccine—with the appropriate waiting period after the second shot—effectively eliminates the risk of Covid-19 death, nearly eliminates the risk of the hospitalization and drastically reduces a person's ability to infect somebody else."[27]

This explanation had the evidence exactly backwards. We couldn't know if the vaccines reduced the risk of death meaningfully, because not enough people at high risk had been enrolled in the trials. We had no evidence at all on long-term efficacy, because the trial data covered a matter of months.

Vaccine advocates ignored those hard facts and instead made promises that would look worse than foolish in a matter of months.

Even at the time, though, the picture was not as rosy as the advocates seemed to think.

As the rollout progressed worldwide in January and February, no one in the United States seemed to be looking at the data out of Israel and the United Kingdom. Those were the two countries where mass vaccination campaigns had started earliest and progressed fastest.

Israel used only the Pfizer vaccine. Britain used both the Pfizer and Moderna mRNA vaccines, as well as the AstraZeneca vaccine, which was more like the Johnson & Johnson vaccine that would eventually become the third vaccine in the United States. While the AstraZeneca and J&J vaccines worked somewhat differently than the mRNA vaccines, they also caused the body to produce the coronavirus spike protein and stimulate an immune response.

Just as I had seen early on that hospitalizations were the key to understanding the course of the epidemic, I realized in January that Israel and Britain would be key to understanding the vaccinations—for better or worse. American data were less trustworthy, for several reasons. The United States was so large that it didn't really have one epidemic. Covid rolled around the country from region to region and season to season.

Britain and Israel were far smaller, making the effects of seasonality easier to track. They both also have national health care systems (in the case of Israel, four health maintenance organizations oversee care, but every Israeli is covered), which vaccinated people quickly and provided better data on Covid hospitalizations and deaths than the fragmented American system. (The data issue would only become more problematic as 2021 progressed and the debate over vaccines in the United States became increasingly politicized.)

So Israel and Britain had a story to tell.

And throughout January and February, it wasn't a good one. As their mass vaccination campaigns ramped up, so did infections and deaths.

By late January, the United Kingdom was averaging more than 1,200 Covid deaths a day—the equivalent of 6,000 a day in the United States.[28] British deaths in those weeks appear to be the highest any big country ever recorded on a per capita basis. European countries such as France and Spain, which were lagging in vaccinations, saw no similar rise. Israel had a similar peak in cases and deaths, which were higher in late January than ever before.[29]

British physicians noticed the connection. On February 1, 2021, Dr. Martin Vernon, the former national clinical director of the British National Health Service, tweeted:

> One month into the care home vaccination programme, I am deeply concerned to be seeing covid-19 infection outbreaks among first dose vaccinated residents within, and beyond 21 days of vaccination. Are any other clinicians seeing this happening?[30]

Yes, they were.

In March, a study from Denmark of almost 380,000 health care workers and nursing home residents given the Pfizer vaccine would confirm the observation. The report showed the vaccines actually had negative effectiveness in the first two weeks after the first dose. In other words, people who received them were more likely to be infected than those who had not. Health care workers were more than twice as likely, and home residents about 40 percent more.[31]

The most probable explanation was that the first vaccine dose temporarily suppressed the immune system, as Pfizer's early clinical work had suggested. Another possibility was that the actual act of immunization raised risks, as people clustered to receive shots and nursing homes opened their doors to visitors for the first time since the epidemic began.

Whatever the reason, the post-first-dose infection spike—which hit country after country—made questions about the overall effectiveness of the vaccines more pressing. We could not be sure the protection found in the clinical trials would last. A short-term rise in risk was acceptable if protection lasted for years or decades, but not if it faded quickly.

In the United States, Covid deaths also peaked in late January, though at levels significantly below those in Britain on a per capita basis. About 3,400 Americans died each day in late January (again, based on a weekly average), with a daily peak of more than 4,000.[32] The rollout of vaccinations probably also played a role in the winter death surge in the United States, though probably a smaller role than in the UK, since the American vaccination campaign took longer to accelerate.

■   ■   ■

The soaring death count only increased the media and public health push for vaccines. "When will the pandemic end?" Bloomberg asked on February 4.[33] "The answer can be measured in vaccinations."

The relentless pressure made another line of reporting around vaccines a subject of contention.

The United States lacked good data on whether vaccinated people were being hospitalized, but it did have the best public database for vaccine side effects anywhere. Since 1990, VAERS, the federal Vaccine Adverse Event Reporting System, had offered the public and medical professionals a way to file descriptions of injuries or deaths that had come after shots.[34]

Doctors, patients, and pharmacists could all add reports. Vaccine manufacturers were legally required to send in any that they received. The database was updated each Friday, and each individual report was publicly available (with names and other identifying details removed).

Almost as soon as the first Covid vaccinations were offered on December 14, the side effect reports flooded in. By January, they far outpaced those for every other vaccine. Though the majority of the side effects were relatively moderate, thousands of reports of deaths and serious injuries also came in.

As of mid-February, VAERS had received 934 death reports on Covid vaccines. At the time, about 52 million doses had been administered, and 15 million people were fully vaccinated with both doses.[35]

By way of comparison, the database received about twenty reports of deaths following 180 million influenza vaccinations in the 2019–2020 flu season. In other words, as of mid-February, people were more than five hundred times as likely to report a death after a completed two-shot Covid vaccine than a flu shot.

But instead of acknowledging that the reports might indicate real safety problems with the vaccines, reporters simply attacked the database—and me, for mentioning its statistics. "Data from vaccine reporting site being misrepresented online," the Associated Press reported on February 4.[36]

Reporters never disputed the figures that I provided, which came directly from VAERS. Instead, they insisted that reports should not be trusted because they didn't *prove* the vaccines had caused the side effects. "Since anyone can submit a report to the system, it is impossible to know if the symptoms were caused by the vaccine," the AP wrote.

The articles were correct in that no individual report could prove causality. In my reporting and tweeting, I was careful to say the side effects were "associated with" or "followed" the vaccinations.

But to pretend that the reports collectively did not present a disturbing picture was bizarre. And I read enough through the winter and spring to know that although some were weakly supported or even false, most were sincere efforts to report problems. Many were very detailed and showed strong evidence of causality. In any case, what was the point of maintaining the database at all if each report would simply be dismissed as anecdotal?

In fact, the CDC would later implicitly acknowledge the system's value when it admitted in June that the mRNA vaccines could cause myocarditis—a potentially serious heart problem—in young men. Side effect reports from VAERS formed the core of the agency's analysis.[37]

Yet even after that finding, the stories dismissing the value of the VAERS reports went on.[38]

■   ■   ■

I am not an "anti-vaxxer." I was vaccinated as a child. My children are also vaccinated with all the standard vaccines. One day in summer 2021 I took time off from raising questions about the mRNA vaccines to take our younger daughter for her two-year-old well-child visit, where she received her recommended shots.

And in the winter and spring, I did not discourage older people from getting the vaccines. On *Tucker Carlson* and on Twitter, I was very clear. I was not sure how well they worked in anyone, especially the elderly. But I believed that for people over sixty-five and certainly seventy, Sars-Cov-2 presented a risk high enough that being vaccinated probably made sense. And the trials did show a real decrease in mild and moderate infections.

But even in those first months, before the public health establishment and governments began to push quasi-mandates and mandates, I thought we were doing ourselves no favors by ignoring the potential problems with these vaccines.

As winter turned to spring, no one wanted to hear any questions. The backlash I faced on Twitter grew more intense by the day. "Grifter" became a relatively mild insult. "I am going to do gene therapy on Alex Berenson using cyanide," someone wrote in March—in a tweet that received eighteen likes.[39] But worse than the anonymous death threats were the comments from people with large audiences.

In May, Michael Eisen, a blue check with fifty-three thousand followers, wrote, "What utterly disgusting murderous POSs all the prominent people in the media spreading anti-vaccine propaganda are. Alex Berenson is a murderer."[40] For people with thousands of followers to accuse me of murder was frankly dangerous to me—and my family. But there wasn't much I could do about it.

Fortunately, even if the conservative elite didn't want to hear my concerns about vaccines, many of my readers on Twitter, whatever their politics, had learned to trust me in 2020. They were willing to consider what I wrote.

I also found a vocal group of new supporters—"anti-vaxxers" like Robert F. Kennedy Jr. and Naomi Wolf. I learned in the months to come that many were good people. Wolf sent me a supportive message even after I criticized her on Twitter.

But my alliance with them was uneasy. They were opposed to all vaccines, not just the mRNAs. And they offered wild conspiracy theories, each more implausible than the last. For a while they obsessed with 5G cellular technology, before moving on to the idea that the vaccines could somehow magnetize the body.

At one point Wolf tweeted about "the conversation I overheard in a restaurant in Manhattan 2 yrs ago in which an Apple employee was boasting about attending a top secret demo: they had a new tech to deliver vaccines w nanoparticles that let you travel back in time. Not kidding."[41]

To state the obvious, this kind of speculation only made it easier to dismiss me and the questions I was raising. My audience, which included many physicians and scientists, knew the difference. But the blue check vaccine fanatics were more than happy to lump me in with Wolf and Kennedy.

Aside from the anti-vaxxers, a few public figures and journalists—most notably Tucker Carlson and Joe Rogan—continued to raise questions about the vaccines. What they had in common was not conservatism but a populist wariness of government bureaucracies, public health experts, and Big Pharma. They might not know the details of the way Merck had hidden Vioxx's problems two decades earlier, but they were naturally skeptical, even cynical. That attitude served them well.

But even with their huge audiences, Carlson and Rogan were outgunned by the media, corporate, and government machine pushing Covid vaccinations. Governments at every level spent billions of dollars to advertise the vaccines,[42] but the public campaigns were only the start. The biggest, most successful retailers and consumer products companies in the world put their skills to work advertising and marketing the shots.[43] "Get back to what you love," promised a Google ad, which ended with the words "covid vaccine near me."[44] Walgreens featured the pianist John Legend telling viewers, "This Is Our Shot."[45]

Pollsters ran surveys and focus groups to test ways to overcome "vaccine hesitancy"—resulting in an Orwellian sameness of language in the ads. "Early on, when vaccine demand outstripped supply, politicians and public health authorities repeated the same message over and over: "Get vaccinated when it's your turn."[46] The vaccines were "safe" and "effective"; side effects were "rare"—and, when that claim became impossible to maintain, "mild" and "expected." The vaccines had not been "rushed," they had been developed over decades.[47] (In fact, while artificial mRNA had been *discussed* as a potential therapeutic mechanism for decades, it had been tested on only a few hundred people before 2020. No mRNA drugs or vaccines were even close to widespread human use when the coronavirus epidemic began.)

The propaganda was impossible to avoid, much less counter. And rather than questioning it, supposedly objective journalists furthered it. I could find no precedent for the government-private-media-academic collaboration here, with the possible exception of the propaganda that accompanied the United States' entry into World War I. So, yeah, I was on lonely ground.

But I believed in John 8:32—famously engraved on the lobby wall of the Central Intelligence Agency's original headquarters building— "And ye shall know the truth, and the truth shall make you free."

33

Truth Leaks Out

The quest for truth-in-Covid did pick up some steam in late spring 2021.

Not about the vaccine, though.

About the origins of the virus.

From the first days of the epidemic, strong circumstantial evidence suggested Sars-Cov-2 had leaked from a Chinese lab. Both the virus itself and the facts around its emergence pointed to human intervention.

Wuhan, the city of ten million people where the first cases were found, was home to China's most important viral research laboratory, the Wuhan Institute of Virology. The institute aggressively researched bat coronaviruses, which China had viewed as a serious risk since the original SARS outbreak in 2003.

In 2017 the institute had opened China's first Biosafety Level 4 laboratory. Level 4 labs are the most secure available, designed to handle deadly pathogens such as Ebola.[1] But just months after the lab opened, U.S. State Department officials visited and reported in a cable to Washington that the new facility was at risk of a serious accident. They found "a serious shortage of appropriately trained technicians and investigators needed to safely operate this high-containment laboratory."[2]

The troubled lab was located only miles from the first cluster of cases in central Wuhan. And it had worked with a virus very similar to Sars-Cov-2 known as RaTG13 (or RaBtCov/4991), which had been found in a cave in 2013 after several miners working there became seriously ill with pneumonia.[3]

That cave—like other caves that had large numbers of the bats that were the original animal hosts for naturally occurring coronaviruses—was nowhere near Wuhan. It was located in southern China, several hundred miles away. And the Chinese couldn't trace a chain of human transmission from that region to Wuhan. They had reported no early cases in the villages and cities around the caves, or between the caves and Wuhan.

Early on, Chinese and international reports had offered a different potential explanation for the fact Sars-Cov-2 had emerged first in Wuhan. They linked the outbreak to a large "wet market" there. Wet markets, which are common in China, sell wild and domesticated live animals for slaughter.[4] An NPR reporter visited a similar market in Hong Kong and reported that "it's quite obvious why the term 'wet' is used.... The countertops of the stalls are red with blood as fish are gutted and filleted."

But the theory was discounted within months, because Chinese researchers could not find Sars-Cov-2 in tissue samples of animals taken from the Wuhan wet market.[5]

Meanwhile, from the start of the epidemic, Chinese authorities at every level behaved as if they had something to hide. Sending police to silence Li Wenliang, the Wuhan doctor who in late December 2020 had first warned about the new pneumonia,[6] was only the first step.

An Associated Press investigation in June 2020 found that China had "sat on releasing the genetic map, or genome, of the virus for more than a week after three different government labs had fully decoded the information.... Chinese government labs only released the genome after another lab published it ahead of authorities on a virologist website on Jan. 11."[7] The next day, China shut that other lab for "rectification."[8]

Beijing also told the World Health Organization it did not believe people could transmit the virus to each other. Five days later, with hospitals in Wuhan filling, China reversed course and acknowledged that people could and did spread Sars-Cov-2.[9]

Still, China refused to give the WHO detailed data on Covid patients for another ten days, according to the Associated Press investigation. Nor would it let international experts visit Wuhan to see what was happening first-hand. On February 7, the *New York Times* reported, "C.D.C. and W.H.O. Offers to Help China Have Been Ignored for Weeks: Privately, Chinese doctors say they need outside expertise. But Beijing, without saying why, has shown no interest so far."[10]

Finally, three days after that article, China allowed an international team inside its borders.

At best, China's attitude revealed badly misplaced national pride. Through 2020 and into 2021, long after the virus had become a far larger problem in the United States and Europe than in China, the People's Republic continued to stonewall.

In January 2021, more than a year after the coronavirus first emerged, China finally allowed a WHO team of scientists to speak to researchers from the Wuhan Institute of Virology for an investigation. But the inquiry faced such severe Chinese-imposed restrictions that no one expected it to investigate aggressively.

■   ■   ■

Meanwhile, Sars-Cov-2 itself had several characteristics that suggested it might not be entirely natural.

From the start, it was both remarkably communicable and surprisingly stable, as if it had been optimized to infect humans. Throughout 2020, it hardly mutated. (The sudden acceleration in variants came alongside widespread vaccinations, and viral mutation is a known risk of vaccinations.)[11]

At the same time, it turned out that civet cats and many other possible "intermediate hosts" for the virus didn't seem vulnerable to Sars-Cov-2.[12] For other coronaviruses, including the original SARS and MERS, intermediate hosts had provided a crucial link between the bats that originally hosted the virus and humans. The lack of a plausible intermediate host was puzzling.

Further, the genome of Sars-Cov-2 contained a very unusual sequence that made it more dangerous, the "furin cleavage site" I mentioned in Chapter 7.[13]

A May 2020 article in *Nature* highlighted the power and danger of furin cleavage: "Robert Garry, a virologist at Tulane University in New Orleans, Louisiana, estimates that [the site] gives SARS-CoV-2 a 100–1,000 times greater chance than SARS-CoV of getting deep into the lungs. 'When I saw SARS-CoV-2 had that cleavage site, I did not sleep very well that night,' he says."[14]

But bat coronaviruses generally do not have furin cleavage sites, raising the question of how Sars-Cov-2 had acquired its own. RaTG13, the virus that the Wuhan Institute had admitted working with, was the closest known viral relative of Sars-Cov-2, but by virology standards it was still relatively distant, and it lacked the furin cleavage site.

One possible answer for how the virus could have added the genes necessary to make the furin cleavage site lay in what scientists called "gain-of-function" research. The phrase is euphemistic, bordering on Orwellian. In plain English, it means *altering a virus's genetic code to make it more dangerous.*

Gain-of-function research can be targeted and complex, with scientists making tiny and precise changes to a virus's RNA and tracking whether they make the virus more infectious. Or it can be as simple as infecting lab animals with different viruses simultaneously and then seeing how the viruses recombine with each other.[15]

Whatever the method, the goal of gain-of-function research is often to figure out how to make a virus more infectious, more lethal, or both. In theory, this work can help scientists and public health experts figure out which viruses are most dangerous and how to manage them. But many scientists have sharply criticized gain-of-function research, saying its risks far outweigh any potential benefits. In 2018, Marc Lipsitch, a Harvard professor who is one of the world's top epidemiologists, argued forcefully against manipulating the flu this way:

> This chapter makes the case against performing exceptionally dangerous gain-of-function experiments that are designed to create potentially pandemic and novel strains of influenza....
>
> The additional scientific value of this so-called gain-of-function research of concern...is relatively modest compared to what can be learned from [gain-of-function] experiments that do not create [viruses potentially capable of causing pandemics], combined with other approaches to experimental and observational influenza studies.[16]

The concerns about gain-of-function research became so serious that in October 2014 the National Institutes of Health imposed a moratorium on it.[17] But researchers with labs in the business of gain-of-function research protested.

Among the most prominent defenders of the research was Ralph Baric of the University of North Carolina, who before the moratorium had worked with Shi Zhengli, a senior scientist at the Wuhan lab, on coronavirus gain-of-function research.[18]

On November 12, 2014, Baric and another scientist would write to express their "profound concerns regarding the recent US Government directive to 'temporarily halt all new funding for experiments...using gain of function strategies that might increase pathogenesis and transmissibility in mammals.'"[19]

Among the other proponents of gain-of-function research was one Anthony Fauci. In December 2011, he was the lead author—along with Dr. Francis Collins, the head of the NIH—of a *Washington Post* opinion piece headlined "A Flu Virus Risk Worth Taking."[20]

A few months later, Fauci went even further. In a commentary for the American Society of Microbiology, in September 2012, he wrote:

> In an unlikely but conceivable turn of events, what if that scientist becomes infected with the virus, which leads to an outbreak and ultimately triggers a pandemic? . . .
>
> Scientists working in this field might say—as **indeed I have said**—that the benefits of such experiments and the resulting knowledge outweigh the risks. [emphasis added] [21]

The view of proponents like Dr. Fauci carried the day. In December 2017, the NIH dropped its restrictions, enabling Baric and others to move forward with gain-of-function research if they chose.[22]

Of course, the Wuhan lab had never been subject to American rules. And documents released in September 2021 appeared to show that it had continued to work on gain-of-function research all along.[23]

So Sars-Cov-2 had been the subject of what could only be called a cover-up at the highest levels of the Chinese government, it had unusual genetic elements, and it had emerged in the city that held a lab performing risky research on coronaviruses.

As I sometimes liked to write on Twitter, *Nothing to see here, folks!*

■   ■   ■

The case for the lab leak theory was compelling—though it was still circumstantial. Meanwhile, with neither Sars-Cov-2 nor any very close viral relative anywhere to be found in the wild, the support for the theory that the coronavirus had emerged naturally was also entirely circumstantial.

Essentially, the natural origins theory went something like this: Lots of coronaviruses exist. They regularly mutate and trade pieces of their genomes with each other. An intermediate host will be found sooner or later, even if some of the obvious candidates haven't panned out. (The path of the original SARS—bats to civets to humans[24]—had been tracked less than a year after that outbreak began in November 2002.)[25]

Or maybe the virus had jumped directly from bats to humans in more or less its current form and was still lurking in a Chinese cave somewhere, waiting to be found. The first two dangerous coronaviruses that had emerged since 2000, SARS and MERS, had had natural origins. This one did too.

■   ■   ■

I found one of these two theories far more plausible than the other.

As an unnamed White House official would tell the *Washington Post* in April, "The idea that it was just a totally natural occurrence is circumstantial. The evidence it leaked from the lab is circumstantial. Right now, the ledger on the side of it leaking from the lab is packed with bullet points and there's almost nothing on the other side."[26]

At the very least, an honest appraisal of the relative strength of the two theories suggested that scientists, journalists, and governments should aggressively investigate the possibility the virus had leaked from a lab.

That's not what happened.

By mid-February 2020, virologists and other scientists had launched a coordinated campaign to squelch any discussion of the lab leak theory. The first shot across the bow came on February 19, when *The Lancet* published its "statement in support of the scientists, public health professionals, and medical professionals of China combatting COVID-19."

A month later, on March 17, five top virologists published a short letter in the journal *Nature Medicine* claiming, "We do not believe that any type of laboratory-based scenario is plausible."[27]

To support their theory, they noted that some features of Sars-Cov-2 could be found in coronaviruses that infect pangolins, an anteater found in Africa. How exactly those pangolin coronaviruses would have traded genes with those found in bats in Chinese caves was a question for another day. (And even the pangolin coronaviruses didn't have furin cleavage sites, as the letter acknowledged.)

The letter was heavy on unsupported conjecture and lacking hard evidence. If the question of the virus's origins were a trial—*The World v. Wuhan Institute of Virology*—the letter would have been no more than an opening statement. Nonetheless, almost four thousand other research papers, an extraordinary number, have cited it.

Major media outlets also leaned heavily on the letter—and the scientists who signed it—to shoot down any discussion of a potential lab leak.

Sometimes journalists deliberately conflated the leak theory with the far more implausible view—offered by a few genuine conspiracy theorists—that the Chinese had created Sars-Cov-2 as a biological weapon and released it *intentionally*. (Given that the coronavirus was generally not dangerous to healthy military-age adults, it would have made a lousy weapon of war.)

But more often they attacked even the potential of an *accidental* lab leak—especially after Trump said at the White House on April 30 that intelligence agencies had evidence of a leak. "We're going to put it all together," Trump said. "I think we will have a very good answer eventually. And China might even tell us."[28]

Reporters roundly attacked this claim.

The Atlantic referred to Trump's statement about "the virus first appearing in a Chinese lab" as "a notion that scientists have dismissed."[29] The *Washington Post* posted a "Fact Checker" on May 1 headlined "Was the New Coronavirus Accidentally Released from a Wuhan lab? It's Doubtful."[30] (This piece ran just weeks after Josh Rogin's column in the *Post* on the State Department's concerns about the Wuhan Institute of Virology.)

But then the *Post* had been insisting on the natural origins theory as early as February, long before anyone had definitive evidence either way. In an attack on Senator Tom Cotton, it called the lab leak idea "a coronavirus conspiracy theory that was already debunked."[31]

Fauci fueled the anti–lab leak sentiment in a May 4 interview with *National Geographic*. Fauci "says the best evidence shows the virus behind the pandemic was not made in a lab in China," the magazine reported.[32]

Some reporters went even further, arguing that the lab leak theory was racist. The online magazine Slate claimed in February 2020 that "rumors of a lab escape or a bioweapon stem from historical amnesia, a caricatured villain, and good old-fashioned racism."[33] More than a year later, Apoorva Mandavilli, who covered the epidemic for the *Times*, would tweet that the theory had "racist roots."[34]

I never understood why pointing out the lab leak theory was considered racist, while mentioning that Chinese people buy wild animals for slaughter in unsanitary markets was fine. No matter. Woke rules are woke rules. The lab leak theory quickly became so toxic that Facebook actively censored it.[35]

As the months passed and neither Chinese authorities nor anyone else found any plausible animal host for the virus, I assumed that the lab leak theory would have to be taken more seriously.

Nope.

By the fall, only a few brave scientists spoke out to call for further inquiry—notably Alina Chan, a junior researcher at the Massachusetts Institute of Technology.[36] For the most part, they were ignored. (I tweeted regularly about the theory too; I couldn't believe how cavalierly reporters had dismissed it.)

After Biden won, I assumed reporters would take a fresh look. I had become so cynical that I assumed that the journalistic consensus was an effort to ensure Trump could not blame China for the crisis. Once again, I was wrong. Most reporters seemed to believe genuinely in the consensus view—just as they believed, in the face of overwhelming evidence, that masks suppressed the virus and school closures protected kids. In February 2021, after Biden's inauguration, Ari Shapiro of NPR's *All Things Considered*—the ultimate voice of the elite media consensus—told listeners, "OK, so it's clear the virus did not come from a lab."[37]

Still, the World Health Organization investigation marked the beginning of the end of the efforts to demonize the lab leak theory, mainly because it proved to be so toothless that it actually provoked a backlash. It came to the wildly implausible conclusion that the virus was more likely to have been *imported into China in frozen food* than to have leaked.[38] A *Wall Street Journal* op-ed on February 21 summed up the skepticism: "WHO Said What about Wuhan? International Investigators Ignore the Lab-Leak Theory but Investigate Frozen Fish."[39]

In fact, when the WHO finally released the formal results of the investigation on March 30, the cover page described it as a "Joint WHO-China Study, January 14–February 10 2021, Joint Report,"[40] a title that suggested the WHO hardly wanted full responsibility for the findings.

But the dam really broke in May 2021, seventeen long months after the virus had emerged. On May 2, Nicholas Wade, a former science reporter for the *New York Times*, self-published a magazine-length piece on Medium headlined "Origin of Covid—Following the Clues."[41]

The article concluded:

> Perhaps the international community of virologists will come to be seen as a false and self-interested guide. The common-sense perception that a pandemic breaking out in Wuhan might have something to do with a Wuhan lab cooking up novel viruses of maximal danger in unsafe conditions could eventually displace the ideological insistence that whatever Trump said can't be true.
>
> And then let the reckoning begin.

Wade's piece was thoughtful and well-written. But it contained almost no points that the lab leak contrarians had not made for more than a year. It simply arrived at the right time.

Just over three weeks later, on May 26, Biden ordered intelligence agencies to review what they knew about the origins of the virus.[42] (That review very predictably came to an inconclusive answer when it was released in August.)[43]

And, in an unapologetic about-face, Facebook announced that it was no longer censoring the theory. Facebook's statement was stunning. Social media companies were now announcing publicly which ideas they found acceptable and which they would prohibit.[44]

A few days later, some real news broke.

It was about a potential cover-up.

Not in China. In the United States.

BuzzFeed published an archive of emails to Fauci's official account at the National Institutes of Health, which the outlet had received through a Freedom of Information Act request. In what might have been the most overt display of bootlicking of Fauci in the entire epidemic (and the competition was fierce), many reporters treated the cache as little more than evidence of how hard he had been working.

"Fauci's Emails from the Pandemic Show His Stress-Filled Days," *People* magazine gushed.[45]

"Thousands of emails from and to Dr. Fauci reveal the weight that came with role as a rare source of frank honesty within the Trump administration's Covid-19 task force," CNN "reported" in a tweet.[46]

CNN was right, the mail dump was revealing. But what it revealed was not *frank honesty.*

Quite the contrary. The emails showed that, within *weeks* after it first emerged, Fauci had been warned that Sars-Cov-2 might have been genetically modified and leaked from a lab. On Friday, January 31, 2020, Kristian Andersen, a California virologist, had emailed Fauci to warn him that the genome of the virus had "unusual features...some of the features (potentially) look engineered."[47]

Within hours, Fauci had set up a conference call for the next day, which was a Saturday, with Andersen and other prominent virologists to discuss the email. Early Saturday morning, he also emailed Dr. Hugh Auchincloss, his deputy, a copy of the 2015 paper in which Ralph Baric had reported his coronavirus gain-of-function research he had conducted with the Wuhan lab's Shi Zhengli.

"Read this paper as well as the email that I will forward to you now," Fauci wrote. "You will have tasks today that must be done." (In one of my favorite Fauci moments, he then ended the email with a breezy "Thanks, Tony.")[48]

Fauci has never disclosed what the "tasks" he gave to Auchincloss were or what he discussed with Andersen and the other virologists on the conference call—which has never been released. But we do know that the coordinated campaign to discredit the lab leak theory began days later.

And the lead author of the March 17 letter published in Nature Medicine *that became the ur-text used against the leak theory was...*

Kristian Andersen. Yes, the same virologist who had told Fauci on January 31 that the virus appeared "engineered."

And the emails contained still more damning evidence, showing the central role that a man named Peter Daszak had played in trying to steer inquiries away from the lab leak. To say Daszak had a conflict of interest was an understatement. His non-profit, EcoHealth Alliance, had helped funnel money from the NIH to fund coronavirus research at the Wuhan lab.[49]

At best, the emails suggested that behind the scenes Fauci and top virologists and infectious disease researchers had had serious concerns about a lab leak—concerns based on a top virologist's observation that parts of the Sars-CoV-2 genome might have been artificially engineered—and acted in bad faith when they publicly dismissed it.

China might never have cooperated with an investigation no matter how much pressure the United States put on it, but our own public health officials had ensured that the scientific and medical community never even came together to demand that the Chinese open their doors. They had ensured China would have plenty of time to destroy whatever evidence it had.

This scandal was genuine, worthy of the world's best investigative reporters.

Who ignored it. The primary contribution of the *New York Times* to the story came on June 14, when it published a "conversation" with Kristian Andersen (calling it an interview would have been too confrontational, I suppose). Over email, Andersen explained that the concerns he had expressed privately to Fauci in January hadn't matched the public letter six weeks later because—well, because science.

But you could trust Andersen. After all, he said so!

"My comments and conclusions are strictly driven by scientific inquiry, and I strongly believe that careful, well-supported public messaging around complex topics is paramount," he claimed.

Best of all, the subhead of the hard-hitting "conversation" was this groundless assertion: "In early 2020, Kristian Andersen wrote to Anthony Fauci about the possibility of an engineered coronavirus. His research has since dispelled those suspicions."[50]

What research? Andersen was no closer to identifying a natural host for Sars-Cov-2 in June 2021 than he had been in January 2020. And any "research" he had done before supposedly changing his mind would have had to take place in a matter of weeks in the winter of 2020. This was not journalism but stenography, the equivalent of the *Vogue Arabia* interview in 2019 when Kayne West interviewed Kim Kardashian, his (then) wife.

But even with outlets such as the *Times* refusing to step forward, I thought the public discussion of the lab leak was a hopeful sign, as was as the fact that Facebook had backed off on its censorship. Media outlets were once again acknowledging realities that I and other skeptics had hammered since the start of the epidemic.

With the fight over Covid vaccines heating up, I hoped I was seeing a new commitment to the truth from both social and legacy media outlets.

I was about to learn how wrong I was.

34

Dodging Bullets

At the risk of sounding like an uncool fifth grader, I thought Twitter was my *frieeend*.

For more than a year, I had used its service to put out scientific studies, government data, news articles, and emails from readers about Covid—with a dollop of cynicism and sarcasm. Sometimes two dollops.

My audience reached roughly a quarter-million followers around Election Day 2020. It shrank for a while as Twitter purged right-wing bots (and live conservatives angrily unfollowed me after I said Trump hadn't won). But by spring 2021 it was growing again.

Twitter didn't pay me. But it gave me access to its audience of 200 million daily users.[1] I could tell them about the *Unreported Truths* booklets—which were not free.

I didn't pay Twitter. But my tweets engaged readers, pro and con, helping Twitter sell ads.

A fair deal, as far as I was concerned.

Most of all, Twitter *let me write*.

After Amazon tried to ban the first *Unreported Truths* booklet in June 2020, I feared big tech and social media censorship. In particular, I knew how Facebook treated users and posts that didn't fit its preferred story line. *There is so much peace to be found in people's faces…. I love people's faces.*[2]

Facebook sure did love faces, especially when Mark Zuckerberg was taking his cut for matching them up. Facts, not so much.

I made halting efforts at a safety valve in case Twitter suppressed me. In late 2020 I set up accounts on Telegram, a secure messaging app, and Parler, a conservative competitor to Twitter. But I used the Telegram account so little I lost it for inactivity. I hardly posted to Parler either. In any case, my account vanished after Amazon pulled Parler's web hosting and forced it offline in January 2021.[3]

Once again Twitter was my only outlet.

I was less worried than I should have been. Twitter seemed to allow unpopular opinions about Covid in a way that Facebook and YouTube did not. I lauded Twitter for doing so, both in tweets and television interviews. I hoped to encourage it.

And I believed Twitter appreciated my presence. My audience was not enormous by the company's standards. Some celebrities had tens of millions of followers. But my readers were very engaged, and my rise to prominence as a lockdown skeptic showed the platform's power. All by itself, my presence on Twitter had given me influence, though I didn't work for the *Times* anymore, or any legacy media company.

As my profile rose in 2020, Brandon Borrman—at the time Twitter's head of communications—emailed me for a productive conversation about Twitter's attitude toward speech and open discussion. Jack Dorsey, Twitter's founder, even followed me for a while (I'm not sure for how long, or if he ever stopped).

Twitter was never easy. I had lots of hate-readers. They pored over my feed, looking for errors and failed predictions.[4] Blue checks I wished I had the time to sue called me a grifter and a liar on a near constant basis—though they rarely offered specific examples of my supposed lies.

The death wishes kept coming too. Those were ugly, but I saw them as the price for speaking out. (Active threats like the one I mentioned in chapter 32 were different. I tried to report those. Twitter generally removed them, if not as quickly as I hoped.)

At the same time, I had a large and loud core of fans. By mid-2021, I often didn't even have to engage with people attacking me. Readers did so on their own. And my email continued to be overwhelmingly positive, almost shockingly so.

I grew to believe that much of the anger that came at me on Twitter was performative, from blue checks who feared I was right but saw no advantage in finding out for sure. How else to explain their attacks, which so often came down to *nah nah grifter, nah nah nah liar, vaccines work—science!*

Readers sometimes encouraged me to move to Gab or Gettr, which became Twitter's top conservative competitors after Amazon vaporized Parler. I would find a friendlier audience there, they said.

But I didn't want to preach only to the converted. The chance to engage and hopefully persuade people who disagreed was another reason staying on Twitter mattered to me. And I knew I was having an impact. Governments and agencies and media outlets responded to my tweets, even if they would not admit doing so.

One example came on June 21, 2021, when I pointed out the World Health Organization's website recommended against Covid vaccinations for anyone under eighteen—in contradiction to American policy advising kids twelve to seventeen to be vaccinated.

The WHO page explained:

Children should not be vaccinated for the moment.
There is not yet enough evidence on the use of vaccines against COVID-19 in children to make recommendations for children to be vaccinated against COVID-19. Children and adolescents tend to have milder disease compared to adults. [emphasis in the original][5]

I tweeted: "Fun fact: @who still recommends AGAINST vaccine for anyone under 18.... In completely unrelated news, Pfizer will not be hiring anyone from WHO this year."[6]

The tweet encapsulated the way I used Twitter. It was factually accurate, and it was from an official source that until now had gone unnoticed, but it also had a cynical streak.

It landed hard. Versions of what I'd written made their way around Instagram and Facebook.

The next day, June 22, the WHO rewrote its webpage in a classic politically motivated walk-back. The new recommendation had muddier language—but reached essentially the same conclusion:

> Children and adolescents tend to have milder disease compared to adults, so unless they are part of a group at higher risk of severe COVID-19, **it is less urgent to vaccinate them than older people,** those with chronic health conditions and health workers.
>
> **More evidence is needed** on the use of the different COVID-19 vaccines in children to be able to make general recommendations on vaccinating children against COVID-19. [emphasis added][7]

Within days, the woke "fact-checkers" showed up. As usual, they could not dispute the accuracy of my original tweet. Instead, they tried to explain it away. They claimed the WHO hadn't meant, "Children should not be vaccinated for the moment. There is not yet enough evidence," when it had used those exact words.

No, supposedly it was just trying to save vaccines for older people.

"The WHO has explained that vaccine supply is scarce in certain countries, which is why the agency made this recommendation," *USA Today* claimed on June 25.[8]

The spin was both shameless and silly. Anyone who knew how to use an internet archive could see first-hand that my original tweet had been correct. This was twenty-first-century journalism at its worst, politicized opinion masquerading as supposedly neutral fact-checking.

Except people weren't fooled. My reach grew and grew. By August I had almost 345,000 followers, and the growth was accelerating.

And month after month, I focused on the vaccines: their effectiveness, their side effects, whether they made sense for children, the logic of mandating them. I tracked the data as closely as I could before I published the fourth *Unreported Truths* booklet in late March—and after, too.

As the spring progressed, the truth, the very heavily reported truth, was that the vaccines seemed to be working.

Again, Israel and Britain proved key. Cases, hospitalizations, and deaths in both countries plunged from March through May. I wasn't entirely convinced the drop was due to the vaccines. Covid had proven strongly seasonal in 2020. And it typically rolled in and out in two- to four-month stretches. The natural ebb and flow of the epidemic might well have been partly responsible for the decline. On Twitter, I compared Israel to Southern California, which had a similar climate and had also seen a sharp drop in cases in late winter following its earlier spike.

Still, the Israeli trends were undeniable and powerful. Positive tests fell from 3,700 a day at the end of February to 33 by mid-May—a 99 percent drop in 10 weeks. Daily deaths went from 25 to 1 over the same span.[9]

Online and off, vaccine advocates crowed about the country's success. As early as mid-March, Israel's health minister referred to the "vaccination miracle."[10] The *New York Times* headlined an April 5 piece "'Like a Miracle': Israel's Vaccine Success Allows Easter Crowds in Jerusalem."[11]

Someone on Twitter asked me on April 4 what evidence out of Israel would convince me the vaccines worked. My answer:

> A big new wave that skips Israel (the current spike in parts of Europe/Middle East does not count as it is likely related to first-dose vaccinations).

The better question is: what will it take for you [**the original tweeter**] to admit I'm right [**that is, the vaccines aren't
working long-term**]? A rise in all-cause mortality? A "variant"
wave in Israel? [Bracketed material added for context]

At the time this response probably seemed defensive.

The good news in the spring wasn't confined to Israel. The CDC
reported on March 29 that the vaccines were more than 90 percent effective in a group of almost four thousand American first responders.
"Authorized mRNA COVID-19 vaccines are effective for preventing
SARS-Cov-2 infection in real world conditions," the agency's scientists
wrote.[12]

Three days later came the nastiest attack on me yet, Derek Thompson's piece in *The Atlantic* calling me "The Pandemic's Wrongest Man."
I had spent a year lampooning the magazine on Twitter. Thompson did
his best to return the favor.

In a four-thousand-word piece, he attacked a series of straw men
that had little to do with my core concerns about the vaccines. As I had
explained repeatedly—including in my new *Unreported Truths*
booklet—Pfizer and Moderna had not enrolled the people most at risk
in their clinical trials. Thus we had no idea if the vaccines would largely
eliminate deaths and serious illnesses as vaccine advocates had
promised.

Further, the companies and advocates had obviously played down
vaccine side effects. Both the clinical trials and the real-world VAERS
data suggested they were more severe than those posed by most other
vaccines, particularly the flu vaccines, the closest benchmark. Given that
Covid posed minimal risks to most healthy adults, a fair discussion of
the cost-benefit analysis of vaccines had to include those side effects.

Instead of addressing my concerns head-on, Thompson swiped near
randomly at them.

He attacked me for saying Covid cases had risen in countries after
vaccination campaigns began—but either failed or pretended not to

understand that I was specifically referring to the first two weeks after the first dose. He spent hundreds of words on a discussion of how the pharmaceutical companies had counted cases during the trials, an issue of almost no interest to me, and one I hadn't even mentioned in the booklet.[13]

Thompson emailed me questions weeks before his piece came out. Though I was sure his motives were unfriendly, I answered them seriously. When he asked if I thought people over or under 50 should be vaccinated, for example, I explained, "For most healthy people under 50—and certainly under 35—the side effects from the shots are likely to be worse than a case of Covid. Over 70, sure. The grey zone is somewhere in the middle and probably depends on personal risk factors."

In general, a first round of questions for an article like this is just that—a first round. When I worked for the *Times*, I never wrote articles without telling their subjects all the questions I intended to raise, in enough detail that nothing would surprise them. The more deeply I was investigating, the more chances to respond I offered.

That's journalism at its most basic.

It used to be, anyway.

Thompson asked no follow-up questions after his initial email. He gave me no chance to clarify answers he found incomplete or baffling. He simply took my first batch of answers and looked for holes in them, even if he had to twist my words to do so. For example, when he referred to my email about the ages of people I thought might need the vaccine, he ignored that I had specified healthy adults—a crucial distinction, and one I was always careful to make.

I gave Thompson credit for being a serious reporter, one who would consider my answers honestly. That's why I answered him. Had he sent more questions, I would have answered those too.

But I was wrong. He wasn't a serious reporter. He had the piece pre-written (in his mind, at least) before he contacted me. I had wasted my time by talking to him at all.

The Team Apocalypse blue checks didn't want to face the reality that I was not shouting about tracking chips or population control. I scored points with sharp-tongued sarcasm on Twitter, but I stuck to the facts—on Twitter, on television, in the booklets, and in this book.

Thompson preferred to argue with a caricature. His piece ended, "The case for the vaccines is built upon a firm foundation of scientific discovery, clinical-trial data, and real-world evidence. The case against the vaccines wobbles because it is built upon a steaming pile of bullshit."

Time—not much time—would prove extremely unkind to these sentences, and to Thompson. His piece came out on April Fool's Day.

Soon enough, that publication date would seem unintentionally ironic.

But for the next couple of months I had to take my lumps.

As the summer approached, the United States followed Israel and the United Kingdom into what I would later call the "happy vaccine valley"—the months after the second mRNA dose when Covid vaccines generated enough antibodies to work, even in older people. (Coincidentally or not, the happy vaccine valley lasted almost exactly as long as the major clinical trials that Pfizer and Moderna had run. Big Pharma is lots of things, but it's not dumb.)

Across the United States, cases, hospitalizations, and deaths plunged. After peaking at 250,000 a day in January, positive tests fell to 70,000 by mid-April, then took another leg down and bottomed around 12,500 a day in mid-June. Deaths fell from 3,500 a day in late January to about 260 at the end of June.[14]

Seasonality likely drove much of the early decline. Vaccines could have played only a small role—deaths fell by almost two-thirds before mid-March, when fewer than one in eight Americans were fully vaccinated. But the spring drop did appear to be vaccine-related.

In any case, vaccine advocates gave the shots all the credit.

Still, they couldn't convince everyone. The number of Americans receiving vaccinations plunged after mid-April. Two factors drove this apparent paradox. The people most willing to be vaccinated had already gotten the shots by that point. And on April 13 regulators briefly suspended use of the Johnson & Johnson vaccine when several young women suffered from a rare blood clotting condition after receiving it.[15]

Though the Johnson & Johnson vaccine used different biotechnology from the Pfizer and Moderna vaccines, the incident highlighted safety concerns about all the vaccines. Those rose further in May, when regulators acknowledged that the mRNA vaccines appeared linked to heart problems in young men. After reaching almost four million a day in mid-April for all three vaccines, vaccinations fell to under one million in late June.[16]

Nonetheless, vaccine advocates grew more excited through the spring. Even the drug companies, which had mostly allowed governments to carry their water while they remained in the background, became more publicly confident.

On April 28, Dr. Ugur Sahin—the chief executive of BioNTech, the German company that had developed the mRNA vaccine that Pfizer sells—said he expected European countries to reach herd immunity by August.

Sahin "cited studies from Israel, which shares medical data on its vaccination campaign with Pfizer, showing that people who have been immunized rarely fall seriously ill and are significantly less likely to transmit the virus."[17]

Three weeks later, Monica Gandhi revisited her January tweet predicting that vaccines prevented both "disease and spreading"[18]—infection and transmission. Pointing to a dozen studies that seemed to show how well the vaccines worked, she wrote,

> Good to see this January 9 tweet has so much evidence behind it now in real world that vaccines block transmission since biological plausibility was ample.[19]

As chest-thumping from vaccine advocates went, Monica's tweet was mild.

May 12: *Fortune* names the chief executives of Pfizer, Moderna, and BioNTech among the "World's Greatest Leaders" "for the mRNA COVID vaccine miracle."[20]

May 20: In an interview headlined "Leadership during Crisis," Fauci tells the *Washington Post*, "I don't think we should be that concerned right now about how long they're effective. I think they will be effective long enough that we will get to the point where we are not going to be necessarily worrying about a surge."[21]

May 22: CNBC says, "Yes, it's going to be a hot vax summer."[22]

May 25: CNN explains "A vaccine marvel is bringing America back.... The near-miraculous vaccines have the virus—which has ravaged the nation—in retreat. Deserted cities that once echoed at night to the wail of ambulance sirens are stirring. Travelers are taking to skies and once again filling un-mothballed jets. Life, nervously for many—and unbelievably for almost all—is being restored."[23]

On and on the hosannahs went.

On and on and on.

Western Europeans complained their governments had fallen behind in the vaccine race and then dutifully lined up for their shots, rapidly closing on the United States.[24] Vaccine equity turned into the next big fight: How quickly would poorer countries share in the miracle?[25]

Still, the vaccine fanatics were not satisfied. In late spring, more than 100 million American adults refused to partake, a fact that annoyed them terribly. Why wouldn't these mouth-breathers trust the science? What would convince them?

"How to Talk to Someone Who's Hesitant to Get the COVID-19 Vaccine," the *US News & World Report* explained to its readers on May 12. "Some people have legitimate reasons for being cautious."[26] This formulation basically meant African Americans were allowed to have extra questions about the vaccine because of the hideous Tuskegee experiment, in which the federal government deliberately left a group of black men with syphilis untreated *for forty years*.[27] But white people had no excuse—especially if they had voted for Trump.

"Tennessee, like much of the nation, is finding that rural, white residents need a little more coaxing," NPR explained in mid-April, dripping with fake folksiness.[28]

"Our best way out of this is clearly vaccines," John Oliver, the HBO host who is the walking, talking embodiment of woke leftist condescension, said on his show on May 2. "We badly need to convince anyone who can be convinced."[29]

"The 'Vaccine Hesitant' Are a Threat to Society. But We Must Show Them Compassion," a column in the *Globe and Mail*—Canada's preeminent newspaper—urged on May 7.[30]

This formulation made little sense. Hospitalizations and deaths were plunging. If the vaccines worked as well as advertised, the unvaccinated threatened only themselves—and the small number of people already too ill to risk the vaccine, or too immunocompromised to have any vaccine response. The argument that unvaccinated adults posed a danger to children was essentially a lie, given Covid's microscopic risk to kids who were not already gravely ill.

Some public health experts claimed unvaccinated people might become walking petri dishes for the virus, allowing it to mutate after they were infected. "Fauci: Vaccinations Will Help Coronavirus Variants from Emerging," a CNN headline reported in January.[31]

This theory ignored the fact that viruses—including coronaviruses—naturally tend to evolve in ways that make them more contagious but less dangerous. Viruses spread most widely when they don't kill or even severely sicken their hosts.

It also ignored that Sars-Cov-2 could mutate in *vaccinated* people too—and, if it did, would almost by definition change in ways that made vaccines less effective. As two (strongly pro-vaccine) physicians had explained in the *Journal of the American Medical Association* in January: "'Escape mutations' typically arise when the virus is put under selective pressure by antibodies that limit but do not eliminate viral replication. Under these conditions, the virus might then find a way to escape this pressure and restore its ability to reproduce more efficiently."[32]

In reality, as with everything else related to Covid, the elite insistence on vaccinations seemed to arise from motivations as much sociological as scientific. *We know what's best, dummies! Don't make us tell you again! If the magic shot is good enough for us, it's good enough for you.*

Spring saw states and companies roll out incentive campaigns to convince the hesitant—each more condescending than the next. Budweiser and the White House promised "a shot and a beer."[33] States offered lotteries, with prizes of up to $5 million.[34] Detroit offered a $50 debit card for anyone who drove someone else to a vaccination site. Uber provided free rides.[35]

I found the campaigns risible, especially the lotteries. The vaccines were still not close to actual Food and Drug Administration approval. Giving people money to take an experimental medical treatment was borderline unethical.

In any case, the campaigns made no difference. Vaccinations kept declining, and a research letter in the *Journal of the American Medical Association* in July found Ohio lottery incentives were not "associated with increased rates of adult COVID-19 vaccinations."[36] People had no interest in trading their medical rights for a bottle of Bud or a scratch-off ticket.

Even as the elites on both left and right grew frustrated with Americans who did not want vaccines, Biden and other top Democrats, as well as public health advocates, made clear they would not impose Covid vaccine mandates or passports.

As early as December 4, 2020, Biden had ruled out requiring vaccines. "I don't think it should be mandatory," he said. "I wouldn't demand it to be mandatory."[37]

Almost five months later, on April 29, 2021, House Speaker Nancy Pelosi said at a press conference, "So here's the thing, we cannot require someone to be vaccinated. That's just not what we can do. It is a matter of privacy to know who is or who isn't.... We can't require vaccinations for the members, much less for the American people."[38]

On June 9, Dr. Vivek Murthy, the surgeon general, told an NPR listener, "We do not anticipate a federal mandate for vaccinations. So I would not anticipate any direction for the federal government telling your university that they should require you to get a vaccine."[39]

The general attitude of the left's political leaders seemed to be that eventually everyone—or nearly everyone—would see the wonder of this scientific miracle and decide to be vaccinated.

After all, the hardcore anti-vaccine community was relatively small. In 2019, more than 90 percent of American kids had received polio, measles, chickenpox, and hepatitis vaccines by the time they were two years old, CDC data showed. Despite warnings about vaccine hesitancy, the percentages had generally increased slightly over the previous five years.[40]

Just keep advertising and marketing and offering incentives to chip away at the "vaccine hesitant." Sooner or later, the controversy would fade as people on the fence saw for themselves how well the vaccines worked, and we'd all have a Hot Vaxxed Summer.

It was a good plan.

It had just one flaw.

The vaccines were failing.

The sudden collapse of mRNA vaccine efficacy in the summer of 2021 belongs as much to Shakespeare or Sophocles as to science. It was hubris meeting nemesis on the biggest possible stage, the best and the brightest outdoing themselves once more, Icarus smirking at thirty thousand feet, waving at the sun as his wings drip away.

Pride goeth before a fall.

The problems first showed up in Israel.

Positive tests bottomed in early June at around fifteen a day, a tiny number in a country of ten million people. But in the second half of June they began rising. On June 30, Israel had almost three hundred positive tests nationwide. On July 15, it had almost a thousand. By July 31, it was near three thousand.[41]

Cases had risen nearly ten-fold in a month, close to two-hundred-fold in two months.

Britain followed the same trend—although the situation was more complicated there because the British had a "casedemic" caused by cheap and widely available non-PCR tests.

As cases rose, vaccine fanatics explained the shots were not really failing. Hospitalizations and deaths were still low, they said. They had never promised that the vaccines would stop infection or transmission, much less eliminate or nearly eliminate Covid.

They were lying. In his May 20 interview with the *Washington Post*—just weeks before the vaccine failure began—Fauci had said the vaccines might allow the United States not just to reduce Covid to a handful of cases but end it entirely: "With good vaccination programs, [countries can] essentially eliminate the presence of a particular pathogen.... That's called elimination, and the other is control. You have a very, very low level in the community . . . enough to know you haven't completely eliminated it.... With Sars-Cov-2 and with COVID-19, I would hope it would be much closer to elimination than just control."[42]

In any case, the new attempt to move the goalposts became "inoperative"—in the famous term from the Nixon White House—soon enough. Hospitalizations of vaccinated people quickly followed cases higher. By early August, deaths did too.

Since they had to admit vaccinated people were becoming ill and dying, the advocates moved the goalposts again. Unvaccinated people were still becoming sick at higher rates than the vaccinated, they said. The vaccines were still somewhat protective.

This statement was correct, but it failed to account for a crucial factor that likely made vaccine protection seem stronger than it was. Vaccination rates were so high among the elderly in Israel and Britain that the unvaccinated and vaccinated populations could not be easily compared—many of the unvaccinated people over seventy or eighty in those two countries had probably not received a shot only because they were so frail that *it was too dangerous to vaccinate them*. And if they were too sick to receive a vaccine, then they were also already at very high risk of dying from Covid—higher risk than the vaccinated people their age.

A similar phenomenon was already known to occur with influenza vaccines. Older people who received the flu shot were less likely to die after they received it than those who didn't get the shot. But a landmark 2006 study in the *International Journal of Epidemiology* found they were also less likely to die *before* they received it. The flu shot was a *marker* for health, not a driver of health. People who got the influenza vaccine were healthier than those who did not.[43]

This was a classic epidemiological problem—and yet another reason why randomized controlled trials are the only foolproof way to judge whether a drug actually works.

As the summer went on, the coronavirus vaccine advocates continued to insist the shots worked very well against severe disease. Yet Britain and Israel belied their claims. Covid deaths in both countries continued to rise—among vaccinated as well as unvaccinated people.

The *total* number of Covid deaths in Britain was far higher in August and September 2021 than in the same months in 2020—when the vaccines hadn't existed at all, except in clinical trials. The vaccine failure was so profound it even overwhelmed Covid's typical seasonality. And British government statistics showed close to 70 percent of the dead were fully vaccinated. Another 5 percent had had at least one dose.[44]

Epidemiologists and virologists scrambled to explain why the vaccines had lost their protective effect so quickly.

The core problem seemed to be that the anti–spike protein antibodies that vaccinations caused the body to produce declined very fast. A paper out of Israel showed they decreased at up to 40 percent per month. Antibodies produced in response to natural infection peaked at lower levels but declined much more slowly.[45]

Meanwhile, the long-term immunity that vaccines provided through B- and T-cells was both weak and narrowly focused. Even narrow mutations in Sars-Cov-2 could overcome it easily. Natural immunity from coronavirus infection and recovery caused appeared far broader and superior. Rockefeller University researchers reported in August:

> While vaccination gives rise to memory B cells that evolve over a few weeks, natural infection births memory B cells that continue to evolve over several months, producing highly potent antibodies adept at eliminating even viral variants.
>
> The findings highlight an advantage bestowed by natural infection rather than vaccination.[46]

A large Israeli study showed that the theoretical advantage Rockefeller had found for natural immunity was very real. Posted on August 25, the study revealed that people who were vaccinated were thirteen times as likely to be infected with Sars-Cov-2 as those who had natural immunity following a previous infection. From June 1 to August 14, only nineteen out of sixteen thousand people with natural immunity were reinfected.[47]

"It's a textbook example of how natural immunity is really better than vaccination," a Swedish researcher told *Science* magazine.[48]

But scientists needed to do much more to understand why the vaccines had failed so badly. The crisis occurred so quickly that even in September they were not sure how much of a role the Delta variant had played and how much was simply a function of waning immunity over time.

As July continued, the United States followed Israel and Britain out of the happy vaccine valley, and the fourth American coronavirus wave began.

As I wrote over and over on Twitter, this trend shouldn't have surprised anyone. Human biology was the same everywhere. In early September, Philip Dormitzer, the chief scientific officer at Pfizer, would call Israel a "laboratory" for the company's vaccine. He added that Israel had "immunized a very high proportion of the population very early—so it's been a way that we can almost look ahead: What we see happening in Israel happens again in the US a couple months later."[49]

And unlike Britain or Israel, the United States—at least the Sunbelt—had seasonality working *against* it in the summer.

Sure enough, new American cases rose relentlessly, jumping from roughly 15,000 positive tests on July 5 to roughly 165,000 in early September. Deaths inevitably followed. After bottoming around 300 a day in mid-July, they topped 1,600 by mid-September.[50]

Vaccine advocates in the United States dealt with this failure in the most disingenuous way possible—by blaming it on unvaccinated people.

They were lying. I don't like using the word lie, but I have to. Nothing else fits. Fauci and Surgeon General Vivek Murthy both pretended that 97 or even 99 percent of American hospitalizations and deaths were in unvaccinated people.[51]

As early as May, this statement was provably untrue. An internal CDC paper reported that 15 percent of deaths in hospitals tracked by the agency were in fully vaccinated people, up from 2 percent in February. The document, reported in the *Washington Post*, found "an increasing percentage of vaccinated persons among those hospitalized."[52] Data from individual states and cities also belied the 99 percent figure, as I reported in late July.[53]

Public health officials created the 99 percent figure by comparing the number of vaccinated people who had died of Covid to *all* deaths that had occurred since vaccinations began in December 2020 (or sometimes January 1, 2021).

This statistical artifice obscured the fact that the vast majority of those deaths had occurred in the winter, when almost no one was vaccinated.

Maybe the vaccines would have protected those people. Maybe not. *No one could know, since they hadn't received them.* The only reason to include their deaths in a comparison purporting to demonstrate how well the vaccines were working six months later was to make the vaccines look better—as even the dumbest public health experts surely knew.

To understand how well the vaccines were or were not working in July and August and September, we needed real-time data from July and August and September. We didn't have it.

While Israel and Britain published transparent figures on vaccinated and unvaccinated infections and deaths on a weekly or even daily basis, the Centers for Disease Control and most state health departments in the United States did not. The CDC had even stopped counting infections in non-hospitalized vaccinated people on May 1, a bizarre decision that made tracking the performance of the vaccines nearly impossible.[54]

Fortunately, we had the international data, which made the reality of vaccine failure impossible to deny.

To be sure, the percentage of people dying of Covid in the United States in September who were unvaccinated was significantly higher than 25 percent, the British figure. But then, the United States had a higher overall percentage of unvaccinated people.

It may also have had an even more severe confounding issue than other countries. In other words, after accounting for age, the people at lowest risk from Covid were probably the *most* likely to be vaccinated. Polls showed that unvaccinated people were *less* afraid to travel, go to the gym, or eat at restaurants than the vaccinated.[55]

But the idea that the summer surge was a "pandemic of the unvaccinated"—as Biden and other Democrats and public health officials said over and over[56]—was simply untrue.

The vast majority of Americans over sixty-five were vaccinated. If vaccines worked nearly as well as public health authorities pretended, we simply wouldn't have had enough vulnerable people to put a strain on the health care system, especially since many unvaccinated people had natural immunity from previous infection.

The effort to deny reality led to absurdities, such as the August 31 *Washington Post* headline about vaccinated people who had so-called "breakthrough" infections: "They're called mild cases. But people with breakthrough covid can still feel pretty sick."[57]

No matter. All the spin in the world could not hide the fact that mRNA vaccine protection eroded a little more each day.

But the endless political and media untruths did have a serious real-world impact. They led to a widening schism, as vaccinated people grew increasingly angry. The vaccinated were no longer complacent and condescending, as they had been in the spring. Now they were frightened, and their fear needed an outlet.

They found it in unvaccinated people. "The Anger toward Unvaccinated People Is Personal for Some Who Got Breakthrough COVID," NPR reported on August 13.[58]

The families of vaccinated people who had died from Covid blamed unvaccinated Americans—*all* unvaccinated Americans, apparently—for the infections. Journalists repeated their complaints without question. "An Iowa woman whose husband died from a breakthrough COVID-19 infection is blaming Americans who refuse to mask or get vaccinated," the Associated Press reported on September 14, and there were many similar articles.[59]

Instead of telling the truth about vaccine failure, Biden and other leaders *encouraged this attitude.*

"Our patience is wearing thin," the man I had come to call "Uncle Joe" said on September 9.[60] Biden seemed willing to blame any problem he faced on the unvaccinated. Six days earlier he had complained that they were responsible for a dismal report about August job growth. As CNBC reported:

> Biden said that group [of unvaccinated people] is prolonging the pandemic and contributing to anxieties that impact the economy.
>
> "This is a continuing pandemic of the unvaccinated," the president said. "Too many have not gotten vaccinated, and it's creating a lot of unease in our economy and around our kitchen tables."

Of course, the United States had suffered similar sorry episodes before. Japanese Americans had been interned by the federal government during World War II. African Americans had been treated as second-class citizens under the laws of southern states for much of the twentieth century.

What made this scapegoating of the unvaccinated astonishing was not just that it ran counter to scientific facts and common sense—if the vaccines worked, why did the vaccinated need protection so desperately? —but that the very people who held themselves up as society's most tolerant were leading it.

For generations, public health leaders had preached tolerance— tolerance for gay men with AIDS, tolerance for drug addicts (a term that was no longer even acceptable), tolerance for alcoholics and smokers and the morbidly obese. Their problems belonged to all of us, we were told. They deserved the best possible care, without a smidgen of judgement.

Yet this tolerance did not extend to people who chose not to take vaccines. *New York Times* contributing writer Frank Bruni demanded that unvaccinated people be segregated in restaurants and elsewhere:

> What if the willfully, proudly, stubbornly unvaccinated —people who have access to shots and no rational medical exemption but still won't get them—were ever more frustrated as they sought their pleasures and ever more inconvenienced as they ran their errands? Would that wear down the resistance of at least a few of them? Isn't it worth trying?[61]

Academics suggested that people who refused to be vaccinated should be denied insurance coverage if they were hospitalized for Covid[62]—or, even more bizarrely, be forced to pay for care for *other people* they had supposedly infected.[63]

Worse, elite media outlets began to debate publicly whether unvaccinated people should be *denied medical care* (though they usually grudgingly answered no.) "Do the unvaccinated deserve scarce ICU beds?" a September 1 *Washington Post* opinion piece asked.[64]

If the vaccine failure was Shakespearean, what happened next came straight out of Joseph Heller.

After almost a year of promising he would not, President Biden decided to mandate vaccines after all. On September 9, he announced that federal workplace safety rules would require businesses with more than one hundred employees to make their employees be vaccinated.[65]

Never mind the patent absurdity of a rule that applied only to large employers. Was Sars-Cov-2 dangerous to greeters at Wal-Mart, but not the clerk at a local bookstore? To associates at big law firms but not the administrative assistant who worked with a sole practitioner?

Never mind the fact that the rule may have overstepped Biden's executive branch authority and faced immediate legal challenges.[66]

Never mind that the science behind the theory—that unvaccinated people represented a special threat to the vaccinated that needed to be neutralized—appeared to be murky. On August 24, researchers in Wisconsin had posted a study showing vaccinated people were just as likely to be carrying infectious virus as the unvaccinated. But the vaccinated were *more* likely to show no symptoms. "Even asymptomatic, fully vaccinated people might shed infectious virus," the authors concluded.[67]

The plan failed to answer a basic question: *If vaccines were failing within months, why had the government decided to push them harder?*

Wouldn't pausing to consider whether using them at all make more sense?

I wanted to view the decision to increase the mandate pressure just when vaccine failure became obvious as ironic, not sinister.

But plenty of my readers did not agree.

Alongside the mandate came a push for "boosters"—and more evidence that the Biden administration had politicized the science around Covid far more than Donald Trump could have dreamed.

Moderna and Pfizer-BioNTech had designed the mRNA vaccines to be administered in two doses, with the doses given three or four weeks apart. The companies had tested the vaccines in their pivotal clinical trials as a two-dose regimen.

Nonetheless, as vaccine efficacy collapsed and Israel's Covid wards began to fill in July, Israel moved abruptly to administer a third "booster" dose. The country pressed boosters not just to the extremely elderly or the immunocompromised, but to everyone.

This strategy was essentially untested.

Neither Pfizer nor Moderna had run placebo-controlled trials on boosters. In fact, at the time Israel began its booster program, the publicly available data about a third dose covered a few *dozen* people. Boosters clearly provided a short-term increase in antibodies against the spike protein. But no one knew how long it might last or what the side effects or long-term risks might be.

Nonetheless, the uncertainties did not stop the Biden administration from unveiling its own plan for a third dose on August 16, only weeks after the Israeli campaign started.[68] The speed with which the White House moved was the surest signal yet that the Biden administration understood how quickly the vaccines were failing.

Originally, the administration said people would need a third dose after eight months. But on August 27, Biden and Fauci said boosters might actually be recommended after *five* months.[69] (In his interview with the *Washington Post* in May, at the height of peak overconfidence in the vaccines, Fauci had said boosters might not be needed at all.) Even the flu vaccine was only offered annually—and it had side effects far less serious than those of the mRNA vaccines. Meanwhile, Israel was already preparing its citizens for a *fourth* dose.[70]

But Biden was not only *recommending* boosters. He had promised they would be available on a specific day—Monday, September 20. Yet when he made the announcement, neither the Food and Drug Administration nor the Centers for Disease Control had approved boosters at all.

Then, on August 31, two top FDA vaccine regulators said they were leaving the agency.[71]

Two weeks later they cosigned a letter to *The Lancet*, perhaps the world's top medical journal, saying they did not believe boosters were needed for most people. "The currently available evidence does not show the need for widespread use of booster vaccination," they wrote.[72]

I could only imagine how the media would have reacted if Trump had promised boosters before regulators signed off. The rules were different for Biden. The fact that his own regulators had quit in the face of his plan somehow became a curiosity rather than a scandal.

The White House plowed ahead, even in the face of rising scientific opposition. Then an FDA advisory panel resoundingly rejected boosters for the general population on September 17—just three days before the Biden administration had said they would be available. Although the panel did recommend them for people over sixty-five, its decision marked a public rebuke for Biden and Dr. Anthony Fauci, who had publicly pushed boosters for everyone.[73]

For the first time since the epidemic began, independent scientists had stood up to Fauci's overreach. But the efforts by Biden and Fauci to push Covid vaccines on everyone—including healthy children and adults—would continue.

By July and August, I had grown more concerned about the vaccines than ever. Alongside their declining effectiveness and the data showing the superiority of natural immunity, their "tail risks" appeared to be rising. A tail risk is one that is unlikely to happen but will have enormous consequences if it does. A plane crash is a tail risk of flying.

For vaccines, two tail risks were clear. The first was a Marek's disease–leaky vaccine scenario in which the vaccinated would become dangerous to the unvaccinated. The second was antibody dependent enhancement, or ADE, the true horror, in which the shots would not just fail but actually increase the dangers of new variants for the vaccinated.

To be clear, both still appeared unlikely—and ADE very unlikely. But the evidence for both was increasing.[74]

As I continued to ask questions on Twitter, I hoped my demonstrated record of accuracy would help protect me. And no one who looked at the data could doubt that, at best, vaccine protection was declining fast.

But I failed to understand how aggressively the White House wanted to censor dissent—and the weakness of Twitter's supposed commitment to free speech.

As late as March 2021, well after I became a leading voice raising questions about the vaccines, I was still in touch with Brandon Borrman of Twitter. On March 1, Twitter announced that it would implement a "five-strike" policy to combat Covid "misinformation." The next day, I emailed Borrman:

> Just following up on this in the wake of Twitter's announcement yesterday. I intend to continue to write about the vaccines—as always, with a heavy reliance on governmental data (whether from Israel, the US, or elsewhere) and published studies.
>
> I appreciate the fact that Twitter has allowed me to provide a risk-benefit analysis that people are generally not seeing elsewhere and I respect that you do not want conspiracy theories, etc, on the site. If your fact-checkers do have questions about something I've written, I hope you will let me know and give me a chance to respond to it before taking any action.

Borrman responded later that day: "Thanks for reaching out. I will say that your name has never come up in the discussions around these policies. If it does I will try to ensure you're given a heads up before an action is taken, but I am not always made aware of them before they're executed. If something happens, please let me know."

With this assurance, over the next four months, I tweeted hundreds (perhaps thousands) of times, about the vaccines: about an African

American college student who had died of heart failure shortly after being vaccinated, about the CDC's data on myocarditis, about the tens of billions of dollars in profits that Pfizer and BioNTech and Moderna were making.

Twitter knew exactly what I was doing. Not only did my tweets regularly attract thousands of likes and retweets and millions of views, blue checks with even larger audiences than mine complained about me. Calls for the service to ban my account were frequent.

Twitter did put a misleading tag on one of my tweets in May. I complained about it to Borrman—in our last conversation before he left the company in June. He said he'd look into it.

But even after Twitter began to tag other tweets of mine as "misleading" (they were not), it did not warn me that I was accumulating strikes under its five-strike rule. Under their rule, the strikes began with a warning, followed by two twelve-hour suspensions. The fourth strike was a week-long suspension, and the fifth the permanent ban.

Then, on Thursday, July 15, at a White House briefing, Biden's press secretary Jen Psaki and Surgeon General Vivek Murthy complained about "misinformation" and "disinformation" on social media.[75] Murthy called explicitly for censorship from Facebook, Twitter, and other social media outlets: "We're saying we expect more from our technology companies. We're asking them to operate with greater transparency and accountability. We're asking them to monitor misinformation more closely. We're asking them to consistently take action against misinformation super-spreaders on their platforms."

In response to a follow-up question, Murthy added, "All of us have an important role here to play, and technology companies have a particularly important role."

On the morning of July 16, *Politico* reported, "Pressure is escalating on Silicon Valley to take action against anti-vaccine posts after top Biden officials chided social media giants."[76]

At a press conference later that same day, Psaki again called for censorship, asking social media companies to "create robust enforcement strategies." She added that the White House wanted different companies to work together to censor. "You shouldn't be banned from one platform and not others if you—for providing misinformation out there."[77]

At almost exactly the same time, in response to a shouted question about "platforms like Facebook," Biden said, "They're killing people.... Look, the only pandemic we have is among the unvaccinated, and that's—they're killing people."[78]

Later that afternoon, Twitter locked my account for the first time, in response to this tweet: "Something really odd is going on. The vaccines are failing. READ THIS THREAD." I had linked to a thread showing that all over Europe, higher levels of vaccination were correlated with higher rates of Covid.[79]

This warning from Twitter was particularly striking for at least four reasons.

First, the original post which I linked to was not tagged as misleading.

Second, *two days earlier* I had used exactly the same language—"the vaccines are failing"—in a tweet about the United Kingdom—and Twitter had not tagged it.

Third, Twitter had never sent me a warning email before, yet it seemed to regard this tweet as my second strike.

Fourth, the warning came one day after Murthy's warning and *the same day* as the Biden and Psaki follow-ups.

Twitter locked my account for twelve hours again on July 27—without specifically explaining to me which tweet had violated its rules. Then it locked my account for seven days on July 30, my fourth strike, in response to this Tweet:

> The pivotal clinical trial for the @pfizer #Covid vaccine shows it does nothing to reduce the overall risk of death. ZERO. 15 patients who received the vaccine died; 14 who received placebo died. The end. The trial blind is broken now. This is all the data we will ever have.

Every single word in this tweet was 100 percent true. On July 28, Pfizer had released updated results from its forty-thousand-person trial, and they said exactly what I reported. To be clear, these were *not* just Covid deaths—and I did not say they were. There were only three Covid-related deaths among people in the trial, two in the placebo arm and one among people who received the drug.[80]

A month later, on the night of Saturday, August 28, Twitter permanently suspended my account, which at the time had almost 345,000 followers. The company did not email me to notify me which tweet had led to my suspension. In fact, it has never actually told me I've been suspended at all. But in response to questions from Fox News, NBC, and elsewhere, Twitter did issue a statement defaming my work:

> The account you referenced has been permanently suspended for repeated violations of our COVID-19 misinformation rules.[81]

As of this writing, I am consulting with lawyers over potential legal claims against Twitter. I am exploring several potential legal avenues. To preserve maximum flexibility, I will not comment further on what actions I may take.

In the meantime, I continue to post on Substack, where I now have over 150,000 readers. But Twitter was a uniquely important platform, and its defamatory action has already emboldened further efforts at censorship. On September 7, Massachusetts senator Elizabeth Warren asked Amazon to suppress my *Unreported Truths* booklets; in support of her "concerns that Amazon is peddling misinformation" by selling my work, her letter specifically cited Twitter's ban.[82]

Warren's effort at censorship backfired. When I wrote about it on Substack on September 13, readers bought so many booklets that Amazon briefly ran out. Within a day, the vaccine booklet had become the top-selling book on Amazon.

People want the truth about Covid. They are desperate for the truth. All I have tried to do for the last two years is offer it to the best of my ability.

For this act of rebellion I have been vilified and now censored. But—thanks to you—not silenced.

The proof is in your hands.

35: IN CONCLUSION

Our Own Shadows

We should be done with Covid.

I don't mean that we should have no cases or deaths. Zero Covid was always a fantasy. We have never come close to eliminating influenza, the most obvious comparison for Sars-Cov-2. Why would we think we could eradicate a respiratory virus that can survive in animals, is highly contagious, and can infect people anywhere in the world?

What I mean is this: This book should not have to exist. Two years on, Covid should no longer be a focus of my life, or your life, or almost anyone's life. It should belong to virologists and epidemiologists and doctors and nurses.

The pandemia should be long past. We should be treating Covid like the manageable medical problem that it is. We should be treating Covid like the flu.

Yes, Covid is worse than the average flu. It kills significantly more people than the flu. But in bad flu years, hospitals sometimes open triage tents. In flu years good and bad, healthy adults sometimes die from influenza. We view these deaths as what they are: isolated tragedies.

We lost all sense of perspective almost two years ago, and we are nowhere close to getting it back. We continue to view Sars-Cov-2 as cause for hysteria. And, worse, as an excuse to mandate vaccines that we already know cannot eliminate it—or, if Israel's experience is any guide, even slow its transmission.

That "we" is unfair, though.

Many Americans—well over 100 million—are indeed long past Covid. They have had it and recovered, or have accepted that they cannot avoid being infected sooner or later and might as well stop worrying.

They don't wear masks except when someone makes them. Whether or not they have taken the vaccine, they know it is no silver bullet. They just want to get on with their lives. They are eating dinner at crowded restaurants, standing shoulder to shoulder by the hundreds of thousands at football stadiums, and sending their kids to school unmasked.

But our political and media class either ignore or demonize them. For the public health mandarins, the Twitter blue checks, and the Democratic elite, every day is Groundhog Day. Every day is another day to count Covid deaths—never other deaths, always and only Covid deaths—and to search coast to coast for crowded ICUs and people under fifty who have been unlucky enough to die from Covid.

All the better if they're unvaccinated.

Are our woke betters genuinely scared of Covid's risks? Maybe—though repeated incidents like the one in September 2021 where San Francisco mayor London Breed was photographed dancing maskless and then complained about the "fun police" suggest they know the real odds as well as the rest of us.[1] But they are certainly aware of Covid's uses as they work to grow the government and thus their power, though.

For more than a year, people who didn't want to pay rent didn't have to—because Covid. They received huge extra unemployment benefits even as jobless rates fell to ordinary levels—because Covid. Teachers didn't have to bother with the hassle of going to school—because Covid.

"Paid leave is infrastructure," a Democratic senator wrote in April 2021, arguing for a multi-trillion-dollar spending package that as of this writing is still under debate in Congress. "Caregiving is infrastructure." It is hardly an exaggeration to joke that from the left's point of view, Covid is infrastructure.[2]

But Covid has also revealed the depth of the crisis in the American health care system—the absurdly expensive American health care system, great at producing tear-jerking ads and making millionaires and even billionaires of hospital and pharmaceutical and insurance company executives. Not so great at helping the sick.

Our hospitals have been pushed to the brink of disaster, or so we are told, by a virus that at the peak of its winter virulence killed 3 in 1,000 of the Americans it infected. That's not according to me or some other "Covid denier," that's according to the National Institutes of Health.[3] Either the media is overstating the strain on hospitals, or we are not getting anything like our money's worth for the $1.3 trillion—$4,000 for every person in the United States—we will spend on hospitals in 2021.[4]

Probably both.

Now the vaccine mandates the Biden administration has forced on hospitals are pushing the system to the brink of collapse. So many nurses are quitting that hospitals are being forced to pay up to $10,000 a week to traveling nurses.[5] This situation is unsustainable. Hospitals around the country are cutting services—including an upstate New York medical center that said in September it would have to stop delivering babies because of staffing shortages caused by the mandate.[6]

But the failure extends past our hospitals.

Almost two years into the crisis, we have not just failed to find really effective new small-molecule drug treatments for Covid, *we do not even know if a long list of cheap drugs that are already widely available might help*. Would ivermectin? Who knows? Hydroxychloroquine? Who knows? (Probably not.) Vitamin D? Who knows? Fluvoxamine? Who knows? Albuterol? Who knows?

The only medicine in this category that we *know* helps reduce mortality is the steroid dexamethasone, and we only know that because of a trial in Britain. Here's something else we know: the medical establishment, and especially the federal health bureaucracy, have been bizarrely reluctant to consider or test older and cheaper drugs.

At every opportunity they have treated these potential therapies with scorn, while lavishing attention on expensive new drugs such as remdesivir, which have so far failed to make any dent in the pandemic. (Monoclonal antibodies do work, and pharmaceutical companies deserve credit for developing those—but they are expensive and difficult to produce, and thus hard to scale widely even in the United States, much less across the world.)

Vaccines—and the mRNA vaccines in particular—are the ultimate example of this obsession with new and expensive biotechnology.

The very word vaccine seems to have a hypnotizing power, for non-scientists and scientists alike. We had good reason in 2020 to predict that a vaccine for Sars-Cov-2 would not work very well. *mRNA therapeutics were not even intended as vaccines.* They were repurposed as vaccines when their developers realized that they had toxicities that would make repeated dosing difficult. The history of vaccines for influenza and other coronaviruses should have been another warning sign. Flu vaccines are notoriously ineffective, while vaccines for other coronaviruses don't exist at all.

Yet from the first, Dr. Fauci had an *idée fixe* that vaccines would save us all. Naturally this easy solution appealed to Donald Trump. Warp Speed! Trump is out, but Biden is even more committed to vaccines. And now, in the face of obvious vaccine failure, Fauci and the White House will not back down. Thus the effort to force boosters even in the face of concerted opposition from the Food and Drug Administration and World Health Organization—and press vaccines for children on reluctant parents.

A third dose has little chance of working for more than few months, and it comes with major risks. But without a third dose, whatever protection the vaccines have offered will likely collapse just as a fall and winter wave hits the United States, making the nonsense about "a pandemic of the unvaccinated" even more impossible to sustain.

Already, a strong argument can be made that the vaccines are *extending* the pandemic. Natural immunity confers extremely strong protection against reinfection; anyone who gets Covid and recovers from it is extremely unlikely to get it again.

In contrast, our currently available vaccines lose their power in a matter of months—as *Pfizer itself now acknowledges*. At the FDA's meeting on September 17, 2021, William Gruber, the Pfizer executive in charge of vaccine development, said the United States would face *more than five million* additional Sars-Cov-2 infections if it did not immediately approve boosters for everyone. "Israel could portend the U.S. Covid-19 future, and soon," Gruber said. The vaccines also appear to have driven the spread of the Delta variant (as Pfizer has *not* acknowledged).

I am not a conspiracy theorist, but many choices public health authorities have made around vaccines are inexplicable, including their unwillingness to acknowledge natural immunity and the rush to force shots on healthy young adults.

Worse, the ultimate risk of the vaccines is not that they fail and efficacy falls to zero. It is far higher—and the unwillingness of Fauci and other public health grandees to acknowledge that reality is sadly unsurprising, given that they have been all in on vaccines from the first.

If we are lucky, the current mess won't do much more than lead to huge profits for Pfizer, Moderna, and BioNTech.[7] Vaccine efficacy will slide towards zero and we will live with Sars-Cov-2 and its variants just as we do with the flu.

If we aren't lucky…

Well, let's hope we're lucky.

If our health care system has failed us, we have also failed it. Like the opioid crisis, the Covid epidemic has highlighted and exacerbated broader societal fractures.

In Western European countries, deaths from Covid are almost exclusively confined to the elderly, especially the extremely elderly. Denmark has almost six million people; during the first eighteen months of the epidemic, twenty-six Danes under the age of fifty died of Covid—barely one per month.[8]

Obese people are at much higher risk of death from Covid than everyone else, as a massive review of British medical records proved.[9] And the United States has markedly more Covid deaths in people under sixty than other advanced nations for one simple reason: our sky-high rates of obesity, especially morbid obesity. For almost two years, the media has refused to acknowledge this simple truth (or the fact that lockdowns likely worsened it).

We need to encourage people to treat their bodies with more respect—a goal easy to articulate but apparently impossible to achieve. We have forgotten the most basic tenet of medicine: *an ounce of prevention is worth a pound of cure.* But there's no money in prevention, not enough to matter, anyway.

But the shortcomings of our health care system pale in comparison to the complete failure of our media outlets to ask even the most basic questions about our response to Covid—and now the vaccines.

When it comes to Covid, the Fourth Estate is now an arm of the First. Even the fact that so many medical professionals would rather quit their jobs than be vaccinated has not prompted the media to reconsider whether the vaccines may not be the miracle we were told.

I shouldn't complain about this fiasco. Despite the vitriol I receive, every day I have more leads than I can even consider reporting, and a worldwide network of people who will offer tips, tell their stories, and analyze data. For free! And I have an audience whose size and passion stuns me.

But my windfall is the world's misfortune. The fact that supposedly reputable news organizations are openly working in concert with governments to craft narratives around Covid—and now to push vaccines and demonize the unvaccinated—is extraordinarily dangerous.

And the fact that Twitter banned me at the open urging of the federal government is a betrayal of American values that is hard to believe in peacetime. The only answer to the questions I've raised for the last two years is to take away my ability to use a platform supposedly intended for free speech?

One of my Twitter strikes came for saying "the vaccines are failing." Two months later Pfizer's top vaccine scientists admitted his company's vaccine is failing. And no one in the legacy media will speak out for me against this censorship, much less admit I was right?

What has happened to journalism? What has happened to journalists?

So here we are, almost two years in. The right "answer" to Covid has not changed since the spring of 2020, when the empty hospital ships sailed out of New York Harbor[10]—proving that even at its worst, Sars-Cov-2 (the original variant, at least) could not collapse our medical system. The right answer has not changed since 2006, when Donald Henderson, who helped eradicate smallpox,[11] and his co-authors explained, "Experience has shown that communities faced with epidemics or other adverse events respond best and with the least anxiety when the normal social functioning of the community is least disrupted."[12]

To say the least, we have not taken Dr. Henderson's advice.

Now the failure of the vaccines has led to a fresh crisis. If they had worked as promised, we would have so few Covid cases now that we would have no choice but to return to normal. The panic governments and the media created in 2020 would be gone.

But the vaccines don't work as promised. We will have to take back our lives for ourselves. I cannot help thinking of John Belushi's speech from *Animal House* (it's a movie, kids, look it up): *Over? Did you say over? Nothing is over until we decide it is.*

Can we decide? Will our governments *allow* us to decide? I want to think so. But then I never imagined the government of the United States of America would try to prevent me and other dissidents from having access to the most important media platforms of our time.

Some countries, such as Britain, do appear to be going back to normal. "Britain is reporting more than 30,000 new coronavirus cases a day, but the public seems to have moved on," the *New York Times* noted (disapprovingly) in late August.[13]

But other countries have gone the other way. Australia is now building internment camps for Covid quarantine. It calls them "centers for national resilience."[14] George Orwell would be proud.

Which way will the United States tip? Will we choose freedom or fear?

We and our allies defeated fascism in World War II. We defeated communism in the Cold War. I am old enough to remember the Berlin Wall falling. No, not falling, *being torn down*—by people who were no longer willing to live under the heel of authoritarian governments.

I believe that for all its many flaws, the United States remains, in the phrase that is attributed to Ronald Reagan but actually dates back to John Winthrop four centuries ago, "a city upon a hill."[15]

I believe we will take back our freedoms from the would-be authoritarians who spent 2020 trying to cage us in our homes, 2021 chipping away at our medical autonomy, and both years censoring our freedom to speak and debate. All for our own good, of course.

I believe in the Constitution and the Bill of Rights and the rule of law. I believe they, and we, are more powerful than this crummy little virus.

I believe truth will prevail.

I have to. We all have to.

The alternative is impossible to imagine.

Acknowledgments

This book has been my most solitary work—and my most communal.

As old friends in journalism and the media turned away, unwilling to deal with the information I presented, others stepped forward. Tucker Carlson, Laura Ingraham, Buck Sexton, Clay Travis, Liz Wheeler, and Joe Rogan are just some of the people who offered me the space to share facts and data. Thank you. Elon Musk spoke out at a crucial moment. I still have never met Elon, and I'm not sure I ever will, but dude—I owe you. Beers on me.

Countless scientists and physicians referred me to papers I wouldn't have seen—and helped me understand them. All errors are mine alone, of course. Nurses and first responders told me the truth about the patients they saw. Parents shared their fury with the way schools treated their children.

And by the thousands, you encouraged me not to worry about the hate from the blue checks—that you stood with me and that my Twitter feed mattered to you. Right back at ya: your words mattered to me, more than you know.

Closer to home, Deneen Howell represents my book deals ably (I am not sure she agrees with everything I write, but she's too good a lawyer to care). When the big publishers ran away, Regnery stepped forward, and having a partner that is committed to this book no matter what has proven to be a blessing. Thanks, Elizabeth and Tom.

Most of all, I have to thank Jackie and our kids. Jackie understood just how overhyped Covid was before almost anyone else. And Lucy, Ezra, and Percy are joys every day (okay, almost every day)—and living reminders of the immorality of sacrificing the young for the old, the future for the past. All four of you have put up with a LOT of tweeting, emailing, substacking, and television trucks in the driveway.

I hope you know the fight is worth the trouble.

Notes

1: Welcome to Pandemia

Alex Berenson (@AlexBerenson), "Against hysteria, satire. Against…," Twitter, April 16, 2020, 4:14 a.m., available at the Wayback Machine, https://web.archive.org/web/20210324020334/https://twitter.com/AlexBerenson/status/1250744283012960258. Twitter has now censored me by suspending my account, which does not just prevent me from tweeting but also makes my older tweets unavailable. Fortunately, I downloaded an essentially complete archive of my tweets and do intend to make them publicly available, unedited. But for the moment they cannot be found on Twitter. When I quote one of my tweets, I note whether I have a screenshot of it in my archive. And where it was captured and is still available elsewhere on the internet, usually at the Internet Archive's Wayback Machine, I give that link.

1. Mirco Nacoti et al., "At the Epicenter of the COVID-19 Pandemic and Humanitarian Crises in Italy: Changing Perspectives on Preparation and Mitigation," *NEJM Catalyst Innovations in Care Delivery*, March 21, 2020, https://catalyst.nejm.org/doi/full/10.1056/CAT.20.0080.

2: Happy New Year

1. "Li Wenliang: Coronavirus Kills Chinese Whistleblower Doctor," BBC News, February 7, 2020, https://www.bbc.com/news/world-asia-china-51403795.
2. Sui-Lee Wee and Vivian Wang, "China Grapples with Mystery Pneumonia-Like Illness," *New York Times*, January 6, 2020, https://www.nytimes.com/2020/01/06/world/asia/china-SARS-pneumonialike.html.
3. Sui-Lee Wee and Donald G. McNeil Jr., "From January 2020: China Identifies New Virus Causing Pneumonialike Illness," *New York Times*, January 8, 2020, https://www.nytimes.com/2020/01/08/health/china-pneumonia-outbreak-virus.html.
4. Xixing Li et al., "Who Was the First Doctor to Report the COVID-19 Outbreak in Wuhan, China?" *Journal of Nuclear Medicine*, 61, no. 6 (June 2020): 782–83, https://doi.org/10.2967/jnumed.120.247262.
5. World Health Organization (WHO) (@WHO), "Preliminary investigations conducted by the Chinese authorities have found no clear evidence of human-to-human transmission of the novel #coronavirus (2019-nCoV) identified in #Wuhan, #China," Twitter, January 14, 2020, 6:18 a.m., https://twitter.com/WHO/status/1217043229427761152.
6. Emily Baumgaertner, "As Coronavirus Outbreak Worsens, China Agrees to Accept Help from WHO," *Los Angeles Times*, January 28, 2020, https://www.latimes.com/science/story/2020-01-28/coronavirus-china-accepts-who-help.
7. Zhuang Pinghui, "Chinese Laboratory That First Shared Coronavirus Genome with World Ordered to Close for 'Rectification,' Hindering Its Covid-19 Research," *South China Morning Post*, February 28, 2020, https://www.scmp.com/news/china/society/article/3052966/chinese-laboratory-first-shared-coronavirus-genome-world-ordered.

8.   "China Confirms Human-to-Human Transmission of 2019n-CoV, Infection of Medical Staff," Xinhua Net, January 20, 2020, http://www.xinhuanet.com/english/2020-01 /20/c_138721762.htm.

9.   Sheridan Prasso, "China's Epic Dash for PPE Left the World Short on Masks," *Bloomberg Businessweek*, September 17, 2020, https://www.bloomberg.com/news/ar ticles/2020-09-17/behind-china-s-epic-dash-for-ppe-that-left-the-world-short-on -masks.

10.   Chris Buckley and Javier C. Hernanández, "China Expands Virus Lockdown, Encircling 35 Million," *New York Times*, January 23, 2020, https://www.nytimes.com /2020/01/23/world/asia/china-coronavirus-outbreak.html.

11.   Gerry Shih, "In China's Coronavirus Crisis, a Fleeting Flicker of Freer Speech," *Washington Post*, February 6, 2020, https://www.washingtonpost.com/world/asia_pa cific/in-chinas-health-crisis-a-fleeting-flicker-of-free-speech/2020/02/06/21e16f8a-48 88-11ea-8a1f-de1597be6cbc_story.html.

12.   Shawn Yuan, "Wuhan Turns to Social Media to Vent Anger at Coronavirus Response," Al Jazeera, March 3, 2020, https://www.aljazeera.com/news/2020/2/3/wuhan-turns -to-social-media-to-vent-anger-at-coronavirus-response.

13.   Justin Harper, "Wuhan Lockdown: How People Are Still Getting Food," BBC News, January 31, 2020, https://www.bbc.com/news/business-51305566.

14.   Stephanie Nebehay, "WHO Says Widespread Travel Bans Not Needed to Beat China Virus," Reuters, February 3, 2020, https://www.reuters.com/article/us-china-healthd -who/who-chief-says-widespread-travel-bans-not-needed-to-beat-china-virus-idUSK BN1ZX1H3.

15.   Iain Marlow, "China Lashes Out at Countries Restricting Travel over Virus," Bloomberg, February 6, 2020, https://www.bloomberg.com/news/articles/2020-02 -06/china-lashes-out-at-countries-restricting-travel-over-virus.

16.   Megan Thielking and Lev Facher, "Health Experts Warn China Travel Ban Will Hinder Coronavirus Response," Stat News, January 31, 2020, https://www.statnews.com/20 20/01/31/as-far-right-calls-for-china-travel-ban-health-experts-warn-coronavirus-res ponse-would-suffer/.

17.   Alice Miranda Ollstein, "Coronavirus Quarantine, Travel Ban Could Backfire, Experts Fear," *Politico*, February 4, 2020, https://www.politico.com/news/2020/02/04/coron avirus-quaratine-travel-110750.

18.   "Naming the Coronavirus Disease (COVID-19) and the Virus That Causes It," World Health Organization, https://www.who.int/emergencies/diseases/novel-coronavirus-20 19/technical-guidance/naming-the-coronavirus-disease-(covid-2019)-and-the-virus-th at-causes-it.

3: In the Beginning

1.   Richard Kent Zimmerman, "If Pneumonia Is the 'Old Man's Friend,' Should It Be Prevented by Vaccination? An Ethical Analysis," *Vaccine* 23, no. 29 (May 31, 2005): 3843–49, https://pubmed.ncbi.nlm.nih.gov/15893623/.

2.   Joe Butash, "How the 1918 Flu Pandemic Stopped Scranton in Its Tracks," PA Homepage, March 6, 2020, https://www.pahomepage.com/news/how-the-1918-flu -pandemic-stopped-scranton-in-its-tracks/.

3.   Christopher Klein, "How America Struggled to Bury the Dead during the 1918 Flu Pandemic," History, February 12, 2020, https://www.history.com/news/spanish-flu -pandemic-dead.

4. Quoted in Gina Kolata, *Flu: The Story of the Great Influenza Pandemic of 1918 and the Search for the Virus That Caused It* (New York: Simon & Schuster, 1999), 13–14.

5. Douglas Jordan with contributions from Terrence Tumpey and Barbara Jester, "The Deadliest Flu: The Complete Story of the Discovery and Reconstruction of the 1918 Pandemic Virus," Centers for Disease Control and Prevention, https://www.cdc.gov /flu/pandemic-resources/reconstruction-1918-virus.html.

6. Kolata, *Flu*, 55–56.

7. "Lesson 1: Introduction to Epidemiology, Section 2: Historical Evolution of Epidemiology," in *Principles of Epidemiology in Public Health Practice: An Introduction to Applied Epidemiology and Biostatistics*, 3rd ed., Centers for Disease Control and Prevention, https://www.cdc.gov/csels/dsepd/ss1978/lesson1/section2 .html.

8. *Second Annual Report of the Registrar-General of Births, Deaths, and Marriages in England* (London: W. Clowes and Sons, 1840), 84, https://babel.hathitrust.org/cgi/pt ?id=njp.32101064041955&view=1up&seq=85.

9. Lawrence Cosentino, "Maskers and 'Slackers,' a Century Ago," *City Pulse*, July 23, 2020, https://www.lansingcitypulse.com/stories/maskers-and-slackers-a-century-ago ,14743.

10. Wilfred H. Kellogg, *Influenza: A Study of Measures Adopted for the Control of the Epidemic* (Sacramento: California State Printing Office, 1919), 3, https://babel.hathit rust.org/cgi/pt?id=uc1.31378008030317&view=1up&seq=7.

11. Aria Nouri, "The Discovery of Bacteria," American Association for the Advancement of Science, July 5, 2011, https://www.aaas.org/discovery-bacteria.

12. Frank L. Horsfall Jr., *Thomas Milton Rivers, 1888–1962* (Washington, D.C.: National Academy of Sciences, 1965), 270, https://books.nap.edu/resource/biomems/trivers.pdf.

4: All the Wrong Lessons

1. Rebecca Kreston, "The Public Health Legacy of the 1976 Swine Flu Outbreak," *Discover*, September 30, 2013, https://www.discovermagazine.com/health/the-public -health-legacy-of-the-1976-swine-flu-outbreak.

2. F. Barre-Sinoussi et al., "Isolation of a T-Lymphotrophic Retrovirus from a Patient at Risk for Acquired Immune Deficiency Syndrome (AIDS)," *Science* 220, no. 4599 (May 1983): 868–71, https://science.sciencemag.org/content/220/4599/868.

3. "Table 1. Number and Percentage of Persons with AIDS, by Selected Characteristics and Period of Report—United States, 1981–2000," Centers for Disease Control, June 8, 2001, https://www.cdc.gov/mmwr/preview/mmwrhtml/mm5021a2.htm#tab1.

4. Jack King, "The Drama That Raged against Reagan's America," BBC, October 19, 2020, https://www.bbc.com/culture/article/20201019-the-drama-that-raged-against -reagans-america.

5. Ben Cohen, "Dr. Fauci Was a Basketball Captain: Now He's America's Point Guard," *Wall Street Journal*, March 29, 2020, https://www.wsj.com/articles/dr-fauci-was-a-b asketball-captain-now-hes-americas-point-guard-11585479601.

6. Ushma S. Neill, "A Conversation with Tony Fauci," *Journal of Clinical Investigation* 124, no. 7 (July 2014): 2814–15, https://www.ncbi.nlm.nih.gov/pmc/articles/PMC40 71403/.

7. Donald G. McNeil Jr., "'We Loved Each Other': Fauci Recalls Larry Kramer, Friend and Nemesis," *New York Times*, May 27, 2020, https://www.nytimes.com/2020/05 /27/health/larry-kramer-anthony-fauci.html.

8. Anne Barber, "NIH Docs Answer Call to Help the Needy of Washington," *NIH Record* 42, no. 11 (May 29, 1990): 1–4, https://nihrecord.nih.gov/sites/recordNIH/files/pdf/1990/NIH-Record-1990-05-29.pdf.

9. "Interview: Larry Kramer," PBS, January 22, 2005, https://www.pbs.org/wgbh/pages/frontline/aids/interviews/kramer.html.

10. Anthony S. Fauci, "The Global Challenge of Infectious Diseases: The Evolving Role of the National Institutes of Health in Basic and Clinical Research," *Nature Immunology* 6, no. 8 (August 2005): 743–47, https://www.ncbi.nlm.nih.gov/pmc/articles/PMC7097332/.

11. Eric Lipton and Jennifer Steinhauer, "The Untold Story of the Birth of Social Distancing," *New York Times*, April 22, 2020, https://www.nytimes.com/2020/04/22/us/politics/social-distancing-coronavirus.html.

12. Richard J. Hatchett et al., "Public Health Interventions and Epidemic Intensity during the 1918 Influenza Pandemic," *Proceedings of the National Academy of Sciences of the United States of America* 104, no. 18 (May 1, 2007): 7582–87, https://www.pnas.org/content/104/18/7582#ref-6.

13. "Interim Pre-Pandemic Planning Guidance: Community Strategy for Pandemic Influenza Mitigation in the United States: Early, Targeted, Layered Use of Nonpharmaceutical Interventions," Centers for Disease Control, February 2007, https://stacks.cdc.gov/view/cdc/11425.

14. "Community Mitigation Guidelines to Prevent Pandemic Influenza—United States, 2017," Centers for Disease Control, April 21, 2017, https://stacks.cdc.gov/view/cdc/45220.

15. "Non-Pharmaceutical Public Health Measures for Mitigating the Risk and Impact of Epidemic and Pandemic Influenza," World Health Organization, 2019, https://apps.who.int/iris/bitstream/handle/10665/329438/9789241516839-eng.pdf.

16. Thomas V. Inglesby et al., "Disease Mitigation Measures in the Control of Pandemic Influenza," *Biosecurity and Bioterrorism: Biodefense Strategy, Practice, and Science* 4, no. 4 (December 2006): 366–375, https://www.liebertpub.com/doi/10.1089/bsp.2006.4.366?url_ver=Z39.88-2003&rfr_id=ori%3Arid%3Acrossref.org&rfr_dat=cr_pub++0pubmed&.

17. The Institute of Medicine, "Modeling Community Containment for Pandemic Influenza," The National Academies of Sciences, Engineering, and Medicine, 2006, https://www.nap.edu/catalog/11800/modeling-community-containment-for-pandemic-influenza-a-letter-report.

5: Globetrotting

1. Ella Ide, "10 Italian Towns in Lockdown over Coronavirus Fears," Yahoo, February 21, 2020, https://www.yahoo.com/now/10-italian-towns-lockdown-over-coronavirus-fears-220635548.html.

2. Holly Ellyatt, "Italians on High Alert as Coronavirus Spreads beyond the North of the Country," CNBC, February 25, 2020, https://www.cnbc.com/2020/02/25/italians-under-lockdown-as-coronavirus-spreads.html.

3. Daniel Wolfe and Daniel Dale, "'It's Going to Disappear': A Timeline of Trump's Claims That Covid-19 Will Vanish," CNN, October 31, 2020, https://www.cnn.com/interactive/2020/10/politics/covid-disappearing-trump-comment-tracker/.

4. Philip Bump, "Which Is Trump More Worried About: Coronavirus Numbers or Coronavirus Patients?" *Washington Post*, March 7, 2020, https://www.washingtonpo

st.com/politics/2020/03/07/which-is-trump-more-worried-about-coronavirus-numbers-or-coronavirus-patients/.

5.   Mike Baker et al., "Washington State Declares Emergency amid Coronavirus Death and Illnesses at Nursing Home," *New York Times*, February 29, 2020, https://www.nytimes.com/2020/02/29/us/coronavirus-washington-death.html.

6.   Scottie Andrew and Jessie Yeung, "Masks Can't Stop the Coronavirus in the US, but Hysteria Has Led to Bulk-Buying, Price-Gouging and Serious Fear for the Future," CNN, February 29, 2020, https://www.cnn.com/2020/02/29/health/coronavirus-mask-hysteria-us-trnd/index.html.

7.   Jacqueline Howard, "Masks May Actually Increase Your Coronavirus Risk If Worn Improperly, Surgeon General Warns," CNN, March 2, 2020, https://www.cnn.com/2020/03/02/health/surgeon-general-coronavirus-masks-risk-trnd/index.html.

8.   Daniele Macchini, "In una delle constanti…," Facebook, March 6, 2020, https://www.facebook.com/photo.php?fbid=3395151233834056&set=a.44236782244576 0&type=3.

9.   Silvia Stringhini (@silviast9), "1/ I may be repeating myself, but I want to fight this sense of security that I see outside of the epicenters, as if nothing was going to happen 'here.' The media in Europe are reassuring, while there's little to be reassured of. #COVID19 #coronavirus," Twitter, March 9, 2020, 4:36 a.m., https://twitter.com/silviast9/status/1236933818654896129?s=20.

10.   Jason Horowitz, "Italy Announces Restrictions over Entire Country in Attempt to Halt Coronavirus," *New York Times*, March 9, 2020, https://www.nytimes.com/2020/03/09/world/europe/italy-lockdown-coronavirus.html.

11.   Rachel Sandler, "How the CDC Botched Its Initial Coronavirus Response with Faulty Tests," *Forbes*, March 2, 2020, https://www.forbes.com/sites/rachelsandler/2020/03/02/how-the-cdc-botched-its-initial-coronavirus-response-with-faulty-tests/?sh=5272 818d670e.

12.   Barbara J. Culliton, "Bush Goes 0 for 2 with Anthony Fauci," *Science* 246, no. 4932 (November 1989), https://science.sciencemag.org/content/246/4932/880.

13.   Barbara J. Culliton, "Help Wanted: Director, NIH," *Science* 245, no. 4923 (September 1989), https://science.sciencemag.org/content/245/4923/1181.

14.   Ushma S. Neill, "A Conversation with Tony Fauci," *Journal of Clinical Investigation* 124, no. 7 (July 2014): 2814–15, https://www.jci.org/articles/view/77277.

15.   "President Bush Honors Presidential Medal of Freedom Recipients," White House website archives, June 19, 2008, https://georgewbush-whitehouse.archives.gov/news/releases/2008/06/20080619-9.html.

16.   Molly Roberts, "Anthony Fauci Built a Truce. Trump Is Destroying It," *Washington Post*, July 16, 2020, https://www.washingtonpost.com/opinions/2020/07/16/anthony-fauci-built-truce-trump-is-destroying-it/.

17.   Denise Grady, "Not His First Epidemic: Dr. Anthony Fauci Sticks to the Facts," *New York Times*, March 8, 2020, https://www.nytimes.com/2020/03/08/health/fauci-coronavirus.html.

6: Fifteen Days

1.   Sam Quinn, "Rudy Gobert Touched Every Microphone at Jazz Media Availability Monday, Now Reportedly Has Coronavirus," CBS, March 12, 2020, https://www.cbssports.com/nba/news/rudy-gobert-touched-every-microphone-at-jazz-media-availability-monday-now-reportedly-has-coronavirus/.

2. Jake Russell, "Rudy Gobert Contracted the Coronavirus in March. He Still Can't Smell Properly," *Washington Post*, June 28, 2020, https://www.washingtonpost.com/sports/2020/06/28/rudy-gobert-contracted-coronavirus-march-he-still-cant-smell-properly/.

3. Jenni Carlson, "Carlson: Yes, Jazz Star Rudy Gobert Was a Goob about COVID, but He's Also Become an Accidental Hero," *The Oklahoman*, March 15, 2020, https://www.oklahoman.com/article/5657635/coronavirus-in-oklahoma-yes-jazz-star-rudy-gobert-was-a-goob-but-hes-also-become-an-accidental-hero.

4. ESPN, "Mark Cuban Reacts to NBA Suspending Season Due to Coronavirus: NBA on ESPN," YouTube, March 11, 2020, https://www.youtube.com/watch?v=b2-wU42KJ0c.

5. Ken Davidoff, "The Night Baseball Returned after 9/11: These People Needed This," *New York Post*, September 11, 2019, https://nypost.com/2019/09/11/two-braves-greats-relive-night-baseball-returned-to-nyc-after-9-11/.

6. Anthony D'Alessandro, "Tom Hanks & Rita Wilson Test Positive for Coronavirus as Outbreak Hits 'Elvis Presley' Film," Deadline, March 11, 2020, https://deadline.com/2020/03/tom-hanks-rita-tom%20h-positive-coronavirus-elvis-presley-movie-1202880431/.

7. "WHO Director-General's Opening Remarks at the Media Briefing on COVID-19—11 March 2020," World Health Organization, March 11, 2020, https://www.who.int/director-general/speeches/detail/who-director-general-s-opening-remarks-at-the-media-briefing-on-covid-19—-11-march-2020.

8. Laurel Wamsley, "March 11, 2020: The Day Everything Changed," NPR, March 11, 2021, https://www.npr.org/2021/03/11/975663437/march-11-2020-the-day-everything-changed.

9. Keith Collins and David Yaffe-Bellany, "About 2 Million Guns Were Sold in the U.S. As Virus Fears Spread," *New York Times*, April 1, 2020, https://www.nytimes.com/interactive/2020/04/01/business/coronavirus-gun-sales.html.

10. Eliza Shapiro, "New York City Public Schools to Close to Slow Spread of Coronavirus," *New York Times*, March 15, 2020, https://www.nytimes.com/2020/03/15/nyregion/nyc-schools-closed.html.

11. Chelsea Bruce Lockhart et al., "The Shocking Coronavirus Study That Rocked the UK and US," *Financial Times*, March 19, 2020, https://www.ft.com/content/16764a22-69ca-11ea-a3c9-1fe6fedcca75.

12. Chloé Hecketsweiler and Cédric Pietralunga, "Coronavirus: Les Simulations Alarmantes des Épidémiologistes pour la France," *Le Monde*, March 15, 2020, https://www.lemonde.fr/planete/article/2020/03/15/coronavirus-les-simulations-alarmantes-des-epidemiologistes-pour-la-france_6033149_3244.html.

13. Joanna Wilson, "Theoretical Physics to Pandemic Modelling: Neil Ferguson on His Life in Science," Imperial College London, September 24, 2020, https://www.imperial.ac.uk/news/205053/theoretical-physics-pandemic-modelling-neil-ferguson/.

14. Kate Wong, "'Mad Cow' Sheep in Britain Could Increase the Human Death Toll," *Scientific American*, January 10, 2002, https://www.scientificamerican.com/article/mad-cow-sheep-in-britain/.

15. "Variant Creutzfeldt-Jakob Disease Current Data (February 2015)," University of Edinburgh, February 13, 2015, available at the Wayback Machine at https://web.archive.org/web/20150226031911/http://www.cjd.ed.ac.uk/documents/worldfigs.pdf.

16. James Sturcke, "Bird Flu Pandemic 'Could Kill 150M," *The Guardian*, September 30, 2005, https://www.theguardian.com/world/2005/sep/30/birdflu.jamessturcke.

17. "Cumulative Number of Confirmed Human Cases for Avian Influenza A(H5N1) Reported to WHO, 2003–2011," World Health Organization, August 19, 2011, https://

www.who.int/influenza/human_animal_interface/EN_GIP_20110819CumulativeN
umberH5N1casesN.pdf?ua=1.

18. "WHO Collaborating Centre for Infectious Disease Modeling," World Health Organization, https://apps.who.int/whocc/Detail.aspx?FJdjEEdrcMNfOU4d+dseSg==.

19. Mark Landler and Stephen Castle, "Behind the Virus Report That Jarred the U.S. and the U.K. to Action," *New York Times*, March 17, 2020, https://www.nytimes.com/20 20/03/17/world/europe/coronavirus-imperial-college-johnson.html.

20. Deirdre Hine, "The 2009 Influenza Pandemic," Pandemic Flu Response Review Team, July 2010, https://assets.publishing.service.gov.uk/government/uploads/system/uploa ds/attachment_data/file/61252/the2009influenzapandemic-review.pdf.

21. "Scientific Advice and Evidence in Emergencies—Science and Technology Committee," Parliament of the United Kingdom, March 2, 2011, https://publications.parliament.uk /pa/cm201011/cmselect/cmsctech/498/49803.htm.

22. Mark Landler and Stephen Castle, "The Secretive Group Guiding the U.K. on Coronavirus," *New York Times*, April 23, 2020, https://www.nytimes.com/2020/04 /23/world/europe/uk-coronavirus-sage-secret.html.

23. Mark Landler and Stephen Castle, "For Boris Johnson's Science Advisers, Pressure, Anxieties and 'Pastoral Support,'" *New York Times*, June 26, 2020, https://www.nyt imes.com/2020/06/26/world/europe/sage-britain-coronavirus-ferguson.html.

24. Bill Bostock, "How 'Professor Lockdown' Helped Save Tens of Thousands of Lives Worldwide—and Carried COVID-19 into Downing Street," Business Insider, April 25, 2020, https://www.businessinsider.com/neil-ferguson-transformed-uk-covid-respo nse-oxford-challenge-imperial-model-2020-4.

25. Ian Sample et al., "Sage Minutes Reveal How UK Advisers Reacted to Coronavirus Crisis," *The Guardian*, May 29, 2020, https://www.theguardian.com/world/2020/may /29/sage-minutes-reveal-how-uk-advisers-reacted-to-coronavirus-crisis.

26. David Adam, "Special Report: The Simulations Driving the World's Response to COVID-19," *Nature*, April 2, 2020, https://www.nature.com/articles/d41586-020-01 003-6.

27. Xihong Lin, "Learning from 26,000 Cases of COVID-19 in Wuhan," Google Docs, March 20, 2020, https://docs.google.com/presentation/d/1-rvZs0zsXF_0Tw8TNsBx KH4V1LQQXq7Az9kDfCgZDfE/edit#slide=id.p1.

28. Landler and Castle, "Behind the Virus Report That Jarred the U.S. and the U.K. to Action."

29. Freddie Sayers, "Neil Ferguson Interview: China Changed What Was Possible," UnHerd, December 26, 2020, https://unherd.com/thepost/neil-ferguson-interview-ch ina-changed-what-was-possible/.

30. William Booth, "A Chilling Scientific Paper Helped Upend U.S. and U.K. Coronavirus Strategies," *Washington Post*, March 17, 2020, https://www.washingtonpost.com/wo rld/europe/a-chilling-scientific-paper-helped-upend-us-and-uk-coronavirus-strategies /2020/03/17/aaa84116-6851-11ea-b199-3a9799c54512_story.html.

31. James Gallagher, "Coronavirus: UK Changes Course amid Death Toll Fears," BBC, March 17, 2020, https://www.bbc.com/news/health-51915302.

32. Jeremy C. Young (@jeremycyoung), "We can now read the Imperial College report on COVID-19 that led to the extreme measures we've seen in the US this week. Read it; it's terrifying. I'll offer a summary in this thread; please correct me if I've gotten it wrong," Twitter, March 17, 2020, 2:03 p.m., https://twitter.com/jeremycyoung/status /1239975682643357696?lang=en.

33. "Field Briefing: Diamond Princess COVID-19 Cases, 20 Feb Update," National Institute of Infectious Diseases, February 21, 2020, https://www.niid.go.jp/niid/en/20 19-ncov-e/9417-covid-dp-fe-02.html.

34. "Sorveglianza Integrata COVID-19 in Italia," Epicentro, February 27, 2020, https://www.epicentro.iss.it/coronavirus/bollettino/Infografica_16marzo%20ITA.pdf.

35. Tina Reed, "NIH's Fauci on Coronavirus: 'The Risk Group Is Very, Very Clear," Fierce Healthcare, March 9, 2020, https://www.fiercehealthcare.com/practices/fauci-offers -update-coronavirus-to-jama-for-clinicans.

36. Andrew Joseph, "U.S. Official Says Data Show Severe Coronavirus among Millennials, Not Just Older Americans," Stat News, March 18, 2020, https://www.statnews.com /2020/03/18/u-s-official-says-data-show-severe-coronavirus-infections-among-millen nials-not-just-older-americans/.

37. Rory Carroll, "Coronavirus Is a Threat to Young People Too, U.S. Official Fauci Tells NBA Star Curry," Reuters, March 26, 2020, https://www.reuters.com/article/us-heal th-coronavirus-curry-fauci/coronavirus-is-a-threat-to-young-people-too-u-s-official-fa uci-tells-nba-star-curry-idUSKBN21D3GN.

38. "Options for Increasing Adherence to Social Distancing Measures," SAGE, March 22, 2020, https://assets.publishing.service.gov.uk/government/uploads/system/uploads/at tachment_data/file/882722/25-options-for-increasing-adherence-to-social-distancing -measures-22032020.pdf.

39. Barry S. Coller, "AIDS and Civil Liberties," *New York Times*, June 26, 1983, https://www.nytimes.com/1983/06/26/nyregion/aids-and-civil-liberties.html.

40. Annika Olson, "An Open Letter to My Peers Partying on the Beach," CNN, March 19, 2020, https://www.cnn.com/2020/03/19/opinions/spring-breakers-coronavirus -warning-olson/index.html.

41. Josh K. Elliott, "COVIDIOTS: New Name for Shaming Ignorant, Selfish Coronavirus Reactions," Global News, March 23, 2020, https://globalnews.ca/news/6717139/covi diots-coronavirus/.

7: Following the Science

1. "UCSC Genome Browser on SARS-Cov-2 Jan. 2020/NC_045512.2 Assembly (wuhCor1)," University of California at Santa Cruz, http://genome.ucsc.edu/cgi-bin/hg Tracks?db=wuhCor1&lastVirtModeType=default&lastVirtModeExtraState=&virt ModeType=default&virtMode=0&nonVirtPosition=&position=NC_045512v2%3A 14916%2D14987&hgsid=1102816655_teyySluTHY4jScJU5DrUZNrvoBTu.

2. Victor M. Corman et al., "Detection of 2019 Novel Coronavirus (2019-nCoV) by Real-Time RT-PCR," *Eurosurveillance* 25, no. 3 (January 2020), https://www.ncbi .nlm.nih.gov/pmc/articles/PMC6988269/pdf/eurosurv-25-3-5.pdf.

3. Kary B. Mullis and Michael Smith, "The Nobel Prize in Chemistry 1993," Nobel Prize website, 1993, https://www.nobelprize.org/prizes/chemistry/1993/summary/.

4. James McGirk, "UCSC Genome Browser Posts the Coronavirus Genome," Baskin School of Engineering, University of California at Santa Cruz, February 7, 2020, https://www.soe.ucsc.edu/news/ucsc-genome-browser-posts-coronavirus-genome.

5. I. Hamming et al., "Tissue Distribution of ACE2 Protein, the Functional Receptor for SARS Coronavirus. A First Step in Understanding SARS Pathogenesis," *Journal of Pathology* 203, no. 2 (June 2004): 631–37, https://pubmed.ncbi.nlm.nih.gov/15141377/.

6. Daniel Wrapp et al., "Cryo-EM Structure of the 2019-nCoV Spike in the Prefusion Conformation," Science 367, no. 6483 (March 2020): 1260–63, https://pubmed.ncbi .nlm.nih.gov/32075877/.

7. Shuai Xia et al., "The Role of Furin Cleavage Site in SARS-CoV-2 Spike Protein-Mediated Membrane Fusion in the Presence or Absence of Trypsin," *Signal Transduction and Targeted Therapy 5*, no. 92 (2020), https://www.nature.com/articl es/s41392-020-0184-0.

8. Charles Calisher et al., letter to the editor, *The Lancet*, February 19, 2020, https://www .thelancet.com/journals/lancet/article/PIIS0140-6736(20)30418-9/fulltext.

9. Angela N. Baldwin, "Doctors Rush to Understand COVID-19's Second Week Crash," ABC News, May 6, 2020, https://abcnews.go.com/Health/doctors-rush-understand -covid-19s-week-crash/story?id=70457111.

10. Martin J. Vincent et al., "Chloroquine Is a Potent Inhibitor of SARS Coronavirus Infection and Spread," *Virology Journal 2*, no. 69 (August 2005), https://www.ncbi .nlm.nih.gov/pmc/articles/PMC1232869/.

11. Jianjun Gao et al., "Breakthrough: Chloroquine Phosphate Has Shown Apparent Efficacy in Treatment of COVID-19 Associated Pneumonia in Clinical Studies," *Biosci Trends* 14, no. 1 (March 2020): 72–73, https://pubmed.ncbi.nlm.nih.gov/32074550/.

12. Lev Facher, "Trump Says His Belief in One Potential Coronavirus Drug Is 'Just a Feeling,'" Stat News, March 20, 2020, https://www.statnews.com/2020/03/20/trump -coronavirus-drug-just-a-feeling/.

13. Ariana Eunjung Cha and Laurie McGinley, "Antimalarial Drug Touted by President Trump Is Linked to Increased Risk of Death in Coronavirus Patients, Study Says," *Washington Post*, May 22, 2020, https://www.washingtonpost.com/health/2020/05 /22/hydroxychloroquine-coronavirus-study/.

14. Mandeep R. Mehra et al., "Retracted: Hydroxychloroquine or Chloroquine with or without a Macrolide for Treatment of COVID-19: A Multinational Registry Analysis," *The Lancet*, May 22, 2020, https://www.thelancet.com/journals/lancet/article/PIIS0 140-6736%2820%2931180-6/fulltext.

15. "NIH Trial of Remdesivir to Treat COVID-19 Begins," National Institutes of Health, February 25, 2020, https://www.nih.gov/news-events/news-releases/nih-clinical-trial -remdesivir-treat-covid-19-begins.

16. "NIH Clinical Trial Shows Remdesivir Accelerates Recovery from Advanced COVID-19," National Institutes of Health, April 29, 2020, https://www.nih.gov/news-events /news-releases/nih-clinical-trial-shows-remdesivir-accelerates-recovery-advanced-co vid-19.

17. Berkeley Lovelace Jr., "Dr. Anthony Fauci Says Gilead's Remdesivir Will Set a New 'Standard of Care' for Coronavirus Treatment," CNBC, April 29, 2020, https://www .cnbc.com/2020/04/29/dr-anthony-fauci-says-data-from-remdesivir-coronavirus-drug -trial-shows-quite-good-news.html.

18. John H. Beigel et al., "Remdesivir for the Treatment of Covid-19—Final Report," *New England Journal of Medicine* 383 (November 2020): 1813–26, https://www.nejm.org /doi/full/10.1056/nejmoa2007764.

19. Noah Higgins-Dunn, "Gilead's $1.5B in Remdesivir Sales Help Buoy Worse-than-Expected Declines for Mainstay HIV, Hepatitis C Drugs," Fierce Pharma, April 30, 2021, https://www.fiercepharma.com/pharma/gilead-s-1-5b-remdesivir-sales-help-bu oy-greater-than-expected-declines-for-mainstay-hiv.

20. Ivan O. Rosas et al., "Tocilizumab in Hospitalized Patients with Severe Covid-19 Pneumonia," *New England Journal of Medicine* 384 (April 2021): 1503–1516, https:// www.nejm.org/doi/full/10.1056/NEJMoa2028700.

21. Elisabeth Mahase, "Covid-19: Low-Dose Steroid Cuts Death in Ventilated Patients by One Third, Trial Finds," *British Medical Journal* 369 (June 2020), https://www.bmj

.com/content/369/bmj.m2422?ijkey=1de0e606079f59110fa314b0a0cb0a159e4cc6ee
&keytype2=tf_ipsecsha.

22. Atul Matta et al., "Timing of Intubation and Its Implications on Outcomes in Critically
Ill Patients with Coronavirus 2019 Infection," *Critical Care Explorations* 2, no. 10
(October 2020), https://journals.lww.com/ccejournal/fulltext/2020/10000/timing_of
_intubation_and_its_implications_on.47.aspx#JCL-P-5.

23. Isaac Sher, "Italian Doctor Who Warned of Medical Supply Shortages to Fight
Coronavirus Has Now Died from the Disease," Business Insider, March 20, 2020,
https://www.businessinsider.com/italian-doctor-dies-from-coronavirus-covid-19-after
-warning-low-supplies-2020-3?op=1.

24. Thomas Kirsch, "What Happens If Health-Care Workers Stop Showing Up?" *The
Atlantic*, March 24, 2020, https://www.theatlantic.com/ideas/archive/2020/03/were
-failing-doctors/608662/.

25. "Coronavirus (COVID-19) Update: FDA Takes Action to Help Increase U.S. Supply
of Ventilators and Respirators for Protection of Health Care Workers, Patients," U.S.
Food & Drug Administration, March 27, 2020, https://www.fda.gov/news-events/press
-announcements/coronavirus-covid-19-update-fda-takes-action-help-increase-us-sup
ply-ventilators-and-respirators.

26. Alex Berenson (@AlexBerenson), "1/ Almost 90% of NYC patients put on ventilators…,"
Twitter, April 23, 2020, 4:16 p.m., https://twitter.com/alexberenson/status/1253
417451754098689?lang=en, including a screenshot of Meredith (@thisismeredith), "One
problem is the sheer number….," Twitter, March 25, 2020, 7:50 a.m. My tweet and
part of the screenshot are available at the Wayback Machine, https://web.archive
.org/web/20210811210154/https://twitter.com/alexberenson/status/12534174517540
98689. The complete screenshot is in my possession.

27. Sharon Begley, "With Ventilators Running Out, Doctors Say the Machines Are
Overused for Covid-19," Stat News, April 8, 2020, https://www.statnews.com/2020
/04/08/doctors-say-ventilators-overused-for-covid-19/.

28. Safiya Richardson et al., "Presenting Characteristics, Comorbidities, and Outcomes
among 5700 Patients Hospitalized with COVID-19 in the New York City Area,"
Journal of the American Medical Association 323, no. 20 (April 2020): 2052–59,
https://jamanetwork.com/journals/jama/fullarticle/2765184.

8: The Star of New York

1. Jeffrey Toobin, "The Albany Chronicles," *New Yorker*, February 9, 2015, https://www
.newyorker.com/magazine/2015/02/16/albany-chronicles.

2. "Coronavirus Pandemic Pushes Cuomo to Record High Ratings; Voters Trust Cuomo
over Trump on NY Reopening 78–16%," April 27, 2020, Siena College Research
Institute, https://scri.siena.edu/2020/04/27/coronavirus-pandemic-pushes-cuomo-to
-record-high-ratings-voters-trust-cuomo-over-trump-on-ny-reopening-78-16/.

3. Jackie Willis, "Andrew Cuomo's Celebrity Admirers: Jada Pinkett Smith, Chelsea
Handler and More," ET Online, April 30, 2020, https://www.etonline.com/andrew
-cuomos-celebrity-admirers-jada-pinkett-smith-chelsea-handler-and-more-145755.

4. Will Feuer et al., "Gov. Cuomo Says New York City Will Not Be Quarantined: 'It
Cannot Happen,'" CNBC, March 17, 2020, https://www.cnbc.com/2020/03/17/gov
-cuomo-says-new-york-city-will-not-be-quarantined-it-cannot-happen.html.

5. Reuters, "'I'm Not Going to Do It,' Cuomo Says of Shelter in Place," *New York Times*,
March 19, 2020, https://www.nytimes.com/video/us/politics/100000007043194/cuo
mo-coronavirus.html.

6. "43 Coronavirus Deaths and Over 5,600 Cases in N.Y.C.," *New York Times*, March 20, 2020, https://www.nytimes.com/2020/03/20/nyregion/coronavirus-new-york-up date.html.

7. Jeremy Berke, "New York City's Mayor Warns April and May Are Going to Be 'a Lot Worse' than March as Coronavirus Cases Surge," Business Insider, March 22, 2020, https://www.businessinsider.com/coronavirus-nyc-mayor-deblasio-april-may-worse-th an-march-2020-3.

8. Associated Press, "U.S. Hospitals Brace for 'Tremendous Strain' from New Virus," WTOP News, March 13, 2020, https://wtop.com/coronavirus/2020/03/u-s-hospitals -brace-for-tremendous-strain-from-new-virus/.

9. Amanda MacMillan, "Hospitals Overwhelmed by Flu Patients Are Treating Them in Tents," *Time*, January 18, 2018, https://time.com/5107984/hospitals-handling-burden -flu-patients/.

10. Tom Kertscher, "No, Empty Hospital Beds Do Not Indicate COVID-19 Is 'Fake Crisis,'" PolitiFact, April 3, 2020, https://www.politifact.com/factchecks/2020/apr/03 /facebook-posts/hospital-beds-being-kept-empty-prepare-covid-influ/.

11. Sam Roberts, "Alan Finder, 72, Unflappable Newspaper Journalist, Dies," *New York Times*, March 27, 2020, https://www.nytimes.com/2020/03/27/obituaries/alan-finder -dead-coronavirus.html.

12. Michael Schulman, "Rage for Terrence McNally," *New Yorker,* March 27, 2020, https://www.newyorker.com/culture/postscript/rage-for-terrence-mcnally.

13. Gwen Aviles, "Terrence McNally, Award-Winning Playwright, Dies from Coronavirus Complications," NBC News, March 24, 2020, https://www.nbcnews.com/pop-cultu re/pop-culture-news/award-winning-playwright-terrence-mcnally-dies-coronavirus-co mplications-n1167856.

14. Daniella Silva, "'So Many Patients Dying': Doctors Say NYC Public Hospitals Reeling from Coronavirus Cases," NBC News, March 30, 2020, https://www.nbcnews.com /news/us-news/so-many-patients-dying-doctors-say-nyc-public-hospitals-reeling-n117 2451.

15. Michael Rothfeld et al., "13 Deaths in a Day: An 'Apocalyptic' Coronavirus Surge at an N.Y.C. Hospital," *New York Times*, March 25, 2020, https://www.nytimes.com /2020/03/25/nyregion/nyc-coronavirus-hospitals.html.

16. Michael Schwirtz, "Nurses Die, Doctors Fall Sick and Panic Rises on Virus Front Lines," *New York Times*, March 30, 2020, https://www.nytimes.com/2020/03/30/ny region/ny-coronavirus-doctors-sick.html.

17. Andrew Jacobs et al., "Amid Desperate Need for Ventilators, Calls Grow for Federal Intervention," *New York Times*, March 25, 2020, https://www.nytimes.com/2020/03 /25/health/ventilators-coronavirus.html.

18. Brian M. Rosenthal et al., "'The Other Option Is Death': New York Starts Sharing of Ventilators," *New York Times*, March 26, 2020, https://www.nytimes.com/2020/03 /26/health/coronavirus-ventilator-sharing.html.

19. Jeremy R. Beitler et al., "Ventilator Sharing during an Acute Shortage Caused by the COVID-19 Pandemic," *American Journal of Respiratory and Critical Care Medicine* 202, no. 4 (August 2020): 600–604, https://www.atsjournals.org/doi/10.1164/rccm .202005-1586LE.

20. Sarah Kliff et al., "There Aren't Enough Ventilators to Cope with the Coronavirus," *New York Times*, March 18, 2020, https://www.nytimes.com/2020/03/18/business /coronavirus-ventilator-shortage.html.

21. Geoff Herbert, "Cuomo Refutes Trump, Insists NY Needs up to 40,000 Ventilators: 'I Operate on Facts,'" Syracuse.com, March 27, 2020, https://www.syracuse.com/co

ronavirus/2020/03/cuomo-refutes-trump-insists-ny-needs-up-to-40000-ventilators-i-o
perate-on-facts.html.

22. Martin Kaste and Rebecca Hersher, "Ventilator Shortages Loom as States Ponder Rules
for Rationing," NPR, April 3, 2020, https://www.npr.org/sections/health-shots/2020
/04/03/826082727/ventilator-shortages-loom-as-states-ponder-rules-for-rationing.

23. Tom Woods (@ThomasEWoods), "As @AlexBerenson points out, 7% of the U.S.
population is about 23 million people. I'd point this out to @MollyJongFast, but she'll
just tell me to wait two weeks," Twitter, May 27, 2020, 9:17 p.m., https://twitter.com
/ThomasEWoods/status/1265814472926650368.

24. Dr. Tom Frieden (@DrTomFrieden), "I hear sirens in NYC all day. @nycHealthy released
today's data: on.nyc.gov/2wKiten. Yesterday 672 deaths, today 776. 104 more of my
neighbors killed by #COVID19. In one day. 104. On average pre-covid 147 deaths/day.
Increase of 60%. Words & tears cannot express the tragedy," Twitter, March 29, 2020,
8:00 p.m., https://mobile.twitter.com/drtomfrieden/status/1244414181048291329.

25. Devon Link, "Fact Check: NYC Is Not Planning to Use Trenches in Parks as Burial
Grounds," *USA Today*, April 11, 2020, https://www.usatoday.com/story/news/factch
eck/2020/04/11/fact-check-nyc-wont-use-local-parks-temporary-burial-grounds/513
3460002/.

26. Greg Allen and Scott Neuman, "New York City Has Contingency Plan for Temporary
Burials of COVID-19 Dead," NPR, April 6, 2020, https://www.npr.org/sections/coro
navirus-live-updates/2020/04/06/828289698/new-york-city-plans-to-temporarily-bu
ry-dead.

27. Matt Hickman, "New York's Javits Center Completes Transformation into 1,200 Bed
Emergency Hospital," *Architect's Newsletter*, March 30, 2020, https://www.archpa
per.com/2020/03/new-york-javits-center-coronavirus-emergency-hospital/.

28. "Samaritan's Purse, in Collaboration with Mount Sinai Health System, Opens
Emergency Field Hospital in New York's Central Park in Response to the Coronavirus
Pandemic," Mount Sinai, April 1, 2020, https://www.mountsinai.org/about/newsro
om/2020/samaritans-purse-in-collaboration-with-mount-sinai-health-system-opens
-emergency-field-hospital-in-new-yorks-central-park-in-response-to-the-coronavirus
-pandemic-pr.

29. Steve Schmidt (@SteveSchmidtSES), "Trump is incompetent, dishonest, and profoundly
indecent. His staggering incapacity for moral leadership in this unprecedented moment
is hard to overstate. His empty boasting, dishonesty, blame gaming, lack of empathy
and fragile ego are a deadly combination of traits right now," Twitter, March 22, 2020,
6:58 p.m., https://twitter.com/SteveSchmidtSES/status/1241861791233212416.

30. Michelle Goldberg (@michelleinbklyn), "Journalists are concentrated in cities that are
being ravaged by a plague that could have been better contained with a competent
president. They're lonely and scared and reporting while homeschooling their kids. No
one feels glee or delight. Some of us feel white hot rage," Twitter, March 29, 2020, 11:25
a.m., https://twitter.com/michelleinbklyn/status/1244284645849681922.

31. Dr. Steven W. Thrasher (@thrasherxy), "Just 'attended' my first Zoom funeral and let
me just say Fuck all of this. Fuck COVID-19. Fuck Trump letting it rip thru our most
vulnerable. Fuck the alienation of a crisis that forbids gathering & touch. & fuck the
racism, transphobia & xenophobia that lead us here," Twitter, March 30, 2020, 9:10
p.m., https://twitter.com/thrasherxy/status/1244794233250349057?lang=en.

32. Andrew Solender, "All the Times Trump Has Promoted Hydroxychloroquine," *Forbes*,
May 22, 2020, https://www.forbes.com/sites/andrewsolender/2020/05/22/all-the-times
-trump-promoted-hydroxychloroquine/?sh=7e7f7aaf4643.

33. Meridith McGraw and Sam Stein, "It's Been Exactly One Year Since Trump Suggested Injecting Bleach. We've Never Been the Same," Politico, April 23, 2021, https://www .politico.com/news/2021/04/23/trump-bleach-one-year-484399.

34. "Coronavirus: Outcry after Trump Suggests Injecting Disinfectant as Treatment," BBC, April 24, 2020, https://www.bbc.com/news/world-us-canada-52407177.

35. Aaron Rupar, "'This Is Just My Hunch': Trump Goes on Fox News and Spreads Misinformation about the Coronavirus," Vox, March 5, 2020, https://www.vox.com /2020/3/5/21166031/trump-hannity-coronavirus-who-death-rate.

36. Quint Forgey, "Trump Floats His Own Coronavirus Hunches on 'Hannity,'" *Politico*, March 5, 2020, https://www.politico.com/news/2020/03/05/trump-disputes-corona virus-death-rate-121892.

37. Philip Bump, "Trump's Habit of Fudging Inconvenient Numbers Enters Dangerous Territory," *Washington Post*, March 5, 2020, https://www.washingtonpost.com/poli tics/2020/03/05/trumps-habit-fudging-inconvenient-numbers-enters-dangerous-terri tory/.

38. "COVID-19 Integrated Surveillance Data in Italy," EpiCentro, https://www.epicentro .iss.it/en/coronavirus/sars-cov-2-dashboard.

39. Zack Jones, "Trump's 2020 Presidential Election Odds Fall as Coronavirus Stalls US Economy," *Forbes*, March 26, 2020, https://www.forbes.com/sites/zackjones/2020/03 /26/trumps-2020-presidential-election-odds-fall-as-recession-fears-grow-amid-coron avirus-pandemic/?sh=4f5cec4b4a44.

40. "Unemployment Rate," Federal Reserve Economic Data, last updated July 2, 2020, https://fred.stlouisfed.org/series/UNRATE#0.

41. Ayesha Rascoe, "Trump Resists Using Wartime Law to Get, Distribute Coronavirus Supplies," NPR, March 25, 2020, https://www.npr.org/2020/03/25/821285204/tru mp-sends-mixed-messages-about-invoking-defense-production-act.

42. Zolan Kanno-Youngs and Ana Swanson, "Wartime Production Law Has Been Used Routinely, but Not with Coronavirus," *New York Times*, March 31, 2020, https:// www.nytimes.com/2020/03/31/us/politics/coronavirus-defense-production-act.html ?smid=tw-nytimes&smtyp=cur.

43. Neil A. Halpern and Kay See Tan, "United States Resource Availability for COVID-19," Society of Critical Care Medicine, May 12, 2020, https://sccm.org/getattachment/Bl og/March-2020/United-States-Resource-Availability-for-COVID-19/United-States-Re source-Availability-for-COVID-19.pdf?lang=en-US.

44. "We're in This Together—Washington State to Send Ventilators," Washington Governor Jay Inslee, April 5, 2020, https://www.governor.wa.gov/news-media/we%E2 %80%99re-together-%E2%80%93-washington-state-send-ventilators.

45. Justin P. Hicks, "Michigan to Get 100 Ventilators from New York, Where Coronavirus Has Hit Hardest," Michigan Live, April 15, 2020, https://www.mlive.com/public -interest/2020/04/michigan-to-get-100-ventilators-from-new-york-where-coronavirus -has-hit-hardest.html.

46. "Study Suggests Possible New COVID-19 Timeline in the U.S.," American Red Cross, December 1, 2020, https://www.redcross.org/about-us/news-and-events/press-release /2020/study-suggests-possible-new-covid-19-timeline-in-the-us.html.

9: Twisting the Kaleidoscope

1. Alex Berenson (@AlexBerenson), "Coronavirus is coming…," Twitter, February 22, 2020, 11:18 a.m., https://twitter.com/alexberenson/status/1231252028417957888?la ng=en. Screenshot in my possession.

2.   *The Health Effects of Cannabis and Cannabinoids: The Current State of Evidence and Recommendations for Research* (Washington, D.C.: National Academies Press, 2017), https://www.ncbi.nlm.nih.gov/books/NBK425748/.

3.   Malcolm Gladwell, "Is Marijuana as Safe as We Think?" *New Yorker*, January 7, 2019, https://www.newyorker.com/magazine/2019/01/14/is-marijuana-as-safe-as-we-think.

4.   "Oral Evidence: UK Science, Research and Technology Capability and Influence in Global Disease Outbreaks, HC 136," Science and Technology Committee, House of Commons, March 25, 2020, https://committees.parliament.uk/oralevidence/237/html/.

5.   Neil M. Ferguson et al., "Report 9: Impact of Non-Pharmaceutical Interventions (NPIs) to Reduce COVID-19 Mortality and Healthcare Demand," Imperial College COVID-19 Response Team, March 16, 2020, https://www.imperial.ac.uk/media/imperial-col lege/medicine/sph/ide/gida-fellowships/Imperial-College-COVID19-NPI-modelling -16-03-2020.pdf.

6.   "Oral Evidence."

7.   David Adam, "UK Has Enough Intensive Care Units for Coronavirus, Expert Predicts," *New Scientist*, March 25, 2020, https://www.newscientist.com/article/2238578-uk -has-enough-intensive-care-units-for-coronavirus-expert-predicts/.

8.   Jemima Kelly, "Let's Flatten the Coronavirus Confusion Curve," *Financial Times*, March 27, 2020, https://www.ft.com/content/64b06b64-1400-426d-a147-075f806b 94e6.

9.   Alex Berenson, "Eli Lilly Said to Play Down Risk of Top Pill," *New York Times*, December 17, 2006, https://www.nytimes.com/2006/12/17/business/17drug.html.

10. Jim Romenesko, "Judge: Berenson's Actions 'Reprehensible' in Lilly Leak Case," Poynter, February 14, 2007, https://www.poynter.org/reporting-editing/2007/judge -berensons-actions-reprehensible-in-lilly-leak-case/.

10: My Father and Me

1.   Maggie Haberman (@maggieNYT), "A view of @AlexBerenson threads, which are making their way around the White House among some senior officials >," Twitter, April 5, 2020, 10:21 a.m., https://twitter.com/maggieNYT/status/124680528762707 9681.

2.   "Health Metrics Institute Receives Groundbreaking Grant," University of Washington Medicine, January 25, 2017, https://newsroom.uw.edu/story/health-metrics-institute -receives-groundbreaking-grant.

3.   Philip Bump, "The Grim Death Toll Projections the White House Offered Monday Have Already Been Revised Upward," *Washington Post*, April 2, 2020, https://www .washingtonpost.com/politics/2020/04/02/grim-death-toll-projections-white-house-of fered-monday-have-already-been-revised-upward/.

4.   Joseph Goldstein, "When Will N.Y.C. Reach the Peak of the Outbreak? Here's What We Know," *New York Times*, April 6, 2020, https://www.nytimes.com/2020/04/06 /nyregion/coronavirus-new-york-peak.html.

5.   G. Scott Thomas, "State Is Just 10 Days Away from Peak Strain on Health-Care System, Says Study," *Business Journals*, March 30, 2020, https://www.bizjournals.com/buffa lo/news/2020/03/30/state-is-just-10-days-away-from-peak-strain-on.html.

6.   Alex Berenson (@AlexBerenson), "Update on the @IMHE_UW model versus reality...," Twitter, April 2, 12:22 p.m., https://twitter.com/alexberenson/status/12457483873597 11234?lang=en. Screenshot in my possession, and available at https://thedenforum.com /t/trusting-science-pandemic-and-global-warming/4445/5.

7.   Goldstein, "When Will N.Y.C. Reach the Peak?"

8.   Carl T. Bergstrom (@CT_Bergstrom), "4. Recall this is a model of successful suppression of the epidemic with no second wave. Still my personal impression is that it's extremely optimistic. The total number of deaths is low and the epidemic passes very quickly," Twitter, March 28, 2020, 4:57 a.m., https://twitter.com/CT_Bergstrom/status/12438 24533632454657.

11: Locked Down

1.   Christopher Spata, "Coronavirus Has People Calling the Police and Shaming Neighbors on Social Media," *Tampa Bay Times*, April 7, 2020, https://www.tampabay.com/ne ws/health/2020/04/07/coronavirus-has-people-calling-the-police-and-shaming-neigh bors-on-social-media/.
2.   Daveen Rae Kurutz, "Police: Don't Call 911 Regarding Face Masks, Social Distancing in Beaver County," *Beaver County Times*, April 21, 2020, https://www.timesonline .com/news/20200421/police-donrsquot-call-911-regarding-face-masks-social-distan cing-in-beaver-county.
3.   Erika Martin, "Officials: Paddleboarder Arrested at Malibu Pier for Flouting State Stay at Home Rule," KTLA5, April 2, 2020, https://ktla.com/news/local-news/officials-pa ddleboarder-arrested-at-malibu-pier-for-flouting-state-stay-at-home-order/.
4.   "'Snitches Get Rewards': Garcetti Issues New Rules for Construction Sites, Encourages Community to Report 'Safer at Home' Violators," KCAL9 CBS Los Angeles, March 31, 2020, https://losangeles.cbslocal.com/2020/03/31/coronavirus-los-angeles-eric-gar cetti-snitches-get-rewards/.
5.   Lisa Rathke and David Goldman, "Rhode Island Door Knocks in Search of Fleeing New Yorkers," Associated Press, March 28, 2020, https://apnews.com/article/gina-ra imondo-ct-state-wire-ri-state-wire-tx-state-wire-westerly-15f7327b48cc94781fb1f8a 04948cc8c.
6.   Thomas Goetz, "A Lot of People Don't Even *Know* They Should Stay Home," *Wired*, April 9, 2020, https://www.wired.com/story/a-lot-of-people-dont-even-know-they-sh ould-stay-home/.
7.   "Mobility Trends: Change in Routing Requests since January 13, 2020," Apple Maps, https://covid19.apple.com/mobility.
8.   Chris Chmura and James Jackson, "Can Coronavirus Survive in Your Refrigerator? Here's What a Renowned Scientist Told Us," NBC Bay Area, April 3, 2020, https:// www.nbcbayarea.com/investigations/consumer/can-coronavirus-survive-in-your-refri gerator-heres-what-a-renowned-scientist-told-us/2265804/.
9.   Colleen Shalby et al., "L.A. County Tells Residents to Stay Inside This Week as Coronavirus Hits New Milestone," *Los Angeles Times*, April 7, 2020, https://www.la times.com/california/story/2020-04-07/l-a-county-tell-residents-to-stay-inside-this-we ek-as-coronavirus-hits-new-milestone.
10. Daniel J. Wakin, "Faces That Can't Be Forgotten," *New York Times*, April 16, 2020, https://www.nytimes.com/2020/04/16/reader-center/coronavirus-obits.html.
11. "Understanding Coronavirus in America," University of Southern California Center for Economic and Social Research, 2020, https://covid19pulse.usc.edu/.
12. M. Gao et al., "Supplementary Appendix" (Supplement to: M. Gao et al., "Associations between Body-Mass Index and COVID-19 Severity in 6.9 Million People in England: A Prospective, Community-Based, Cohort Study"), *Lancet Diabetes & Endocrinology*, April 28, 2021, https://www.thelancet.com/cms/10.1016/S2213-8587(21)00089-9/at tachment/88cb76d8-d2d5-4b73-9a05-fffefad4de8d/mmc1.pdf.

13. "COVID-19 Pandemic Planning Scenarios," Centers for Disease Control, March 19, 2021, https://www.cdc.gov/coronavirus/2019-ncov/hcp/planning-scenarios.html.

14. Jennifer Rubin, "Opinion: We Must Hold Politicians Responsible for Deaths They Could Have Prevented," *Washington Post*, April 1, 2020, https://www.washingtonpost.com/opinions/2020/04/01/we-must-hold-politicians-responsible-deaths-they-could-have-prevented/.

15. David Leonhardt, "Florida, Finally," *New York Times*, April 2, 2020, https://www.nytimes.com/2020/04/02/opinion/coronavirus-desantis-trump.html.

16. Erik Augustin Palm, "I Just Came Home to Sweden. I'm Horrified by the Coronavirus Response Here," Slate, April 29, 2020, https://slate.com/news-and-politics/2020/04/sweden-coronavirus-response-death-social-distancing.html.

17. Alex Berenson (@AlexBerenson), "My city in ruins...," Twitter, April 17, 2020. Screenshot in my possession, and available at https://www.google.com/search?q=@alexberenson+%22my+city+in+ruins%22&tbm=isch&source=iu&ictx=1&fir=NW2jNT5C5UlMUM%252CJIxzTej7jy0xFM%252C_&vet=1&usg=AI4_-kT-AIUF23sUmbXT2Ngjqt_wCpLY5A&sa=X&ved=2ahUKEwizn4rMyIzzAhVhGVkFHSmSBlEQ9QF6BAgVEAE#imgrc=NW2jNT5C5UlMUM.

18. Angus Johnston (@studentactivism), "'My city in ruins.' Fuck you, you weasel," Twitter, April 17, 2020, 8:40 p.m., https://twitter.com/studentactivism/status/1251309651695673345.

19. Chase Mitchell (@ChaseMit), "best it's ever looked," Twitter, April 17, 2020, 9:23 p.m., https://twitter.com/ChaseMit/status/1251320339562246145.

20. Greg Gonsalves (@greggonsalves), "As a friend of mine said this weekend: 'There are no natural or social laws preventing us from remaking the economy for the next 18 months, the next 18 years, or forever in a way that prioritizes providing people with food, shelter, health care, education, and information . . .' 12/," Twitter, March 23, 2020, 6:10 a.m., https://twitter.com/greggonsalves/status/1242030950063759361.

21. Michael Hiltzik, "Column: COVID-19 May Make Universal Basic Income More Palatable. That's a Good Thing," *Los Angeles Times*, May 22, 2020, https://www.latimes.com/business/story/2020-05-22/covid-19-universal-basic-income.

22. Brian Flood, "Jane Fonda Says Coronavirus Is 'God's Gift to the Left' because It Could Help Biden Defeat Trump," Fox News, October 7, 2020, https://www.foxnews.com/entertainment/jane-fonda-says-coronavirus-gods-gift-left-help-biden-defeat-trump.

23. Facebook App, "We're Never Lost If We Can Find Each Other," YouTube, March 31, 2020, https://www.youtube.com/watch?v=nWwVFywBCeY.

24. Ads of Brands, "Apple: Creativity Goes On," YouTube, April 15, 2020, youtube.com/watch?v=BbCe_5kSmxI&t=2s.

25. Google, "Thank You Healthcare Workers," YouTube, March 29, 2020, https://www.youtube.com/watch?v=-rtuEgAHWw0.

26. Thomas Beaumont and Hannah Fingerhut, "AP-NORC Poll: Few Americans Support Easing Virus Protections," Associated Press, April 22, 2020, https://apnews.com/article/public-health-health-us-news-ap-top-news-virus-outbreak-9ed271ca13012d3b77a2b631c1979ce1?utm_source=pushnotification.

27. Jonathan Oosting, "What Michigan's New Coronavirus Stay-at-Home Executive Order Means," Bridge Michigan, April 10, 2020, https://www.bridgemi.com/michigan-government/what-michigans-new-coronavirus-stay-home-executive-order-means.

28. Paul Egan and Kara Berg, "Thousands Converge on Lansing to Protest Whitmer's Stay Home Order," *Detroit Free Press*, April 15, 2020, https://www.freep.com/story/news/local/michigan/2020/04/15/lansing-capitol-protest-michigan-stay-home-order/5136842002/.

29. Allan Smith, "'Lock Her Up!': Anti-Whitmer Coronavirus Lockdown Protestors Swarm Michigan Capitol," NBC News, April 15, 2020, https://www.nbcnews.com/politics /politics-news/lock-her-anti-whitmer-coronavirus-lockdown-protestors-swarm-michi gan-capitol-n1184426.

30. Meagan Flynn, "Chanting 'Lock Her Up,' Michigan Protesters Waving Trump Flags Mass against Gov. Gretchen Whitmer's Coronavirus Restrictions," *Washington Post*, April 16, 2020, https://www.washingtonpost.com/nation/2020/04/16/michigan-whit mer-conservatives-protest/.

31. "Protests Not Allowed during Pandemic, Say NYC Mayor and Police Commissioner," Fox5 New York, May 4, 2020, https://www.fox5ny.com/news/protests-not-allowed -during-pandemic-say-nyc-mayor-and-police-commissioner.

12: The Perfect Storm

1. Samples that gave a cycle threshold (Ct) value <40 for both N1 and N2 targets were considered positive. See Nicholas M. Moore et al., "Comparison of Two Commercial Molecular Tests and a Laboratory-Developed Modification of the CDC 2019-nCOV RT-PCR Assay for the Qualitative Detection of SARS-CoV-2 from Upper Respiratory Tract Specimens," medRxiv, May 6, 2020, https://www.medrxiv.org/content/10.110 1/2020.05.02.20088740v1.full and "CDC 2019-Novel Coronavirus (2019-nCoV) Real-Time RT-PCR Diagnostic Panel," Federal Drug Administration, July 21, 2021, https://www.fda.gov/media/134922/download, 35: "All clinical samples should exhibit fluorescence growth curves in the RNase P reaction that cross the threshold line within 40.00 cycles....When all controls exhibit the expected performance, a specimen is considered negative if all 2019-nCoV marker (N1, N2) cycle threshold growth curves DO NOT cross the threshold line within 40.00 cycles (< 40.00 Ct) AND the RNase P growth curve DOES cross the threshold line within 40.00 cycles (< 40.00 Ct)."

2. Will Feuer and Noah Higgins-Dunn, "Cuomo Orders Most New Yorkers to Stay Inside—'We're All under Quarantine,'" CNBC, March 20, 2020, https://www.cnbc .com/2020/03/20/new-york-gov-cuomo-orders-100percent-of-non-essential-businesses -to-work-from-home.html.

3. Noah Higgins-Dunn and Will Feuer, "Gov. Cuomo Says NY Needs Ventilators Now, Help from GM and Ford 'Does Us No Good,'" CNBC, March 24, 2020, https://www .cnbc.com/2020/03/24/gov-cuomo-says-new-york-needs-ventilators-now-help-from -gm-ford-does-us-no-good.html.

4. "Daily Deaths in New York," Worldometers, https://www.worldometers.info/corona virus/usa/new-york/#graph-deaths-daily.

5. Michael Buczyner, "AHCA: 65% of Adult ICU Beds Occupied in Palm Beach County," WPTV, April 2, 2020, https://www.wptv.com/news/region-c-palm-beach-county/ah ca-65-of-adult-icu-beds-occupied-in-palm-beach-county?_amp=true.

6. Zac Anderson, "Delayed Lockdown Decision Could Haunt Gov. DeSantis," *Tallahassee Democrat*, April 3, 2020, https://www.tallahassee.com/story/news/2020/04/03/delay ed-lockdown-decision-could-haunt-gov-desantis/2938720001/.

7. Scott Powers, "Key COVID-19 Model Now Forecasting Earlier Peak in Florida," Florida Politics, April 6, 2020, https://floridapolitics.com/archives/326936-key-covid -19-model-now-forecasting-earlier-peak-in-florida/.

8. Screenshots from the website of the Florida Agency for Health Care Administration, at https://ahca.myflorida.com/, in the author's possession.

9.   Dylan Scott, "Why the Worst Fears about Florida's Covid-19 Outbreak Haven't Been Realized (So Far)," *Vox*, April 24, 2020, https://www.vox.com/2020/4/24/21234641/florida-coronavirus-covid-19-stay-at-home.

10. Arian Campo-Flores and Alex Leary, "Smart or Lucky? How Florida Dodged the Worst of Coronavirus," *Wall Street Journal*, May 3, 2020, https://www.wsj.com/articles/smart-or-lucky-how-florida-dodged-the-worst-of-coronavirus-11588531865.

11. James Glanz et al., "Where America Didn't Stay Home Even as the Virus Spread," *New York Times*, April 2, 2020, https://www.nytimes.com/interactive/2020/04/02/us/coronavirus-social-distancing.html?action=click&module=Top%20Stories&pgtype=Homepage.

12. Dan Margolies, "Private Hospital in Overland Park and Its Clinics Close, Citing Disruption Caused by COVID-19," High Plains Public Radio, April 14, 2020, https://www.hppr.org/post/private-hospital-overland-park-and-its-clinics-close-citing-disrup tion-caused-covid-19.

13. Alia Paavola, "266 Hospitals Furloughing Workers in Response to COVID-19," Becker's Hospital CFO Report, August 31, 2020, https://www.beckershospitalreview.com/finance/49-hospitals-furloughing-workers-in-response-to-covid-19.html.

14. Miriam Jordan and Annie Correal, "Foreign Doctors Could Help Fight Coronavirus. But U.S. Blocks Many," *New York Times*, April 13, 2020, https://www.nytimes.com/2020/04/13/us/coronavirus-foreign-doctors-nurses-visas.html.

15. "Potential Impact of Behavioural and Social Interventions on a Covid-19 Epidemic in the UK," SAGE, March 4, 2020, https://assets.publishing.service.gov.uk/government/uploads/system/uploads/attachment_data/file/887449/21-potential-impact-behavioural-social-interventions-04032020.pdf.

16. Alex Berenson (@AlexBerenson), "Craaazy theory coming: what if…," Twitter, April 4, 2020, 7:08 p.m., https://twitter.com/AlexBerenson/status/1246585434496524288, embedding World Health Organization (WHO), "Live from WHO Headquarters—Coronavirus—COVID-19 Daily Press Briefing 30 March 2020," YouTube, March 30, 2020, https://www.youtube.com/watch?v=2v3vlw14NbM&t=2998s. Screenshot in my possession, and available at the Wayback Machine at https://web.archive.org/web/20210425225158/https:/twitter.com/AlexBerenson/status/1246585434496524288.

17. Chris Riotta, "Ohio Governor Forced to Deny Rumors of 'Coronavirus Camps' as Unfounded Conspiracy Theories Go Viral," *The Independent*, September 8, 2020, https://www.independent.co.uk/news/world/americas/us-politics/ohio-fema-camps-co ronavirus-mandatory-quarantine-mike-dewine-b420727.html.

18. Paul M. McKeigue et al., "Relation of Severe COVID-19 in Scotland to Transmission-Related Factors and Risk Conditions Eligible for Shielding Support: REACT-SCOT Case-Control Study," MedRxiv, March 3, 2020, https://www.medrxiv.org/content/10.1101/2021.03.02.21252734v1.full.

19. Michael Schuit et al., "Airborne SARS-CoV-2 Is Rapidly Inactivated by Simulated Sunlight," *Journal of Infectious Diseases* 222, no. 4 (August 2020): 564–71, https://academic.oup.com/jid/article/222/4/564/5856149.

20. David Leonhardt, "A Misleading C.D.C. Number," *New York Times*, May 11, 2021, https://www.nytimes.com/2021/05/11/briefing/outdoor-covid-transmission-cdc-number.html.

21. "Stay Home. Save Lives," GovStatus, https://govstatus.egov.com/stayhomesavelives.

22. Gregory Pratt, "Mayor Lori Lightfoot Launches Humorous 'Stay Home, Save Lives' Anti-Coronavirus Public Service Announcements," *Chicago Tribune*, March 30, 2020, https://www.chicagotribune.com/coronavirus/ct-coronavirus-chicago-lightfoot-psa-20 200331-nhtlpne7ifbh3adl2hlari7oq4-story.html.

23. "#JimmyKimmelLiveFromHisHouse," Twitter, https://twitter.com/search?q=%23Jim myKimmelLiveFromHisHouse&src=typed_query.

24. "Coronavirus: Germany Hails Couch Potatoes in New Videos," BBC, November 16, 2020, https://www.bbc.com/news/world-europe-54959871.

25. "New Hard-Hitting National TV Ad Urges the Nation to Stay at Home," Department of Health and Social Care (UK), January 22, 2021, https://www.gov.uk/government /news/new-hard-hitting-national-tv-ad-urges-the-nation-to-stay-at-home.

26. Bess Kalb (@bessbell), "If you are lucky enough to make it off a ventilator (the equivalent exertion required for that is running a marathon without training), you will likely get put on dialysis and a feeding tube next. It's a nightmare. It's hell. It's what you're risking on your beach day," Twitter, May 3, 2020, 5:28 p.m., https://twitter.com/bessbell/sta tus/1257059600777408513.

27. Bess Kalb (@bessbell), "Send this thread to any idiot fucker who posts an Instagram at the beach or a crowded park. Tell them my dad says see you later," Twitter, May 3, 2020, 6:25 p.m., https://twitter.com/bessbell/status/1257073852330283008.

28. Erin McCarthy, "New Jersey Closes All State and County Parks to Stop Spread of the Coronavirus," *Philadelphia Inquirer*, April 7, 2020, https://www.inquirer.com/health /coronavirus/coronavirus-new-jersey-state-parks-forests-closed-covid-19-murphy-202 00407.html.

29. Hannah Fry et al., "L.A. Mayor Orders Masks to Be Worn Outdoors; County Sets No End Date for Stay-at-Home Rules but Eases More Restrictions," *Los Angeles Times*, May 13, 2020, https://www.latimes.com/california/story/2020-05-13/beaches-reopen -in-l-a-but-dont-expect-to-go-to-restaurants-or-malls-soon.

30. Peter Lane Taylor, "America's Beaches Are Open for Summer. Here's What You Need to Know State by State," *Forbes*, May 15, 2020, https://www.forbes.com/sites/peterta ylor/2020/05/15/americas-beaches-have-re-opened-for-memorial-day-weekend-heres -what-you-need-to-know-state-by-state/?sh=4894600f7f28.

31. Julia Paskin, "Why the Venice Beach Skate Park Now Looks like This," LAist, April 19, 2020, https://laist.com/news/venice-beach-skate-park-sand-filled.

32. Greg B. Smith, "Lincoln Hospital under Investigation over Patient Who Went into Coma Hours after ER Staff Lost Track of Him," *Daily News*, September 26, 2017, https://www.nydailynews.com/new-york/bronx/lincoln-hospital-investigation-losing -er-patient-article-1.3523728.

33. Howard W. French, "At Least 12 Deaths in Bronx Hospital Linked to Poor Care," *New York Times*, October 28, 1988, https://www.nytimes.com/1988/10/28/nyregion/at-le ast-12-deaths-in-hospital-in-bronx-linked-to-poor-care.html.

34. Joan Gralla, "Nursing Homes Can't Reject Patients Just over Coronavirus, State Says," *Newsday*, March 29, 2020, https://www.newsday.com/news/health/coronavirus/coro navirus-nursing-homes-1.43491608.

35. Bill Hammond and Ian Kingsbury, "COVID-Positive Admissions Were Correlated with Higher Death Rates in New York Nursing Homes," Empire Center, February 18, 2021, https://www.empirecenter.org/publications/covid-positive-admissions-higher-de ath-rates/.

36. Tracey Tully et al., "70 Died at a Nursing Home as Body Bags Piled Up. This is What Went Wrong," *New York Times*, April 19, 2020, https://www.nytimes.com/2020/04 /19/nyregion/coronavirus-nj-andover-nursing-home-deaths.html.

37. Riley Yates, "Nursing Home Deaths Devastated N.J. See Which Parts of the State Were Hit the Hardest," NJ.com, March 12, 2021, https://www.nj.com/coronavirus/2021/03 /nursing-home-deaths-devastated-nj-see-which-parts-of-the-state-were-hit-the-hardest .html.

38. Caroline Lewis, "21 Percent of NYC Residents Tested in State Study Have Antibodies from COVID-19," Gothamist, April 23, 2020, https://gothamist.com/news/new-york -antibody-test-results-coronavirus.

39. J. David Goodman and William K. Rashbaum, "N.Y.C. Death Toll Soars Past 10,000 in Revised Virus Count," *New York Times*, April 14, 2020, https://www.nytimes.com /2020/04/14/nyregion/new-york-coronavirus-deaths.html.

13: How Deadly?

1.   Brooke Baldwin, "How Fighting Coronavirus Taught Me about the Gift of Connection," CNN, April 19, 2020, https://www.cnn.com/2020/04/19/health/coron avirus-diary-sickness-brooke-baldwin/index.html.

2.   Jessica Lustig, "What I Learned When My Husband Got Sick with Coronavirus," *New York Times*, March 24, 2020, https://www.nytimes.com/2020/03/24/magazine/coro navirus-family.html.

3.   "COVID-19 Alert No. 2: New ICD Code Introduced for COVID-19 Deaths," National Vital Statistics System, Centers for Disease Control, March 24, 2020, https://www.cdc .gov/nchs/data/nvss/coronavirus/Alert-2-New-ICD-code-introduced-for-COVID-19 -deaths.pdf.

4.   "Quality Assurance Steps for COVID-19 Data," Virginia Department of Health, June 17, 2021, https://www.vdh.virginia.gov/coronavirus/category/methods/.

5.   Cole Lauterbach, "Maricopa County Clarifies How Officials Classify a 'COVID-Attributed' Death," The Center Square, September 2, 2020, https://www.thecentersq uare.com/arizona/maricopa-county-clarifies-how-officials-classify-a-covid-attributed -death/article_8269def2-ed63-11ea-872c-d7fbb82999a4.html.

6.   Amy Golden, "Coroner: State Included a Murder-Suicide in Grand's COVID Deaths," Sky-Hi News, December 15, 2020, https://www.skyhinews.com/news/coroner-state -included-a-murder-suicide-in-grands-covid-deaths/.

7.   Brian Maass, "New COVID-19 Death Dispute: Colorado Coroner Says State Mischaracterized Death," 4 CBS Denver, May 14, 2020, https://denver.cbslocal.com/20 20/05/14/coronavirus-montezuma-county-coroner-alcohol-poisoning-covid-death/.

8.   Adi V. Gundlapalli et al., "Death Certificate–Based ICD-10 Diagnosis Codes for COVID-19 Mortality Surveillance—United States, January–December 2020," Centers for Disease Control, April 9, 2021, https://www.cdc.gov/mmwr/volumes/70/wr/mm7 014e2.htm.

9.   "Characteristics of Persons Who Died with COVID-19—United States, February 12–May 18, 2020," Centers for Disease Control, July 17, 2020, https://www.cdc.gov /mmwr/volumes/69/wr/mm6928e1.htm.

10. "Provisional Death Counts and Excess Mortality, January to September 2020," Statistics Canada, November 26, 2020, https://www150.statcan.gc.ca/n1/daily-quoti dien/201126/dq201126c-eng.htm.

11. "COVID-19 Daily Epidemiology Update," Government of Canada, https://health-in fobase.canada.ca/covid-19/epidemiological-summary-covid-19-cases.html.

12. "Underlying Medical Conditions Associated with High Risk for Severe COVID-19: Information for Healthcare Providers," Centers for Disease Control, May 13, 2021, https://www.cdc.gov/coronavirus/2019-ncov/hcp/clinical-care/underlyingconditions .html#ref_3.

13. Anne Kelly et al., "Length of Stay for Older Adults Residing in Nursing Homes at the End of Life," *Journal of the American Geriatrics Society* 58, no. 9 (September 2010): 1701–1706, http://dx.doi.org/10.1111/j.1532-5415.2010.03005.x.

14. "Characteristics of SARS-CoV-2 Patients Dying in Italy Report Based on Available Data on April 28th, 2021," Epicentro, April 28, 2021, https://www.epicentro.iss.it/en /coronavirus/bollettino/Report-COVID-2019_28_april_2021.pdf.

15. "Public Data: Deaths in Milwaukee County under Medical Examiner's Jurisdiction," Milwaukee County, https://county.milwaukee.gov/EN/Medical-Examiner/ Public-Data.

16. Kelly Crowe, "Flu Deaths Reality Check," CBC News, November 25, 2012, https:// www.cbc.ca/news/health/flu-deaths-reality-check-1.1127442.

17. Kenneth D. Kochanek et al., "Mortality in the United States, 2019: NCHS Data Brief No. 395," Centers for Disease Control, December 2020, https://www.cdc.gov/nchs/da ta/databriefs/db395-H.pdf.

18. Farida B. Ahmad et al., "Provisional Mortality Data—United States, 2020," Morbidity and Mortality Weekly Report 70, no. 14 (April 2021): 519–22, https://www .ncbi.nlm.nih.gov/pmc/articles/PMC8030985/.

19. Allison Jones, "Delayed Cardiac Surgeries due to Coronavirus May Have Caused 35 Deaths in Ontario: Minister," Global News (Canada), April 28, 2020, https://globalne ws.ca/news/6879082/coronavirus-delayed-surgeries-ontario-deaths/.

20. Nick Coltrain, "Fact Check: Does COVID-19 Have a Mortality Rate of 1%–2%?" *USA Today*, May 5, 2020, https://www.usatoday.com/story/news/factcheck/2020/05 /05/covid-19-fact-check-coronavirus-mortality-rate-misleading/3019503001/.

21. Jude Joffe-Block, "COVID-19 Survival Rate Not Proof Vaccine Unnecessary," Associated Press, August 31, 2020, https://apnews.com/article/archive-fact-checking -9313631457.

22. "Fact Check: Misleading Comparison between COVID-19 Morality Rate and Vaccine Efficiency," Reuters, November 20, 2020, https://www.reuters.com/article/uk-factche ck-vaccine-comparison/fact-check-misleading-comparison-between-covid-19-morta lity-rate-and-vaccine-efficiency-idUSKBN2802H4.

23. "Second Round of COVID-19 Community Testing Completed; Miami-Dade County and the University of Miami Miller School of Medicine Announce Initial Findings," Miami-Dade County, April 24, 2020, https://www.miamidade.gov/releases/2020-04 -24-sample-testing-results.asp.

24. "USC-LA County Study: Early Results of Antibody Testing Suggest Number of COVID-19 Infections Far Exceeds Number of Confirmed Cases in Los Angeles County," County of Los Angeles Public Health, April 20, 2020, http://publichealth.la county.gov/phcommon/public/media/mediapubhpdetail.cfm?prid=2328.

25. Eran Bendavid et al., "COVID-19 Antibody Seroprevalence in Santa Clara County, California," MedRxiv, April 17, 2020, https://www.medrxiv.org/content/10.1101/20 20.04.14.20062463v1.

26. "Results Released for Antibody and COVID-19 Testing of Boston Residents," City of Boston, May 18, 2020, https://www.boston.gov/news/results-released-antibody-and -covid-19-testing-boston-residents.

27. Mark Eichmann, "Researchers at MIT's Biobot Use Fecal Matter to Track Coronavirus in Delaware," WHYY PBS, April 23, 2020, https://whyy.org/articles/researchers-at-mi ts-biobot-use-fecal-matter-to-track-coronavirus-in-delaware/.

28. Frederick J. Angulo et al., "Estimation of US SARS-CoV-2 Infections, Symptomatic Infections, Hospitalizations, and Deaths Using Seroprevalence Surveys," *Journal of the American Medical Association Network Open* 4, no. 1 (January 4, 2021), https://ja manetwork.com/journals/jamanetworkopen/fullarticle/2774584.

29. "COVID 19 Coronavirus Pandemic: United States," Worldometer, https://www.worl dometers.info/coronavirus/country/us/.

30. Sunil S. Bhopal et al., "Children and Young People Remain at Low Risk of COVID-19 Morality," *The Lancet*, March 10, 2021, https://www.thelancet.com/journals/lanchi /article/PIIS2352-4642(21)00066-3/fulltext.

31. Olivia V. Swann et al., "Clinical Characteristics of Children and Young People Admitted to Hospital with Covid-19 in United Kingdom: Prospective Multicentre Observational Cohort Study," *British Medical Journal* 370 (August 17, 2020), https://www.bmj.com /content/370/bmj.m3249.

32. Olga Khazan, "A Failure of Empathy Led to 20,000 Deaths. It Has Deep Roots," *The Atlantic*, September 22, 2020, https://www.theatlantic.com/politics/archive/2020/09 /covid-death-toll-us-empathy-elderly/616379/.

14: Hitting Bottom

1.   Stephanie Armour, "Biden Administration to Give Hospitals More Time to Spend Covid-19 Relief Money," *Wall Street Journal*, June 11, 2021, https://www.wsj.com/ar ticles/biden-administration-to-give-hospitals-more-time-to-spend-covid-19-relief-mo ney-11623427200.

2.   "State Employment and Unemployment—April 2020," Bureau of Labor Statistics, May 22, 2020, https://www.bls.gov/news.release/archives/laus_05222020.pdf.

3.   Sheela Tobben, "Oil for Less than Nothing? Here's How That Happened," Bloomberg, April 21, 2020, https://www.bloomberg.com/news/articles/2020-04-20/negative-pri ces-for-oil-here-s-what-that-means-quicktake.

4.   Sanya Mansoor, "'The Food Supply Chain Is Breaking.' Tyson Foods Warns of Meat Shortage as Plants Close Due to COVID19," *Time*, April 26, 2020, https://time.com /5827631/tyson-foods-meat-shortage/.

5.   Hollie Silverman, "More than 370 Workers at a Pork Plant in Missouri Tested Positive for Coronavirus. All Were Asymptomatic," CNN, May 4, 2020, https://www.cnn.com /2020/05/04/us/triumph-foods-outbreak-missouri/index.html.

6.   Jeanna Smialek, "The Fed Goes All In with Unlimited Bond-Buying Plan," *New York Times*, March 23, 2020, https://www.nytimes.com/2020/03/23/business/economy/co ronavirus-fed-bond-buying.html.

7.   "Unemployment Insurance Relief during COVID-19 Outbreak," Department of Labor, https://www.dol.gov/coronavirus/unemployment-insurance.

8.   Alan Rappeport and Niraj Chokshi, "Crippled Airline Industry to Get $25 Billion Bailout, Part of It as Loans," *New York Times*, April 14, 2020, https://www.nytimes .com/2020/04/14/business/coronavirus-airlines-bailout-treasury-department.html.

9.   "State Actions on Coronavirus Relief Bills," National Conference of State Legislatures, https://www.ncsl.org/research/fiscal-policy/state-actions-on-coronavirus-relief-funds .aspx.

10. Michael Collins and Deirdre Shesgreen, "The $2 Trillion Stimulus Is the Biggest in History. How Does It Compare to 9/11, Financial Crisis Bills?" *USA Today*, March 25, 2020, https://www.usatoday.com/story/news/politics/2020/03/25/coronavirus-emer gency-bill-how-does-it-compare-9-11-financial-crisis/5010452002/.

11. "Coronavirus: Trump Orders Meatpacking Plants to Stay Open," BBC, April 29, 2020, https://www.bbc.com/news/world-us-canada-52466502.

12. "The Florida Department of Economic Opportunity Announces the Pensacola Area December 2020 Employment Data," Florida Department of Economic Opportunity, January 22, 2021, https://www.floridajobs.org/news-center/DEO-Press/2021/01/22 /the-florida-department-of-economic-opportunity-announces-the-pensacola-area-de cember-2020-employment-data.

13. "Gross Domestic Product, 4th Quarter and Year 2020 (Advance Estimate)," Bureau of Economic Analysis, January 28, 2021, https://www.bea.gov/news/2021/gross-do mestic-product-4th-quarter-and-year-2020-advance-estimate.

15: Apocalypse Not

1. Amanda Mull, "Georgia's Experiment in Human Sacrifice," *The Atlantic*, April 29, 2020, https://www.theatlantic.com/health/archive/2020/04/why-georgia-reopening -coronavirus-pandemic/610882/.
2. Dana Millbank, "Georgia Leads the Race to Become America's No. 1 Death Destination," *Panama City News Herald*, April 25, 2020, https://www.newsherald .com/opinion/20200425/dana-milbank-georgia-leads-race-to-become-americas-no -1-death-destination.
3. "Models Project Sharp Rise in Deaths as States Reopen," *New York Times*, May 4, 2020, https://www.nytimes.com/2020/05/04/us/coronavirus-live-updates.html.
4. Allison Chiu and Kate Shephard, "Trump Wanted a Coronavirus Victory Event: It Ended When He Stalked Off after Clashing with Two Female Reporters," *Washington Post*, May 12, 2020, https://www.washingtonpost.com/nation/2020/05/12/trump-me ltdown-coronavirus-testing/.
5. Steve Holland and Jeff Mason, "White House to Wind Down Coronavirus Task Force as Focus Shifts to Aftermath: Trump," Reuters, May 5, 2020, https://www.reuters.com /article/us-health-coronavirus-usa-task-force-idUSKBN22H2KJ.
6. Brian Naylor and Tamara Keith, "Trump Says Coronavirus Task Force to Stay 'Indefinitely,' after Signaling Wind-Down," NPR, May 5, 2020, https://www.npr.org /sections/coronavirus-live-updates/2020/05/05/850959187/white-house-cornoavirus -task-force-to-wind-down.
7. Jorge L. Ortiz, "When Will US Reach 100,000 Deaths? After a Horrific April, Grim Milestone Could Hit in May," *USA Today*, May 4, 2020, https://www.usatoday.com /story/news/nation/2020/05/01/coronavirus-us-may-hit-10000-deaths-record-cases -may/3062216001/.
8. Charlotte Klein, "Trump, Maskless, Goes Golfing as Coronavirus Death Toll Nears 100,000," *Vanity Fair*, May 24, 2020, https://www.vanityfair.com/news/2020/05/tru mp-maskless-goes-golfing-as-coronavirus-death-toll-nears-100000.
9. Jay Greene, "Case of Man Found Dead in Car Off of I-380 in Cedar Rapids Ruled a Homicide, Police Say," 9 ABC KCRG, March 20, 2020, kcrg.com/content/news/Case -of-man-found-dead-in-car-off-of-I-380-in-Cedar-Rapids-ruled-a-homicide-police-say -568966831.html.
10. Alex Berenson (@AlexBerenson), "Serious question: anyone wonder how far down the list…," Twitter, May 23, 2020, 8:37 p.m., https://twitter.com/AlexBerenson/status/12 64354723374739459. Screenshot in my possession.

16: Musk, Bezos, and Me

1. Brian Flood, "Free Speech Advocates Call YouTube's Removal of Coronavirus-Related Video 'Egregious Censorship Effort,'" Fox News, April 29, 2020, https://www.foxne ws.com/media/youtube-video-removed-coronavirus-free-speech.
2. "YouTube's Political Censorship," *Wall Street Journal*, September 14, 2020, https:// www.wsj.com/articles/youtubes-political-censorship-11600126230.

3. David Bondy, "Facebook Shuts Down Group Page Critical of Michigan Stay-at-Home Order," NBC 25 News, May 13, 2020, https://nbc25news.com/news/coronavirus/organizer-of-anti-michigan-quarantine-says-facebook-shut-down-their-group-page.
4. Ava Kofman, "The Hate Store: Amazon's Self-Publishing Arm Is a Haven for White Supremacists," ProPublica, April 7, 2020, https://www.propublica.org/article/the-hate-store-amazons-self-publishing-arm-is-a-haven-for-white-supremacists.
5. Charles Duhigg, "Is Amazon Unstoppable?" *New Yorker*, October 10, 2019, https://www.newyorker.com/magazine/2019/10/21/is-amazon-unstoppable.
6. Alex Berenson (@AlexBerenson), "THEY CENSORED IT! It is based...," Twitter, June 4, 2020, 9:09 a.m., https://twitter.com/AlexBerenson/status/1268530222946758656. Screenshot in my possession, and available at the Wayback Machine at https://web.archive.org/web/20210804135453/https:/twitter.com/AlexBerenson/status/126853022 2946758656.
7. Glenn Greenwald (@ggreenwald), "I've most definitely found Alex Berenson's Covid commentary inaccurate and reckless, but book banning by corporate tech giants is a far worse danger than whatever threats his book supposedly presents," Twitter, June 4, 2020, 3:09 p.m., https://twitter.com/ggreenwald/status/1268620912791744512?lang=en.
8. Andrew Sullivan (@sullydish), "I think this guy is nuts. But denying him access to Amazon because of the content of his book is appalling," Twitter, June 4, 2020, 10:25 a.m., https://twitter.com/sullydish/status/1268549557975158786.
9. Brit Hume (@brithume), ".Amazon.com is refusing to sell @AlexBerenson's booklet on Covid 19. He has been a leading—perhaps THE leading—dissenter on the paralyzing Covid 19 lockdowns. He draws his information from studies and official data.," Twitter, June 4, 2020, 10:33 a.m., https://twitter.com/brithume/status/1268551341519110145 ?lang=en.
10. Elon Musk (@elonmusk), "Time to break up Amazon. Monopolies are wrong!" Twitter, June 4, 2020, 2:01 p.m., https://twitter.com/elonmusk/status/1268603809409888256.
11. Jodi Kantor (@jodikantor), "One phone call and you're done," Twitter, May 24, 2018, 4:33 p.m., https://twitter.com/jodikantor/status/999750330014285824.
12. Reeves Wiedeman, "Times Change: In the Trump Years, the New York *Times* Became Less Dispassionate and More Crusading, Sparking a Raw Debate over the Paper's Future," Intelligencer, *New York*, November 9, 2020, https://nymag.com/intelligencer/2020/11/inside-the-new-york-times-heated-reckoning-with-itself.html.

17: Attention Citizens!

1. Alex Berenson (@AlexBerenson), "Attention citizens: Your Dept. of Pandemia requires 10,000 New York citizens to report to hospitals...," Twitter, April 6, 2020. Screenshot in my possession.
2. Michael Powell (@powellnyt), "Not sure you and @AlexBerenson Berenson fully grasp how appallingly obnoxious you are in a moment of maximum pain for so many people. There is a path to raise questions and there's another to be an asshole...," Twitter, April 7, 2020, 7:35 p.m., https://twitter.com/powellnyt/status/1247669275420221442.
3. Bruce Arthur (@bruce_arthur), "Alex, hi, she cares about people's lives, you're a stupid insane ghoul who should be ashamed every second you're alive, hope this helps," Twitter, June 19, 2020, 9:40 p.m., https://twitter.com/bruce_arthur/status/12741550 15423361025.
4. Bess Kalb (@bessbell), "You fucking ghoul," Twitter, May 6, 2020, 12:32 p.m., https://mobile.twitter.com/bessbell/status/1258072189909135360.

5. Talia Lavin (@chick_in_kiev), "eat shit you death ghoul," Twitter, July 19, 2020, 3:22 a.m., https://twitter.com/chick_in_kiev/status/1284750332472500224.

6. b-boy-bouiebaisse (@jbouie), "This pandemic killed my grandfather but yes, I am sorry you have not been able to get your haircut," Twitter, May 2, 2020, 8:34 p.m., https://twitter.com/jbouie/status/1256743817224392706.

7. Alex Berenson (@AlexBerenson), "Very sorry to hear about your grandfather. My grandparents died of…," Twitter, May 2, 2020, 6:05 p.m. Screenshot in my possession.

8. Alex Berenson (@AlexBerenson), "Went back to see all the blue-check hate I got over the weekend…," Twitter, May 6, 2020, 10:26 p.m. Screenshot in my possession.

9. Alex Berenson, (@AlexBerenson), "Hey @Neil_Ferguson, fuck you: You shut down the world but ignored the lockdown to have an affair with a married woman?" Twitter, May 5, 2020, 2:46 p.m. Screenshot in my possession.

10. Alex Berenson (@AlexBerenson), "Wondering what's really happening in Texas?…," Twitter, June 29, 2020, 6:17 p.m. Screenshot in my possession, and available at the Wayback Machine at https://web.archive.org/web/20200630012014/https://twitter.com/AlexBerenson/status/1277773344625119234.

11. Frank Cerabino, "Wellington Equestrian Estate Prompts Pandemic Political Potshots at Illinois Governor," *Palm Beach Post*, May 2, 2020, https://www.palmbeachpost.com/news/20200502/cerabino-wellington-equestrian-estate-prompts-pandemic-political-potshots-at-illinois-governor.

12. T. R. Allen et al., "An Outbreak of Common Colds at an Antarctic Base after Seventeen Weeks of Complete Isolation," *Journal of Hygiene* 71, no. 4 (1973): 657–67, https://www.ncbi.nlm.nih.gov/pmc/articles/PMC2130424/?page=10.

13. David Freedlander, "Does the King of the COVID-19 Contrarians Have a Case?" *Vanity Fair*, April 16, 2020, https://www.vanityfair.com/news/2020/04/does-the-king-of-the-covid-19-contrarians-have-a-case; Laura Wagner, "Here Are the Questions the Right's Favorite Coronavirus Truther Isn't Willing to Answer," Vice, April 16, 2020, https://www.vice.com/en/article/jge7g4/here-are-the-question-the-rights-favorite-coronavirus-truther-isnt-willing-to-answer.

18: Masking, Unmasked

1. J. Edward Moreno, "Ocasio-Cortez Dismisses Proposed $1B Cut: 'Defunding Police Means Defunding Police,'" *The Hill*, June 30, 2020, https://thehill.com/homenews/house/505307-ocasio-cortez-dismisses-proposed-1b-cut-defunding-police-means-defunding.

2. Mariame Kaba, "Yes, We Mean Literally Abolish the Police," *New York Times*, June 12, 2020, https://www.nytimes.com/2020/06/12/opinion/sunday/floyd-abolish-defund-police.html.

3. John Aguilar, "Many Health Officials Are OK with Police Protests despite COVID-19," *Denver Post*, June 15, 2020, https://www.denverpost.com/2020/06/15/coronavirus-protests-health-racism/.

4. Jingyi Xiao et al., "Nonpharmaceutical Measures for Pandemic Influenza in Nonhealthcare Settings—Personal Protective and Environmental Measures," *Emerging Infectious Diseases* 26, no. 5 (May 2020): 967–975, https://wwwnc.cdc.gov/eid/article/26/5/19-0994_article.

5. C. Raina MacIntyre et al., "A Cluster Randomised Trial of Cloth Masks Compared with Medical Masks in Health Workers," *BMJ Open* 5 (April 22, 2015), https://bmjopen.bmj.com/content/bmjopen/5/4/e006577.full.pdf.

6.   Ontario Nurses' Association, "ONA Wins Landmark Influenza Vaccine-or-Mask Grievance," Cision, September 10, 2015, https://www.newswire.ca/news-releases/ona -wins-landmark-influenza-vaccine-or-mask-grievance-526265811.html.

7.   "In the Matter of an Arbitration between Sault Area Hospital ('SAH' or 'Hospital') and Ontario Hospital Association ('OHA') and Ontario Nurses' Association ('Union' or 'ONA')," Canadian Legal Information Institute, September 2015, https://www.can lii.org/en/on/onla/doc/2015/2015canlii62106/2015canlii62106.pdf.

8.   "In the Matter of an Arbitration between St. Michael's Hospital and The Ontario Hospital Association and The Ontario Nurses' Association," Ontario Nurses' Association, September 6, 2018, https://www.ona.org/wp-content/uploads/ona_kapla narbitrationdecision_vaccineormask_stmichaelsoha_20180906.pdf.

9.   Samy Rengasamy et al., "Filtration Performance of FDA-Cleared Surgical Masks," *Journal of the International Society for Respiratory Protection* 26, no. 3 (2009): 54–70, https://www.ncbi.nlm.nih.gov/pmc/articles/PMC7357397/.

10. "Understanding the Difference," Centers for Disease Control, https://www.cdc.gov/ni osh/npptl/pdfs/understanddifferenceinfographic-508.pdf.

11. Joe Carlson and Christopher Snowbeck, "Walz Urged to Require Minnesotans to Wear Masks in COVID-19 Fight," *Star Tribune*, July 2, 2020, https://www.startribune.com /gov-walz-is-urged-to-require-minnesotans-to-wear-masks-in-covid-19-fight/571593 692/.

12. "Advice on the Use of Masks in the Community, during Home Care and in Health Care Settings in the Context of the Novel Coronavirus (2019-nCoV) Outbreak," World Health Organization, January 29, 2020, https://apps.who.int/iris/bitstream/handle/10 665/330987/WHO-nCov-IPC_Masks-2020.1-eng.pdf?sequence=1&isAllowed=y.

13. Brit McCandless Farmer, "March 2020: Dr. Anthony Fauci Talks with Dr. John Lapook about COVID-19," CBS News, March 8, 2020, https://www.cbsnews.com/ne ws/preventing-coronavirus-facemask-60-minutes-2020-03-08/.

14. Michael Klompas et al., "Universal Masking in Hospitals in the Covid-19 Era," *New England Journal of Medicine* 382, no. 21 (May 21, 2020), https://www.nejm.org/doi /full/10.1056/NEJMp2006372.

15. Judy Woodruff et al., "What Dr. Fauci Wants You to Know about Face Masks and Staying Home as Virus Spreads," PBS, April 3, 2020, https://www.pbs.org/newshour /show/what-dr-fauci-wants-you-to-know-about-face-masks-and-staying-home-as-vi rus-spreads.

16. Daniel Lippman and Meredith McGraw, "Inside the National Security Council, a Rising Sense of Dread," *Politico*, April 2, 2020, https://www.politico.com/news/2020 /04/02/nsc-coronavirus-white-house-162530.

17. "Remarks by President Trump, Vice President Pence, and Members of the Coronavirus Task Force in Press Briefing," Trump White House Archives, April 3, 2020, https://tr umpwhitehouse.archives.gov/briefings-statements/remarks-president-trump-vice-pre sident-pence-members-coronavirus-task-force-press-briefing-18/.

18. Henning Bundgaard et al., "Effectiveness of Adding a Mask Recommendation to Other Public Health Measures to Prevent SARS-CoV-2 Infection in Danish Mask Wearers," *Annals of Internal Medicine* 174, no. 3 (March 2021): 335–43, https://www.acpjour nals.org/doi/10.7326/m20-6817.

19. Xiaowen Wang et al., "Association Between Universal Masking in a Health Care System and SARS-CoV-2 Positivity among Health Care Workers," *Journal of the American Medical Association* 324, no. 7 (July 2020): 703–4, https://jamanetwork .com/journals/jama/fullarticle/2768533.

20. M. Joshua Hendrix et al., "Absence of Apparent Transmission of SARS-CoV-2 from Two Stylists after Exposure at a Hair Salon with a Universal Face Covering Policy—Springfield, Missouri, May 2020," *Morbidity and Mortality Weekly Report 69*, no. 28 (July 17, 2020): 930–32, https://www.cdc.gov/mmwr/volumes/69/wr/mm6928e2.htm.

21. Katherine Ross, "Why Weren't We Wearing Masks from the Beginning? Dr. Fauci Explains," TheStreet, June 12, 2020, https://www.thestreet.com/video/dr-fauci-masks-changing-directive-coronavirus.

22. Jack Nicas, "He Has 17,700 Bottles of Hand Sanitizer and Nowhere to Sell Them," *New York Times*, March 14, 2020, https://www.nytimes.com/2020/03/14/technology/coronavirus-purell-wipes-amazon-sellers.html.

23. Joanne Kenen, "What the Best Public Health Minds Know—and Don't Know—about the Wuhan Coronavirus," *Politico*, January 28, 2020, https://www.politico.com/news/2020/01/28/wuhan-coronavirus-health-108197.

24. "Transmission of SARS-CoV-2: Implications for Infection Prevention Precautions," World Health Organization, July 9, 2020, https://www.who.int/news-room/commentaries/detail/transmission-of-sars-cov-2-implications-for-infection-prevention-precautions.

25. Rahul Subramanian et al., "Quantifying Asymptomatic Infection and Transmission of COVID-19 in New York City Using Observed Cases, Serology, and Testing Capacity," *Proceedings of the National Academy of Sciences of the United States of America 118*, no. 9 (March 2021), https://www.pnas.org/content/118/9/e2019716118.

26. Quint Forgey, "Fauci Says He Wears Mask as 'Symbol' of Good Behavior," *Politico*, May 27, 2020, https://www.politico.com/news/2020/05/27/fauci-wears-mask-as-symbol-of-good-behavior-283847.

27. Jessica Castillo, "How to Talk to People Who Won't Wear Face Masks," *Teen Vogue*, July 8, 2020, https://www.teenvogue.com/story/how-to-talk-to-people-who-wont-wear-face-masks.

28. Allyson Chiru, "Some Covid-19 Rule Breakers Could Be Narcissists, Experts Say. Here's How to Approach Them," *Washington Post*, September 25, 2020, https://www.washingtonpost.com/lifestyle/wellness/narcissism-mask-covid-psychology/2020/09/25/d3de1b32-fe9c-11ea-9ceb-061d646d9c67_story.html.

29. Angela Betsaida B. Laguipo, "Sociopaths Less Likely to Comply with COVID Mask, Hygiene and Social Distancing," Medical Life Sciences News, August 24, 2020, https://www.news-medical.net/news/20200824/Sociopaths-less-likely-to-comply-with-COVID-mask-hygiene-and-social-distancing.aspx.

30. Stephanie Kramer, "More Americans Say They Are Regularly Wearing Masks in Stores and Other Businesses," Pew Research Center, August 27, 2020, https://www.pewresearch.org/fact-tank/2020/08/27/more-americans-say-they-are-regularly-wearing-masks-in-stores-and-other-businesses/.

31. Matt Gertz, "Masks Work. Fox Keeps Hosting Alex Berenson to Claim They Don't," Media Matters, September 11, 2020, https://www.mediamatters.org/coronavirus-covid-19/masks-work-fox-keeps-hosting-alex-berenson-claim-they-dont.

19: Another Brick in the Wall

1. Eric Lipton et al., "He Could Have Seen What Was Coming: Behind Trump's Failure on the Virus," *New York Times*, April 11, 2020, https://www.nytimes.com/2020/04/11/us/politics/coronavirus-trump-response.html.

2. "National School Lunch Program," U.S. Department of Agriculture Economic Research Service, https://www.ers.usda.gov/topics/food-nutrition-assistance/child-nutrition-programs/national-school-lunch-program.
3. Amanda Eisenberg and Madina Touré, "De Blasio: NYC Schools Will Close as of Monday, May Not Reopen This Year," *Politico*, March 15, 2020, https://www.politico.com/states/new-york/albany/story/2020/03/15/de-blasio-nyc-schools-will-close-as-of-monday-may-not-reopen-this-year-1267141.
4. Lauren Camera, "Bill de Blasio: New York City Schools to Stay Open—for Now," *U.S. News & World Report*, March 14, 2020, https://www.usnews.com/news/education-news/articles/2020-03-14/bill-de-blasio-new-york-city-schools-to-stay-open-for-now.
5. Eisenberg and Touré, "De Blasio: NYC Schools Will Close."
6. "Education Systems' Response to COVID19," World Bank, April 3, 2020, https://pubdocs.worldbank.org/en/857971586182572110/COVID19EducationSectorBriefApril3.pdf.
7. Liz Bowie, "'We Feel Like We Are Drowning': Baltimore-Area Parents Struggle to Guide Kids' Schooling from Home," *Baltimore Sun*, May 8, 2020, https://www.baltimoresun.com/coronavirus/bs-md-families-work-remote-learning-20200508-fwxqvp4a6rawdhq4maowwikeoi-story.html.
8. "Stress in America 2020," American Psychological Association, May 2020, https://www.apa.org/news/press/releases/stress/2020/report.
9. Jamie Goldberg, "Oregon School Closures Strain Single-Parent Families during Coronavirus Outbreak," *The Oregonian*, April 18, 2020, https://www.oregonlive.com/coronavirus/2020/04/oregon-school-closures-strain-single-parent-families-during-coronavirus-outbreak.html.
10. Usha Ranji et al., "Women, Work, and Family during COVID-19: Findings from the KFF's Women's Health Survey," Kaiser Family Foundation, March 22, 2021, https://www.kff.org/womens-health-policy/issue-brief/women-work-and-family-during-covid-19-findings-from-the-kff-womens-health-survey/.
11. Alec MacGillis, "The Students Left Behind by Remote Learning," ProPublica, September 28, 2020, https://www.propublica.org/article/the-students-left-behind-by-remote-learning.
12. Ariel Gilreath, "Thousands of Students in SC Aren't Doing Their School Work. Some Have Completely Ghosted," *Greenville News*, May 4, 2020, https://www.greenvilleonline.com/story/news/2020/05/04/coronavirus-thousands-students-sc-not-doing-their-school-work/3040883001/.
13. Veronique Mintz, "Why I'm Learning More with Distance Learning Than I Do in School," *New York Times*, May 5, 2020, https://www.nytimes.com/2020/05/05/opinion/coronavirus-pandemic-distance-learning.html.
14. Jeb Bush, "Opinion: It's Time to Embrace Distance Learning—and Not Just Because of the Coronavirus," *Washington Post*, May 3, 2020, https://www.washingtonpost.com/opinions/2020/05/03/jeb-bush-its-time-embrace-distance-learning-not-just-because-coronavirus/.
15. "Coronavirus: German Easing of Lockdown to Start with Schools on May 4," Deutsche Welle, April 15, 2020, https://www.dw.com/en/coronavirus-german-easing-of-lockdown-to-start-with-schools-on-may-4/a-53127607.
16. "Schools Reopen in Some Parts of Japan after Pandemic Shutdown," *Japan Times*, May 7, 2020, https://www.japantimes.co.jp/news/2020/05/07/national/schools-reopen-coronavirus/.

17. Kostas Danis et al., "Cluster of Coronavirus Disease 2019 (COVID-19) in the French Alps, February 2020," *Clinical Infectious Diseases* 71, no. 15 (August 1, 2020): 825–32, https://academic.oup.com/cid/article/71/15/825/5819060.

18. Qin Wu et al., "Coinfection and Other Clinical Characteristics of COVID-19 in Children," *Pediatrics* 146, no. 1 (July 2020), https://pediatrics.aappublications.org/content/146/1/e20200961.long.

19. "Research Results Based on Data from Municipal Public Health Services (GGDs)," National Institute for Public Health and the Environment (Netherlands), https://www.rivm.nl/en/coronavirus-covid-19/children-and-covid-19/data-from-municipal-public-health-services.

20. Alex Berenson (@AlexBerenson), "From California: not one #coronavirusdeath among the…," Twitter, July 14, 2020, 1:19 p.m. Screenshot in my possession.

21. Clare Smith et al., "Deaths in Children and Young People in England following SARS-CoV-2 Infection during the First Pandemic Year: A National Study Using Linked Mandatory Child Death Reporting Data," Research Square, https://assets.researchsquare.com/files/rs-689684/v1/3e4e93fb-4e98-4081-9315-16143c2bbd2b.pdf?c=1625678600.

22. Nick Coatsworth, "Getting Our Kids Back to School—a Matter of Trust," Australian Government Department of Health, May 3, 2020, https://www.health.gov.au/news/getting-our-kids-back-to-school-a-matter-of-trust.

23. Kyle Swenson, "New D.C. Hospital Numbers Suggest Kids Do Face Some Risk of Coronavirus Hospitalization," *Washington Post*, April 25, 2020, https://www.washingtonpost.com/local/new-dc-hospital-numbers-suggest-kids-do-face-some-risk-of-coronavirus-hospitalization/2020/04/25/5e78c268-86fe-11ea-878a-86477a724bdb_story.html.

24. Eli Saslow, "Voices from the Pandemic," *Washington Post*, August 23, 2020, https://www.washingtonpost.com/nation/2020/08/23/brothers-coronavirus-virginia/.

25. Joseph Goldstein and Pam Belluck, "Children Are Falling Ill with a Baffling Ailment Related to Covid-19," *New York Times*, May 5, 2020, https://www.nytimes.com/2020/05/05/nyregion/kawasaki-disease-coronavirus.html?action=click&module=Top%20Stories&pgtype=Homepage.

26. Sammy Turner and Brad Streicher, "Deadly Illness in Children Linked to COVID-19 Confirmed in Austin Hospital, More Cases Suspected," KVUE, June 3, 2020, https://www.kvue.com/article/news/health/coronavirus/multisystem-inflammatory-syndrome-dell-childrens-austin-coronavirus/269-ef12525f-213c-437a-ad9a-094f422c2f99.

27. "PIMS-TS Inflammation in Children," The UK Kawasaki Disease Foundation, May 15, 2020, https://www.societi.org.uk/kawasaki-disease-covid-19/pims-ts/.

28. Claire Cain Miller and Margot Sanger-Katz, "How 132 Epidemiologists Are Deciding When to Send Their Children to School," *New York Times*, June 12, 2020, https://www.nytimes.com/2020/06/12/upshot/epidemiologists-decisions-children-school-coronavirus.html.

29. "Covid-19 in Schoolchildren: A Comparison between Finland and Sweden," The Public Health Agency of Sweden, 2020, https://www.folkhalsomyndigheten.se/contentassets/c1b78bffbfde4a7899eb0d8ffdb57b09/covid-19-school-aged-children.pdf.

30. "Remarks by President Trump in Roundtable Discussion on Fighting for America's Seniors," Trump White House Archives, June 15, 2020, https://trumpwhitehouse.archives.gov/briefings-statements/remarks-president-trump-roundtable-discussion-fighting-americas-seniors/.

31. Mark Moore, "Randi Weingarten: 'No Way' Schools Can Return This Fall without More Funding," *New York Post*, July 12, 2020, https://nypost.com/2020/07/12/weinga rten-no-way-schools-open-this-fall-without-funding/.

32. Edmund DeMarche, "LA Teachers Union Wants More Money by Defunding the Police, Calls for Medicare for All," Fox News, July 13, 2020, https://www.foxnews.com/us/ los-angeles-teachers-union-calls-on-defunding-police-before-reopening.

33. Melissa Klein, "COVID-19 School Construction Delays Lead to Prolonged Overcrowding," *New York Post*, May 22, 2021, https://nypost.com/2021/05/22/covid -19-school-construction-delays-lead-to-prolonged-overcrowding/.

34. Oriol Güell, "Major Coronavirus Study in Spanish Summer Camps Shows Low Transmission among Children," *El País*, August 26, 2020, https://english.elpais.com /society/2020-08-26/major-coronavirus-study-in-spanish-summer-camps-shows-low -transmission-among-children.html.

35. Ibid.

36. Apoorva Mandavilli, "Older Children Spread the Coronavirus Just as Much as Adults, Large Study Finds," *New York Times*, July 18, 2020, https://www.nytimes.com/2020 /07/18/health/coronavirus-children-schools.html.

37. Apoorva Mandavilli, "Older Children and the Coronavirus: A New Wrinkle in the Debate," *New York Times*, August 14, 2020, https://www.nytimes.com/2020/08/14 /health/older-children-and-the-coronavirus-a-new-wrinkle-in-the-debate.html.

38. Mairead McArdle, "NYC Teachers' Union Threatens Strike Unless 'Every Single Person' Who Enters a School Receives COVID Test," *National Review*, August 19, 2020, https://www.nationalreview.com/news/nyc-teachers-union-threatens-strike-un less-every-single-person-who-enters-a-school-receives-covid-test/.

39. Emily Bloch, "Teachers Are Drafting Wills along with Lesson Plans; One Even Wrote Her Own Obituary," *USA Today*, August 13, 2020, https://www.usatoday.com/story /news/education/2020/08/13/florida-teachers-writing-wills-obituaries-school-reopeni ng-coronavirus/3362679001/.

40. Rebecca Martinson, "I Won't Return to the Classroom, and You Shouldn't Ask Me To," *New York Times*, July 18, 2020, https://www.nytimes.com/2020/07/18/opinion /sunday/covid-schools-reopen-teacher-safety.html.

41. Lizzie Widdicombe, "Should You Send Your Child Back to School during the Pandemic?" *New Yorker*, August 26, 2020, https://www.newyorker.com/news/news -desk/should-you-send-your-child-back-to-school-during-the-pandemic.

42. Dana Goldstein, "She Fought to Reopen Schools, Becoming a Hero and a Villain," *New York Times*, June 22, 2021, https://www.nytimes.com/2021/06/22/us/emily-os ter-school-reopening.html.

43. Talia Lavin (@chick_in_kiev), "this is NOT parenting-shaming good god. i don't have a kid and if i did i'd be going insane right now. on the other hand. the far right fucking loves chaos. a nazi tried to bomb a covid-laden hospital yesterday," Twitter, March 26, 2020, 9:25 p.m., https://twitter.com/chick_in_kiev/status/1243348414450085889.

44. "15 Schools, Rec Centers to Host City Students for In-Person Virtual Learning," WBAL-TV 11, September 10, 2020, https://www.wbaltv.com/article/student-learning -centers-baltimore-schools-recreation-centers-in-person-virtual-learning/33897548#.

45. Laurel Wamsley, "Florida Orders Schools to Reopen in the Fall for in-Person Instruction," NPR, July 7, 2020, https://www.npr.org/sections/coronavirus-live-upda tes/2020/07/07/888320203/florida-orders-schools-to-reopen-in-the-fall-for-in-person -instruction.

46. "Burbio's K–12 School Opening Tracker," Burbio, https://cai.burbio.com/school-open ing-tracker/.

47. Reese Oxner, "Texas Students' Standardized Test Scores Dropped Dramatically during the Pandemic, Especially in Math," *Texas Tribune*, June 28, 2021, https://www.texas tribune.org/2021/06/28/texas-staar-test-results/.

48. Evie Fordham, "Randi Weingarten Faces Backlash for Claiming AFT Tried to Reopen Schools Starting April 2020," Fox News, July 1, 2021, https://www.foxnews.com/po litics/weingarten-american-federation-teachers-reopening-2020-coronavirus.

20: Another Brick in the Wall (College Remix)

1. Nikki Krize, "Travel Restrictions at Bucknell University," WNEP 16, September 18, 2020, https://www.wnep.com/article/news/local/union-county/travel-restrictions-at -bucknell-university/523-467860ff-1ca4-4962-8109-063193e25f6a.

2. Angela Ruggiero, "UC Berkeley Bans Campus Residents from Outdoor Exercise as Part of Clampdown after COVID Surge," *Mercury News*, February 11, 2021, https:// www.mercurynews.com/2021/02/11/uc-berkeley-bans-outdoor-exercise-in-tighter-co vid-19-restrictions-on-campus/.

3. Nicole Acevedo, "Coronavirus Rules Lead Northeastern University to Dismiss 11 Students over a Gathering," NBC News, September 5, 2020, https://www.nbcnews .com/news/us-news/coronavirus-rules-lead-northeastern-university-dismiss-11-studen ts-over-gathering-n1239419.

4. Troy Closson, "'Nobody Likes Snitching': How Rules against Parties Are Dividing Campuses," *New York Times*, September 2, 2020, https://www.nytimes.com/2020 /09/02/nyregion/colleges-universities-covid-parties.html.

5. Jan Wolfe and Daphne Psaledakis, "As Some U.S. College Students Party, Others Blow the Whistle," Reuters, September 16, 2020, https://www.reuters.com/article/us-health -coronavirus-usa-colleges-idUSKBN2671TW.

6. Anna Silman, "You Could Get Us All Sent Home," The Cut, *New York*, September 10, 2020, https://www.thecut.com/article/college-students-parties-campus-covid.html.

7. Penelope Gardner, "Save a Life: Be a Snitch," *University News* (St. Louis University), September 30, 2020, https://unewsonline.com/2020/09/save-a-life-be-a-snitch/.

8. "West Virginia Univ. President Apologizes for Maskless Photo," Associated Press, September 15, 2020, https://apnews.com/article/media-social-media-gordon-gee-west -virginia-virus-outbreak-a4c6f7d7992314cb0d5388a650183649.

9. Dennis Dodd, "Coronavirus in College Football: Hospitalizations, Deaths Predicted by Data Analysts if FBS Plays in 2020," CBS Sports, June 30, 2020, https://www.cbss ports.com/college-football/news/coronavirus-in-college-football-hospitalizations-dea ths-projected-by-data-analysts-if-fbs-plays-in/.

10. Elizabeth Cooney, "Covid-19 Infections Leave an Impact on the Heart, Raising Concerns about Lasting Damage," Stat News, July 27, 2020, https://www.statnews .com/2020/07/27/covid19-concerns-about-lasting-heart-damage/.

11. John Mandrola et al., "Setting the Record Straight: There Is No 'Covid Heart,'" Stat News, May 14, 2021, https://www.statnews.com/2021/05/14/setting-the-record-stra ight-there-is-no-covid-heart/.

12. Juan Perez Jr., "'Play College Football!' Trump Demands as Fall Season Collapses," *Politico*, August 10, 2020, https://www.politico.com/news/2020/08/10/trump-gop-col lege-football-393135.

13. Chris Solari and David Jesse, "Big Ten Football Reinstated; 9-Game Season to Begin October 24," *Detroit Free Press*, September 16, 2020, https://www.freep.com/story/sp orts/college/2020/09/16/big-ten-football-update-vote-2020/5814647002/.

14. Ibid.

15. Jonathan Haidt and Greg Lukianoff, *The Coddling of the American Mind: How Good Intentions and Bad Ideas Are Setting Up a Generation for Failure* (New York: Penguin, 2019), 30.
16. "Motor Vehicle Deaths in 2020 Estimated to Be Highest in 13 Years, Despite Dramatic Drops in Miles Driven," National Safety Council, March 4, 2021, https://www.nsc .org/newsroom/motor-vehicle-deaths-2020-estimated-to-be-highest.
17. Kate Bayless, "What Is Helicopter Parenting?" December 5, 2019, *Parents*, https:// www.parents.com/parenting/better-parenting/what-is-helicopter-parenting/.
18. Ellen Yard et al., "Emergency Department Visits for Suspected Suicide Attempts among Young Persons Aged 12–25 Years before and during the COVID Pandemic—United States, January 2019–May 2021," *Morbidity and Mortality Weekly Report* 70, no. 24 (June 2021): 888–94, https://www.cdc.gov/mmwr/volumes/70/wr/mm7024e1.htm.
19. Abbey Machtig, "Nationally, Many Students Are Unwilling to Receive COVID-19 Testing, UMN Expert Says," *Minnesota Daily*, September 18, 2020, https://mndaily .com/262376/news/nationally-many-students-are-unwilling-to-receive-covid-19-testi ng-umn-expert-says/.
20. Lauren Myers and Amanda Hara, "'COVID-19 Pacts' Happening among UT Students," WVLT 8, September 15, 2020, https://www.wvlt.tv/2020/09/15/covid-19 -pacts-happening-among-ut-students/.
21. Veneta Rizvic, "Mizzou Will Go Back to Virtual Learning after Thanksgiving Break," *St. Louis Business Journal*, November 13, 2020, https://www.bizjournals.com/stlouis /news/2020/11/13/mizzou-will-go-back-to-virtual-learning.html.
22. Graham Rapier, "New College Enrollments Plunged 16% This Fall as Incoming Freshmen Opted for Gap Years over Virtual Learning," Business Insider, October 15, 2020, https://www.businessinsider.com/college-enrollment-numbers-decrease-during -covid-coronavirus-virtual-learning-data-2020-10.

21: Deaths of Despair

1. Mackenzie Bean, "Suicides Fell in 2020, Early CDC Data Shows," *Becker's Hospital Review*, April 1, 2021, https://www.beckershospitalreview.com/public-health/suicides -fell-in-2020-early-cdc-data-shows.html.
2. "Provisional Drug Overdose Death Counts," National Center for Health Statistics, July 4, 2021, https://www.cdc.gov/nchs/nvss/vsrr/drug-overdose-data.htm.
3. "Drug-Related Deaths and Mortality in Europe," European Monitoring Cetre for Drugs and Drug Addiction, May 2021, https://www.emcdda.europa.eu/system/files /publications/13762/TD0221591ENN.pdf.
4. "Opioid- and Stimulant-Related Harms in Canada," Government of Canada, June 23, 2021, https://health-infobase.canada.ca/substance-related-harms/opioids-stimulants/.
5. William Wan and Heather Long, "'Cries for Help': Drug Overdoses Are Soaring during the Coronavirus Pandemic," *Washington Post*, July 1, 2020, https://www.washington post.com/health/2020/07/01/coronavirus-drug-overdose/.
6. Emily Feng, "'We Are Shipping to the U.S.': Inside China's Online Synthetic Drug Networks," NPR, November 17, 2020, https://www.npr.org/2020/11/17/916890880 /we-are-shipping-to-the-u-s-china-s-fentanyl-sellers-find-new-routes-to-drug-user.
7. "Opioid- and Stimulant-Related Harms in Canada."
8. "Olivia Dalton Had Been Sober for over a Year. Then the Pandemic Hit, She Lost Her Job, Relapsed and Overdosed," Canadian Broadcasting Corporation, November 4, 2020, https://www.cbc.ca/news/canada/british-columbia/langley-parents-call-for -increased-supports-following-daughter-s-overdose-death-1.5788261.

9.   Julie Small and Mohar Chatterjee, "Fentanyl Is Killing More People during the Pandemic. In Santa Clara County, Victims Are Getting Younger," KQED, May 24, 2021, https://www.kqed.org/news/11874651/fentanyl-is-killing-more-people-in-the -pandemic-in-santa-clara-county-victims-are-getting-younger.

10.   Denise Coffey, "Significant Increase in Opioid-Related Overdoses on Cape Cod Blamed on COVID-19," *Cape Cod Times*, January 10, 2021, https://www.capecodtimes.com /story/news/2021/01/10/increase-opioid-related-overdoses-blamed-covid-19/6599127 002/.

11.   Aubrey Whelan, "Philadelphia May Be on the Way to a Record for Fatal Drug Overdoses in 2020, Another COVID Consequence," December 6, 2020, *Philadelphia Inquirer*, https://www.inquirer.com/health/opioid-addiction/overdoses-philadelphia -covid-opioid-fentanyl-20201206.html.

12.   "Overdose Deaths in Philadelphia Reach 2nd-Highest Number Ever Recorded in 2020," CBS 3 Philly, June 3, 2021, https://philadelphia.cbslocal.com/2021/06/03/phi ladelphia-overdose-deaths-2020/.

13.   Maria Pulcinella, "Philly Museums Begin Reopening after City Eases COVID-19 Restrictions," WHYY, January 4, 2021, https://whyy.org/articles/philly-museums-be gin-reopening-after-city-eases-covid-19-restrictions/.

14.   Josh Skluzacek, "Nearly 1K Minnesota Alcohol-Related Deaths in 2020, MDH Says," KSTP 5, April 16, 2021, https://kstp.com/minnesota-news/alcohol-related-deaths-inc rease-in-2020-minnesota-department-health-report/6077265/#:~:text=New%20data %20released%20by%20the,171%20deaths%20compared%20to%202019.

15.   "Alcohol Deaths Highest for 20 Years in England and Wales," BBC, May 6, 2021, https://www.bbc.com/news/health-57008067#:~:text=Alcohol%20killed%20more %20people%20in,Office%20for%20National%20Statistics%20says.

16.   "Drug Overdose Deaths in the United States, 1999–2019," National Center for Health Statistics, Centers for Disease Control and Prevention, December 2020, https://www .cdc.gov/nchs/products/databriefs/db394.htm.

17.   "Weekly Updates by Select Demographic and Geographic Characteristics," National Center for Health Statistics, Centers for Disease Control and Prevention, https://www .cdc.gov/nchs/nvss/vsrr/covid_weekly/index.htm.

18.   "Video, Audio, Photos, & Rush Transcript: Governor Cuomo Signs the 'New York State on Pause' Executive Order," New York State Governor website, https://www .governor.ny.gov/news/video-audio-photos-rush-transcript-governor-cuomo-signs-new -york-state-pause-executive-order.

22: Sunbelt Spike

1.   Lidia Ryan, "CT Malls and Major Retailers That Have Reopened," *Connecticut Post*, May 19, 2020, https://www.ctpost.com/news/coronavirus/slideshow/CT-malls-and -major-retailers-opening-in-phase-1-202512.php.

2.   Alex Berenson (@alexberenson), "Flew today. Turns out that even when face diapers are required…they're not really required. I had a mask, of course, and if the flight attendants had wanted me to wear it I would have…but they didn't. Non-Karens are well aware they're viral theater," Twitter, July 1, 2020, 5:42 p.m. Screenshot in my possession, and available at the Wayback Machine at https://web.archive.org/web/20 210324021734/https://twitter.com/alexberenson/status/1278489115516964864.

3.   Norah O'Donnell, "Dr. Fauci Says, 'With All Due Modesty, I Think I'm Pretty Effective,'" *InStyle*, July 15, 2020, https://www.instyle.com/news/dr-fauci-says-with -all-due-modesty-i-think-im-pretty-effective.

4. Alex Berenson (@AlexBerenson), "And there's Dr. Anthony Fauci showing us all he knows exactly how well masks work! Thanks for the lesson, doc," Twitter, July 23, 2020. Screenshot in my possession, and available at the Wayback Machine at https://web.archive.org/web/20210721230239/https://twitter.com/alexberenson/status/1417983356365680640.

5. Travis Pittman, "Fauci Calls Criticism over Photo of Him with Mask Down 'Mischievous,'" WUSA 9, July 24, 2020, https://www.wusa9.com/article/news/health/coronavirus/anthony-fauci-face-mask-down-photo-coronavirus/507-e33379cb-d79e-479b-9960-13293c96572f.

6. Charles Ornstein and Mike Hixenbaugh, "'All the Hospitals Are Full': In Houston, Overwhelmed ICUs Leave COVID-19 Patients Waiting in ERs," ProPublica, July 10, 2020, https://www.propublica.org/article/all-the-hospitals-are-full-in-houston-overwhelmed-icus-leave-covid-19-patients-waiting-in-ers.

7. Alex Berenson (@AlexBerenson), "Update from Houston…," Twitter, July 20, 2020, https://twitter.com/alexberenson/status/1285251820655308804?lang=en. Screenshot in my possession.

8. Alex Berenson (@AlexBerenson), "CASE MIX: The age of the infected…," Twitter, July 16, 2020, https://twitter.com/alexberenson/status/1283754372569194498?lang=en. Screenshot in my possession.

9. Alexis C. Madrigal, "A Second Coronavirus Death Surge Is Coming," *The Atlantic*, July 15, 2020, https://www.theatlantic.com/health/archive/2020/07/second-coronavirus-death-surge/614122/.

10. Thomas Chatterton Williams, "Do Americans Understand How Badly They're Doing? In France, Where I Live, the Virus Is under Control. I Can Hardly Believe the News Coming Out of the United States," *The Atlantic*, July 2, 2020, https://www.theatlantic.com/ideas/archive/2020/07/america-land-pathetic/613747/.

11. Jonathan Chait, "American Death Cult: Why Has the Republican Response to the Pandemic Been So Mind-Bogglingly Disastrous?" *New York*, July 20, 2020, https://nymag.com/intelligencer/2020/07/republican-response-coronavirus.html.

12. Margherita Stancati and Bojan Pancevski, "How Europe Kept Coronavirus Cases Low Even after Reopening," *Wall Street Journal*, July 20, 2020, https://www.wsj.com/articles/how-europe-slowed-its-coronavirus-cases-from-a-torrent-to-a-trickle-11595240731.

13. "Why Has Europe Better Contained the Virus Than the US? Here's What Fauci Says," CNN, July 31, 2020, https://www.cnn.com/politics/live-news/fauci-coronavirus-testimony-07-31-20/h_7b051587c9b0584a6f83d07211a8792b.

14. Thomas V. Inglesby et al., "Disease Mitigation Measures in the Control of Pandemic Influenza," *Biosecurity and Bioterrorism* 4, no. 4 (2006), http://www.upmc-biosecurity.org/website/resources/publications/2006/2006-09-15-diseasemitigationcontrolpandemicflu.html.

15. David Leonhardt, "America's Death Gap," *New York Times*, September 1, 2020, https://www.nytimes.com/2020/09/01/briefing/coronavirus-kenosha-massachusetts-your-tuesday-briefing.html.

16. See Kwok et al., "Obesity: A Critical Risk Factor in the COVID-19 Pandemic," *Clinical Obesity* 10, no. 6 (December 2020), https://pubmed.ncbi.nlm.nih.gov/32857454/.

17. Ivan Pereira, "How New York Has Been Able to Keep Coronavirus at Bay While Other States See Surges," ABC News, July 17, 2020, https://abcnews.go.com/Health/york-coronavirus-bay-states-surges/story?id=71772507.

18. "How Fauci Says the U.S. Can Get Control of the Pandemic," PBS NewsHour, July 17, 2020, https://www.pbs.org/newshour/show/how-fauci-says-the-u-s-can-get-control-of-the-pandemic.

19. Tom Davis, "Gov. Murphy to Reopen NJ Libraries, Museums, Indoor Recreation," *Patch*, June 24, 2020, https://patch.com/new-jersey/holmdel-hazlet/watch-live-gov-murphy-nj-coronavirus-reopen-update-6-24-20.
20. Chris Francescani et al., "100 Days in 'Hell': Gov. Andrew Cuomo on His Pandemic Performance," ABC News, June 17, 2021, https://abcnews.go.com/GMA/News/100-days-hell-gov-andrew-cuomo-pandemic-performance/story?id=71289534.
21. "Video, Audio, Photos & Rush Transcript: Governor Cuomo on President Trump's Failure to Take Responsibility for COVID-19 Crisis: 'This Has Been Gross Negligence,'" New York State Governor website, July 13, 2020, https://www.governor.ny.gov/news/video-audio-photos-rush-transcript-governor-cuomo-president-trumps-failure-take-responsibility.

23: The Forever Lockdowners

1. Andy Slavitt (@ASlavitt), "COVID Update July 26: We can virtually eliminate the virus any time we decide to. 1/," Twitter, July 26, 2020, 7:04 p.m., https://twitter.com/ASlavitt/status/1287524301499965441.
2. Andy Slavitt (@ASlavitt), "So let's define the kitchen sink: 1. Start with universal mask wearing. We didn't do this in Mar–April and let's chalk it up to faulty instructions. But we know better now. 2. Keep the bars & restaurants & churches & transit closed. All hot spots. 3. Prohibit interstate travel10/," Twitter, July 26, 2020, 7:04 p.m., https://twitter.com/ASlavitt/status/1287524334429507585.
3. Andy Slavitt (@ASlavitt), "6. Instead of 50% lockdown (which is what we did in March in April), let's say it's a 90% lockdown. Meaning most of the Americans who couldn't stay home in April because they were picking crops or driving trucks or working in health care would stay home with us. 12/," Twitter, July 26, 2020, 7:04 p.m., https://twitter.com/ASlavitt/status/1287524336249835520.
4. Michael T. Osterholm and Neel Kashkari, "Here's How to Crush the Virus Until the Vaccines Arrive," *New York Times*, August 7, 2020, https://www.nytimes.com/2020/08/07/opinion/coronavirus-lockdown-unemployment-death.html.
5. Michael T. Osterholm and Mark Olshaker, "Opinion: Facing Covid-19 Reality: A National Lockdown Is No Cure," *Washington Post*, March 21, 2020, https://www.washingtonpost.com/opinions/2020/03/21/facing-covid-19-reality-national-lockdown-is-no-cure/.
6. Ritu Prasad, "Coronavirus: How Did Florida Get So Badly Hit by Covid-19?" BBC, July 14, 2020, https://www.bbc.com/news/world-us-canada-53357742.
7. Shawn Radcliffe, "How Contact Tracing Can Stop COVID-19," Healthline, May 4, 2020, https://www.healthline.com/health-news/everything-to-know-about-contact-tracing#What-is-contact-tracing?.
8. Andrew Joseph, "Contact Tracing Could Help Avoid Another Lockdown. Can It Work in the United States?" Stat News, May 29, 2020, https://www.statnews.com/2020/05/29/contact-tracing-can-it-help-avoid-more-lockdowns/.
9. Lisette Voytko, "NY Will Hire Contact Tracing 'Army' of 17,000 to Battle Coronavirus, Cuomo Says," *Forbes*, April 30, 2020, https://forbes.com/sites/lisettevoytko/2020/04/30/ny-will-hire-contact-tracing-army-of-17000-to-battle-coronavirus-cuomo-says/.
10. Franco Ordoñez, "Ex-Officials Call for $46 Billion for Tracing, Isolating in Next Coronavirus Package," NPR, April 27, 2020, https://www.npr.org/2020/04/27/845165404/ex-officials-call-for-46-billion-for-tracing-isolating-in-next-coronavirus-packa.
11. Brian Chasnoff, "'Really Exasperating'—S.A. Officials Struggle to Pinpoint Sources of COVID Infections," *San-Antonio Express News*, June 23, 2020, https://www.ex

pressnews.com/news/local/politics/article/Really-exasperating-S-A-officials-15361645
.php.

12. Matt Arco, "N.J.'s Big Hangup in Coronavirus Fight Gets Worse. Contact Tracers Find 74% Unwilling to Cooperate," NJ.com, December 8, 2020, https://www.nj.com/coro navirus/2020/12/njs-big-hangup-in-coronavirus-fight-gets-worse-contact-tracers-find -74-unwilling-to-cooperate.html.

13. "Kentucky Couple Who Refused Isolation Order on House Arrest after Positive COVID-19 Test," *Courier-Journal*, July 20, 2020, https://www.courier-journal.com /story/news/2020/07/20/kentucky-couple-house-arrest-coronavirus-isolation-order/54 70378002/.

14. Nicoletta Lanese, "Why Hasn't Contact Tracing Managed to Slow the Massive Surge of Coronavirus in the US?" Live Science, July 21, 2020, https://www.livescience.com /covid19-contact-tracing-us-states.html.

15. Mirjam E. Kretzschmar et al., "Impact of Delays on Effectiveness of Contact Tracing Strategies for COVID-19: A Modelling Study," *The Lancet 5*, no. 8 (August 2020), https://www.thelancet.com/journals/lanpub/article/PIIS2468-2667(20)30157-2/full text.

16. Ari Shapiro and Maureen Pao, "California and Texas Health Officials: Mistrust a Major Hurdle for Contact Tracers," NPR, August 10, 2020, https://www.npr.org/sec tions/coronavirus-live-updates/2020/08/10/901064505/california-and-texas-health-of ficials-on-challenges-they-face-in-contact-tracing.

17. "Crowds Seen at Motorcycle Rally Raise Fears of Super Spreader Event," CNN, August 11, 2020, https://www.cnn.com/videos/us/2020/08/11/motorcycle-rally-sturgis-ryan -young-lklv-nr-ldn-vpx.cnn.

18. Ella Lee, "Fact Check: Post Online Misstates Sturgis Rally's Coronavirus Cases," USA Today, September 17, 2020, https://www.usatoday.com/story/news/factcheck/2020/09 /17/fact-check-sturgis-rallys-covid-19-cases-misstated-online-post/3458606001/.

19. Colton Hall, "SDHP: Fatal Motorcycle Crashes, Fatalities Doubled during 2020 Sturgis Motorcycle Rally," NewsCenter1, August 16, 2020, https://www.newscenter1.tv/sdhp -fatal-motorcycle-crashes-fatalities-doubled-during-2020-sturgis-motorcycle-rally/.

20. Damien Gayle et al., "Coronavirus: Police Break Up Anti-Lockdown Protest in London," *The Guardian*, September 26, 2020, https://www.theguardian.com/world /2020/sep/26/london-lockdown-protesters-urged-to-follow-covid-rules.

21. "Hundreds Protest, Clash with Police in Naples over New Coronavirus Curfew," France24, October 24, 2020, https://www.france24.com/en/europe/20201024-hund reds-protest-clash-with-police-in-naples-over-new-coronavirus-curfew.

22. "Thousands Protest Anti-Coronavirus Restrictions in Germany over Weekend," Reuters, October 4, 2020, https://www.reuters.com/article/us-health-coronavirus-ger many-protest-idUKKBN26P0G1.

23. Christine Armario, "Colombia's Long Virus Lockdown Fuels Anxiety and Depression," Associated Press, August 5, 2020, https://apnews.com/article/virus-outbreak-caribbe an-anxiety-health-south-america-0e47524f0453c382c8c652de340b178c.

24. Luis Jaime Acosta, "Colombian Unions, Students Seek to Revive Mass Protests against Government, Police Violence," Reuters, September 22, 2020, https://www.reuters.com /article/colombia-protests-idUSKCN26D0BQ.

25. "Colombia Riots: Several Dead in Protests over Police Violence," Deutsche Welle, September 11, 2020, https://www.dw.com/en/colombia-protests/a-54888415.

26. Rajiv Kalkod, "Bengaluru Cops Say Majority of Rioters Lost Jobs and Had No Income," *Times of India*, August 14, 2020, https://timesofindia.indiatimes.com/city

/bengaluru/post-lockdown-frustrations-proved-fertile-ground-for-riots/articleshow/77 533074.cms.

27. "Thousands of Anti-Government Protesters Rally in Thailand's Capital," *The Guardian*, July 18, 2020, https://www.theguardian.com/world/2020/jul/18/thousan ds-of-anti-government-protesters-rally-in-thailands-capital.

28. Tim Lister and Stefano Pozzebon, "Protests across Latin America Reflect a Toxic Cocktail of Pandemic and Recession," CNN, August 20, 2020, https://www.cnn.com /2020/08/20/americas/latam-covid-19-protests-intl/index.html.

29. "Germany Coronavirus: Anger after Attempt to Storm Parliament," BBC, August 30, 2020, https://www.bbc.com/news/world-europe-53964147.

24: This Is Only a Test

1. Apoorva Mandavilli, "Your Coronavirus Test Is Positive. Maybe It Shouldn't Be," *New York Times*, August 29, 2020, https://www.nytimes.com/2020/08/29/health/corona virus-testing.html.

2. "DNA Evidence: Basics of Analyzing," National Institute of Justice, August 8, 2012, https://nij.ojp.gov/topics/articles/dna-evidence-basics-analyzing.

3. Leonardo Castañeda, "Coronavirus: Here's What It's Really Like to Get a Nasal Swab Test," *Mercury News*, May 9, 2020, https://www.mercurynews.com/2020/05/09/co ronavirus-heres-what-its-really-like-to-get-a-nasal-swab-test/.

4. "COVID-19 and PCR Testing," Cleveland Clinic, https://my.clevelandclinic.org/heal th/diagnostics/21462-covid-19-and-pcr-testing.

5. Sarah Tiner, "The Science behind the Test for the COVID-19 Virus," Discovery's Edge, March 27, 2020, https://discoverysedge.mayo.edu/2020/03/27/the-science-behind-the -test-for-the-covid-19-virus/.

6. Reed Magleby et al., "Impact of Severe Acute Respiratory Syndrome Coronavirus 2 Viral Load on Risk of Intubation and Mortality among Hospitalized Patients with Coronavirus Disease 2019," *Clinical Infectious Diseases*, June 30, 2020, https://aca demic.oup.com/cid/advance-article/doi/10.1093/cid/ciaa851/5865363.

7. Mandavilli, "Your Coronavirus Test Is Positive."

8. "An Overview of Cycle Threshold Values and Their Role in SARS-CoV-2 Real-Time PCR Test Interpretation," Public Health Ontario, September 17, 2020, https://www .publichealthontario.ca/-/media/documents/ncov/main/2020/09/cycle-threshold-valu es-sars-cov2-pcr.pdf?la=en.

9. Anika Singanayagam et al., "Duration of Infectiousness and Correlation with RT-PCR Cycle Threshold Values in Cases of COVID-19, England, January to May 2020," *Eurosurveillance* 26, no. 7 (February 18, 2021), https://pubmed.ncbi.nlm.nih.gov/327 94447/.

10. Rachel Schraer, "Coronavirus: Tests 'Could Be Picking Up Dead Virus,'" BBC, September 5, 2020, https://www.bbc.com/news/health-54000629.

11. Jennifer Abbasi, "Anthony Fauci, MD, on COVID-19 Vaccines, Schools, and Larry Kramer," *Journal of the American Medical Association* 324, no. 3 (June 8, 2020): 220–22, https://jamanetwork.com/journals/jama/fullarticle/2767208.

12. "COVID-19 with Dr. Anthony Fauci," *This Week in Virology*, American Society for Microbiology, https://asm.org/Podcasts/TWiV/Episodes/COVID-19-with-Dr-Antho ny-Fauci-TWiV-641.

13. "Novel Coronavirus (SARS-CoV-2)," European Centre for Disease Prevention and Control, https://www.ecdc.europa.eu/sites/default/files/documents/COVID-19-Disch arge-criteria.pdf, 2.

14. "Reporting of COVID-19 Ct Values Can Better Shape Public Policy," Rhode Island Center for Freedom and Prosperity, December 11, 2020, https://rifreedom.org/2020/12/covid-19-ct-values-better-public-policy/.
15. Mandavilli, "Your Coronavirus Test Is Positive."
16. Ibid.
17. "COVID-19 Integrated Surveillance Data in Italy," Epicentro, https://www.epicentro.iss.it/en/coronavirus/sars-cov-2-dashboard.
18. "Ellume's COVID-19 Home Test Shows 96% Accuracy in Multi-Site US Clinical Study," Ellume, https://www.ellumehealth.com/2020/12/10/ellumes-covid-19-home-test-shows-96-accuracy-in-multi-site-us-clinical-study/.
19. "Technical Advisory Cell," Welsh Government, July 15, 2020, https://gov.wales/sites/default/files/publications/2020-07/core-principles-for-utilisation-of-rt-pcr-tests-for-detection-of-sars-cov-2.pdf.
20. Allison Martell and Ned Parker, "The U.S. Has More Covid-19 Testing Than Most. So Why Is It Falling So Short?" Reuters, July 27, 2020, https://www.reuters.com/article/us-health-coronavirus-usa-testing-insigh-idUSKCN24S19H.
21. Kate Sheridan, "U.S. Needs 193 Million Covid-19 Tests per Month to Reopen Schools and Keep Up with Pandemic, New Report Says," Stat News, September 9, 2020, https://www.statnews.com/2020/09/09/193-million-covid-19-tests-per-month-report/.

25: Long, Long Covid

1. Dylan Byers, "The Atlantic Thrived through Trump and the Pandemic. The Future Is Harder," NBC News, July 13, 2021, https://www.nbcnews.com/media/atlantic-thrived-trump-pandemic-future-harder-rcna1398.
2. Ed Yong, "Long-Haulers Are Redefining Covid-19," *The Atlantic*, August 19, 2020, https://www.theatlantic.com/health/archive/2020/08/long-haulers-covid-19-recognition-support-groups-symptoms/615382/.
3. Ike Swetlizt, "Persistent Lyme Disease Symptoms Aren't Helped by Long-Term Antibiotics," Stat News, March 30, 2016, https://www.statnews.com/2016/03/30/chronic-lyme-antibiotics/.
4. "Post-Treatment Lyme Disease Syndrome," Centers for Disease Control, https://www.cdc.gov/lyme/postlds/index.html.
5. Ross McGuiness, "The 16 Symptoms of 'Long COVID' as Study Reveals 60,000 People Have Been Ill for Three Months," Yahoo, September 8, 2020, https://www.yahoo.com/news/symptoms-long-covid-ill-months-coronavirus-115240083.html.
6. Yong Huang et al., "COVID Symptoms, Symptom Clusters, and Predictors for Becoming a Long-Hauler: Looking for Clarity in the Haze of the Pandemic," medRxiv, March 5, 2021, https://www.ncbi.nlm.nih.gov/pmc/articles/PMC7941647/.
7. Matt Reynolds, "They Never Officially Had Covid-19. Months Later They're Living in Hell," *Wired*, September 11, 2020, https://www.wired.co.uk/article/coronavirus-long-haulers-negative-tests-covid-19; Gina Assaf et al., "Report: What Does COVID-19 Recovery Actually Look Like?" Patient-Led Research Collaborative, May 11, 2020, https://patientresearchcovid19.com/research/report-1/.
8. Ed Hornick, "'I Fear That I Will Never Be the Same Again': What It's Really Like to Be a COVID Long-Hauler," Yahoo, September 1, 2020, https://uk.style.yahoo.com/i-fear-that-i-will-never-be-the-same-again-heres-what-its-really-like-to-be-a-covid-longhauler-185358665.html.
9. Jayne O'Donnell and Khrysgiana Pineda, "Long-Lasting COVID Symptoms from Lungs to Limbs Linger in Coronavirus 'Long-Haulers,'" *USA Today*, July 25, 2020,

https://www.usatoday.com/in-depth/news/health/2020/07/25/covid-19-long-haulers
-fight-months-lingering-symptoms/5420534002/.

10. "National Safety Council: 97 Percent of Workers Report Fatigue Factors," Compliance Signs, August 3, 2017, https://www.compliancesigns.com/blog/national-safety-council-97-percent-of-workers-report-fatigue-factors/.

11. Adam Hampshire et al., "Cognitive Deficits in People Who Have Recovered from COVID-19 Relative to Controls: An N=84,285 Study," medRxiv, October 21, 2020, https://www.medrxiv.org/content/10.1101/2020.10.20.20215863v1.full-text.

12. Katie Gibbons, "Coronavirus Could Age the Brain by 10 Years or Cause IQ to Fall," *The Times* (London), October 27, 2020, https://www.thetimes.co.uk/article/coronavirus-could-age-the-brain-by-10-years-or-cause-iq-to-fall-v9s273rbs.

13. Nidhi Subbaraman, "US Health Agency Will Invest $1 Billion to Investigate 'Long COVID,'" *Nature*, March 4, 2021, https://www.nature.com/articles/d41586-021-00586-y.

14. Sara Berg, "More Resources Needed to Help Millions Living with 'Long COVID,'" American Medical Association, June 16, 2021, https://www.ama-assn.org/delivering-care/public-health/more-resources-needed-help-millions-living-long-covid.

15. Survivor Corps, https://www.survivorcorps.com/.

16. Haley Bull, "Long COVID Highlighted as It Relates to the Americans with Disabilities Act," ABC Action News WFTS Tampa Bay, July 26, 2021, https://www.abcactionnews.com/news/coronavirus/long-covid-highlighted-as-it-relates-to-the-americans-with-disabilities-act.

17. Katharine Q. Seelye, "Clinton Book Draws Cheers as Publisher Holds Breath," *New York Times*, June 22, 2004, https://www.nytimes.com/2004/06/22/us/clinton-book-draws-cheers-as-publisher-holds-breath.html.

18. "Multiplier Project Spotlight: National Science Policy Network," https://multiplier.org/.

19. David M. Morens and Anthony S. Fauci, "Emerging Pandemic Diseases: How We Got COVID-19," *Cell* 182 (September 3, 2020), https://www.cell.com/cell/pdf/S0092-8674(20)31012-6.pdf.

20. Karina Piser, "The Trap Doors and Dead Ends of Trying to Get Treated for Long Covid," *New Republic*, July 27, 2021, https://newrepublic.com/article/163036/long-covid-treatment-dead-ends.

21. Melba Newsome, "New Long-Haul COVID Clinics Treat Mysterious and Ongoing Symptoms," *Scientific American*, June 30, 2021, https://www.scientificamerican.com/article/new-long-haul-covid-clinics-treat-mysterious-and-ongoing-symptoms/.

22. "Amphetamines," Better Health Channel, https://www.betterhealth.vic.gov.au/health/healthyliving/amphetamines#long-term-effects-of-amphetamines.

23. M. J. Nuñez et al., "Effects of Amphetamine on Influenza Virus Infection in Mice," *Life Sciences* 52, no. 10 (1993): PL73–78, https://www.sciencedirect.com/science/article/abs/pii/002432059390520D.

24. "Report: Aspirin Taken Daily with Bottle of Bourbon Reduces Awareness of Heart Attacks," *The Onion*, June 10, 1998, https://www.theonion.com/report-aspirin-taken-daily-with-bottle-of-bourbon-redu-1819564746.

26: Herd Immunity

1. Amanda Watts and Naomi Thomas, "New White House Coronavirus Adviser Says He's a 'Straight Shooter,'" CNN, September 4, 2020, https://www.cnn.com/2020/09/04/health/coronavirus-atlas-straight-shooter/index.html.

2. Yasmeen Abutaleb and Josh Dawsey, "New Trump Pandemic Adviser Pushes Controversial 'Herd Immunity' Strategy, Worrying Public Health Officials," *Washington Post*, August 30, 2020, https://www.washingtonpost.com/politics/trump-coronavirus-scott-atlas-herd-immunity/2020/08/30/925e68fe-e93b-11ea-970a-64c73a1c2392_story.html.

3. "Coronavirus Disease (COVID-19): Herd Immunity, Lockdowns and COVID-19," World Health Organization, December 31, 2020, https://www.who.int/news-room/q-a-detail/herd-immunity-lockdowns-and-covid-19.

4. "Coronavirus 'Herd Immunity' Is Just Another Way to Say 'Let People Die,'" *Los Angeles Times*, September 5, 2020, https://www.latimes.com/opinion/story/2020-09-02/coronavirus-herd-immunity-trump.

5. Brian Resnick, "The Worst Idea of 2020," Vox, December 30, 2020, https://www.vox.com/science-and-health/22202758/herd-immunity-natural-infection-worst-idea-of-2020.

6. Geoff Brumfiel and Tamara Keith, "President Trump's New COVID-19 Adviser Is Making Public Health Experts Nervous," NPR, September 4, 2020, https://www.npr.org/sections/health-shots/2020/09/04/909348915/president-trumps-new-covid-19-advisor-is-making-public-health-experts-nervous.

7. Monica Alba, "Redfield Voices Alarm over Influence of Trump's New Coronavirus Task Force Adviser," NBC News, September 28, 2020, https://www.nbcnews.com/politics/politics-news/redfield-voices-alarm-over-influence-trump-s-new-coronavirus-task-n1241221.

8. Matt Wilstein, "Dr. Anthony Fauci Calls Out Fox News and Scott Atlas in CNN Interview," The Daily Beast, September 29, 2020, https://www.thedailybeast.com/dr-anthony-fauci-calls-out-fox-news-and-scott-atlas-in-cnn-interview-with-brian-stelter.

9. "New Adviser Giving Trump Bad Information on Virus, Top Officials Say," Reuters, September 28, 2020, https://www.reuters.com/article/health-coronavirus-usa-cdc-idUSKBN26K07E.

10. Greg Allen, "Florida's Governor Lifts All COVID-19 Restrictions on Businesses Statewide," NPR, September 25, 2020, https://www.npr.org/sections/coronavirus-live-updates/2020/09/25/916969969/floridas-governor-lifts-all-covid-19-restrictions-on-businesses-statewide.

11. Joe McLean and Ana Ceballos, "Florida Education Commissioner Mandates All Schools Must Reopen Campuses This Fall," News4Jax, July 6, 2020, https://www.news4jax.com/news/local/2020/07/06/florida-education-commissioner-mandates-all-schools-must-reopen-campuses-in-fall/.

12. "Fauci Says Florida's Decision to Fully Reopen Bars and Restaurants 'Very Concerning,'" *Tampa Bay Times*, September 29, 2020, https://www.tampabay.com/news/health/2020/09/29/fauci-says-floridas-decision-to-fully-reopen-bars-and-restaurants-very-concerning/.

13. "Great Barrington Declaration," https://gbdeclaration.org/.

14. Tunku Varadarajan, "Epidemiologists Stray from the Covid Herd," *Wall Street Journal*, October 23, 2020, https://www.wsj.com/articles/epidemiologists-stray-from-the-covid-herd-11603477330.

15. Gregg Gonsalves (@gregggonsalves), "This fucking Great Barrington Declaration is like a bad rash that won't go away," Twitter, October 12, 2020, 5:34 p.m., https://twitter.com/gregggonsalves/status/1315767761398890496?lang=en.

16. Noah Higgins-Dunn, "Dr. Fauci Says Letting the Coronavirus Spread to Achieve Herd Immunity Is 'Nonsense' and 'Dangerous,'" CNBC, October 15, 2020, https://www.cnbc.com/2020/10/15/dr-fauci-says-letting-the-coronavirus-spread-to-achieve-herd-immunity-is-nonsense-and-dangerous.html.

17. Carlie Porterfield, "Dr. Fauci on GOP Criticism: 'Attacks on Me Quite Frankly, Are Attacks on Science,'" *Forbes*, June 9, 2021, https://www.forbes.com/sites/carlieporter field/2021/06/09/fauci-on-gop-criticism-attacks-on-me-quite-frankly-are-attacks-on -science/?sh=39aac9ee4542.
18. Virginia Chamlee, "Dr. Fauci Tells Rand Paul, 'You Do Not Know What You Are Talking About,'" *People*, July 21, 2021, https://people.com/politics/anthony-fauci-ra nd-paul-heated-exchange-covid/.
19. Rhett Jones, "Conservatives Pull Google into Their Plans to Let People Die," Gizmodo, October 14, 2020, https://gizmodo.com/conservatives-pull-google-into-their-plan-to -let-people-1845371054.
20. Ethan Yang, "Reddit's Censorship of the Great Barrington Declaration," American Institute for Economic Research, October 8, 2020, https://www.aier.org/article/reddi ts-censorship-of-the-great-barrington-declaration/.

27: Trump

1. Tom Porter, "Trump Is Such a Germaphobe That Aides Aren't Allowed to Cough in His Presence and Visitors Must Wash Their Hands before Entering the Oval Office, Report Says," Business Insider, July 8, 2019, https://www.businessinsider.com/germa phobe-trump-hates-people-coughing-and-sneezing-in-his-presence-2019-7.
2. Lisa J. Adams Wagner, "Former GOP Presidential Hopeful Herman Cain Dies of COVID-19," Associated Press, July 30, 2020, https://apnews.com/article/virus-outbre ak-election-2020-herman-cain-ap-top-news-ok-state-wire-8173fe14f7cf7095ced3b55 fdc65581e.
3. Jeremy W. Peters, "Will Herman Cain's Death Change Republican Views on the Virus and Masks?" *New York Times*, July 30, 2020, https://www.nytimes.com/2020/07/30 /us/politics/herman-cain-gop-coronavirus.html.
4. Patrick Stout, "Trump Killed Herman Cain," *McDonough County Voice*, August 4, 2020, https://www.mcdonoughvoice.com/story/opinion/columns/2020/08/04/trump -killed-herman-cain/42817567/.
5. John Fritze and Maureen Groppe, "Trump Rallies 2.0: Behind the Curtain at the President's Campaign Events in the Covid-19 Era," *USA Today*, September 12, 2020, https://www.usatoday.com/story/news/politics/elections/2020/09/12/election-2020-wh at-trumps-rallies-look-like-era-covid-19/5768172002/.
6. Sam Gringlas, "At Least 8 People Test Positive for Coronavirus after Rose Garden Event for Barrett," NPR, October 3, 2020, https://www.npr.org/sections/latest-updates-tru mp-covid-19-results/2020/10/03/919851907/at-least-7-people-test-positive-for-coron avirus-after-rose-garden-event-for-barr.
7. Maggie Haberman and Michael D. Shear, "Trump Says He'll Begin 'Quarantine Process' after Hope Hicks Tests Positive for Coronavirus," *New York Times*, October 1, 2020, https://www.nytimes.com/2020/10/01/us/politics/hope-hicks-coronavirus .html.
8. Aatif Sulleyman, "Donald Trump Tests Positive for COVID-19: What Is the Risk for Over-70s?" *Newsweek*, October 2, 2020, https://www.newsweek.com/donald-trump -tests-positive-coronavirus-what-risk-over-70s-1535846.
9. Kate Proctor and Nazia Parveen, "Boris Johnson: It Was 50–50 Whether to Put Me on a Ventilator," *The Guardian*, May 3, 2020, https://www.theguardian.com/world/2020 /may/03/boris-johnson-it-was-50-50-whether-to-put-me-on-ventilator-coronavirus.

10. Zachary B. Wolf, "Here's What Happens If Trump Gets Too Sick to Govern," CNN, October 9, 2020, https://www.cnn.com/2020/10/02/politics/trump-covid-line-of-suc cession-governance/index.html.
11. Sam Gringlas, "White House Official Calls Next 48 Hours 'Critical' for Trump's Care," NPR, October 3, 2020, https://www.npr.org/sections/latest-updates-trump-covid-19 -results/2020/10/03/919869461/watch-live-white-house-doctor-briefs-on-president-tr umps-condition.
12. Alexandra Alper, "After Mixed Messages from White House, Trump Says 'Real Test' Ahead in His COVID Fight," Reuters, October 3, 2020, https://www.reuters.com/ar ticle/health-coronavirus-trump/after-mixed-messages-from-white-house-trump-says -real-test-ahead-in-his-covid-fight-idUSKBN26P02B.
13. Brianna Abbott et al., "Trump Received Experimental Antibody and Remdesivir for Coronavirus," *Wall Street Journal*, October 3, 2020, https://www.wsj.com/articles/tr umps-weight-age-gender-make-severe-covid-19-more-likely-11601660627.
14. Barbara Sprunt, "'Don't Be Afraid of It': Trump Dismisses Virus Threat as He Returns to White House," NPR, October 5, 2020, https://www.npr.org/sections/latest-updates -trump-covid-19-results/2020/10/05/920412187/trump-says-he-will-leave-walter-reed -medical-center-monday-night.
15. Julie Bosman et al., "Most Patients' Covid-19 Care Looks Nothing like Trump's," *New York Times*, October 6, 2020, https://www.nytimes.com/2020/10/06/us/trump-coro navirus-care-treatment.html.
16. Marilynn Marchione, "Ethicists Say Trump Special Treatment Raises Fairness Issue," Associated Press, October 7, 2020, https://apnews.com/article/virus-outbreak-donald -trump-us-news-ap-top-news-international-news-a2f8d343085407a9209ed3c2c230 a6f7.
17. Dan Mangan and Kevin Breuninger, "Trump Tests Negative for the Coronavirus on Consecutive Days, White House Doctor Says," CNBC, October 12, 2020, https://www .cnbc.com/2020/10/12/trump-tests-negative-for-the-coronavirus-on-consecutive-days -white-house-doctor-says.html.
18. Kathryn Watson and Steven Portnoy, "Fauci Says Data on Masks 'Speaks for Itself' after 'Super-Spreader' White House Event," CBS News, October 9, 2020, https://www .cbsnews.com/news/dr-fauci-on-masks-super-spreader-covid-event-interview/.
19. Ronan McGreevy, "Covid-19: World in 'for a Hell of a Ride' in Coming Months, Dr Mike Ryan Says," *Irish Times*, October 2, 2020, https://www.irishtimes.com/news/ire land/irish-news/covid-19-world-in-for-a-hell-of-a-ride-in-coming-months-dr-mike-ry an-says-1.4370626.
20. Sophie Uyoga et al., "Seroprevalance of Anti-SARS-CoV-2 IgG Antibodies in Kenyan Blood Donors," medRxiv, July 29, 2020, https://www.medrxiv.org/content/10.1101/20 20.07.27.20162693v1.full.pdf.
21. Gina Kolata and Roni Caryn Rabin, "'Don't Be Afraid of Covid,' Trump Says, Undermining Public Health Messages," *New York Times*, October 8, 2020, https:// www.nytimes.com/2020/10/05/health/trump-covid-public-health.html.

28: A House Divided

1. Michael McFaul, "The Election of '96," Hoover Institution, *Hoover Digest*, October 1, 1997, https://www.hoover.org/research/election-96.
2. Becky Little, "When a Russian President Ended Up Drunk and Disrobed outside the White House," History, August 30, 2018, https://www.history.com/news/bill-clinton -boris-yeltsin-drunk-1994-russian-state-visit.

3. Emma Newburger, "Biden Leads Trump by 10 Points in Final Days before Election: NBC/WSJ Poll," CNBC, November 1, 2020, https://www.cnbc.com/2020/11/01/biden-leads-trump-by-10-points-in-final-days-before-election-nbc-wsj-poll.html.
4. Stephen Collinson and Maeve Reston, "Biden Defeats Trump in an Election He Made about Character of the Nation and the President," CNN, November 7, 2020, https://www.cnn.com/2020/11/07/politics/joe-biden-wins-us-presidential-election/index.html.
5. "Victory for Joe Biden, at Last," *New York Times*, November 7, 2020, https://www.nytimes.com/2020/11/07/opinion/joe-biden-president-winner.html.
6. Sylvie Corbet, "Paris Mayor Reelected, Green Wave in France Local Elections," Associated Press, June 28, 2020, https://apnews.com/article/europe-virus-outbreak-rachida-dati-ap-top-news-elections-16e161a4349cd2712c5cb084259f1ece; Glenn Kessler, "Trump's Assertion That Only Two European Nations Allow Mail-in Voting," *Washington Post*, December 4, 2020, https://www.washingtonpost.com/politics/2020/12/04/trumps-assertion-that-only-two-european-nations-allow-mail-in-voting/.
7. Emily Badger and Quoctrung Bui, "How the Suburbs Moved Away from Trump," *New York Times*, November 6, 2020, https://www.nytimes.com/interactive/2020/11/06/upshot/suburbs-shifted-left-president.html.
8. "Tucker: How 'Defund the Police' Movement Backfired on Democrats," Fox News, November 10, 2020, https://www.foxnews.com/transcript/tucker-how-defund-the-police-movement-backfired-on-democrats.
9. Deborah Jordan Brooks and Lydia Saad, "The COVID-19 Responses of Men vs. Women," Gallup, October 7, 2020, https://news.gallup.com/opinion/gallup/321698/covid-responses-men-women.aspx.
10. Audie Cornish and Maureen Pao, "To Tackle Racial Disparities in COVID-19, California Enacts New Metric for Reopening," NPR, October 6, 2020, https://www.npr.org/sections/coronavirus-live-updates/2020/10/06/920814386/to-tackle-racial-disparities-in-covid-19-california-enacts-new-metric-for-reopen.
11. Queenie Wong, "Twitter Permanently Bans Trump's Account," CNET, January 9, 2021, https://www.cnet.com/news/twitter-permanently-bans-trumps-account/.
12. "Permanent Suspension of @realDonaldTrump," Twitter, January 8, 2021, https://blog.twitter.com/en_us/topics/company/2020/suspension.
13. Sarah Frier, "Twitter's Trump Ban Deemed Necessary, Derided as Long Overdue," Bloomberg, January 9, 2021, https://www.bloomberg.com/news/articles/2021-01-09/twitter-s-trump-ban-deemed-necessary-derided-as-long-overdue.

29: Here We Go Again

1. "Newsom: State 'Pulling Emergency Brake' on Virus Reopenings," NBC Bay Area, November 16, 2020, https://www.nbcbayarea.com/news/california/new-restrictions-possible-as-gov-newsom-updates-states-virus-response/2400357/.
2. Jill Cowan et al., "California Will Impose Its Strongest Virus Measures since the Spring," *New York Times*, December 3, 2020, https://www.nytimes.com/2020/12/03/us/california-stay-at-home-order.html.
3. Whet Moser, "California Has Lost Control," *The Atlantic*, December 21, 2020, https://www.theatlantic.com/health/archive/2020/12/covid-hospitalizations-california-will-break-records/617455/.
4. Elaine Godfrey, "Iowa Is What Happens When Government Does Nothing," *The Atlantic*, December 3, 2020, https://www.theatlantic.com/politics/archive/2020/12/how-iowa-mishandled-coronavirus-pandemic/617252/.

5. Elaine Godfrey, "Iowans Were Scared into Taking the Virus Seriously," *The Atlantic*, February 6, 2020, https://www.theatlantic.com/politics/archive/2021/02/why-didnt-io wa-have-post-holiday-covid-19-surge/617920/.

6. Brian Melley and Stefanie Dazio, "California Hospitals at 'Brink of Catastrophe' as Many Run Out of ICU Beds," CTV News, December 31, 2020, https://www.ctvnews .ca/world/california-hospitals-at-brink-of-catastrophe-as-many-run-out-of-icu-beds -1.5249919.

7. Cheri Mossburg and Madeline Holcombe, "Oxygen Supply Issues Force Five Los Angeles–Area Hospitals to Declare an 'Internal Disaster,'" CNN, December 29, 2020, https://www.cnn.com/2020/12/29/us/california-hospital-oxygen-covid/index.html.

8. "California's Emergency Field Hospitals Provided Little Help during Height of COVID-19 Surge," KTLA 5, July 31, 2021, https://ktla.com/news/coronavirus/californias-emer gency-field-hospitals-provided-little-help-during-height-of-covid-19-surge/.

9. Corky Siemaszko, "Experts Warn of 'Twindemic' as Covid Cases Rise and Flu Seasons Loom," NBC News, September 21, 2020, https://www.nbcnews.com/news/us-news/ experts-warn-twindemic-covid-cases-rise-flu-seasons-looms-n1240623.

10. Sonja J. Olsen et al., "Decreased Influenza Activity during the COVID-19 Pandemic—United States, Australia, Chile, and South Africa, 2020," *Morbidity and Mortality Report* 69, no. 37 (September 18, 2020): 1305–1309, https://www.cdc.gov/mmwr/vo lumes/69/wr/mm6937a6.htm.

11. "Covid-19: France Moves to Night-Time Curfew from 15 December," BBC, December 10, 2020, https://www.bbc.com/news/world-europe-55266332.

12. "Timeline of UK Coronavirus Lockdowns, March 2020 to March 2021," Institute for Government (UK), https://www.instituteforgovernment.org.uk/sites/default/files/time line-lockdown-web.pdf.

13. "Travel to New Zealand during Covid-19: What You Need to Know before You Go," CNN, https://www.cnn.com/travel/article/new-zealand-travel-covid-19/index.html.

14. "New Zealand in Coronavirus Lockdown as U.K. Variant Cases Reported," Reuters, February 14, 2021, https://www.reuters.com/article/us-health-coronavirus-newzeala nd-idUSKBN2AE0R8.

15. Daniel Wittenberg, "New Zealand Lockdown: Jacinda Ardern Announces Lifting of All Restrictions outside Auckland," *The Independent*, September 21, 2020, https:// www.independent.co.uk/news/world/australasia/new-zealand-lockdown-coronavirus -restrictions-jacinda-ardern-auckland-b511204.html.

16. Matthew S. Schwartz, "New Zealand PM Ardern Wins Re-Election in Best Showing for Labour Party in Decades," NPR, October 17, 2020, https://www.npr.org/2020/10 /17/924934728/new-zealand-pm-ardern-wins-re-election-in-best-showing-for-labour -party-in-decad.

17. Praveen Menon, "New Zealand's Ardern Wins 'Historic' Re-Election for Crushing COVID-19," Reuters, October 16, 2020, https://www.reuters.com/article/uk-newzea land-election/new-zealands-ardern-wins-historic-re-election-for-crushing-covid-19-idU SKBN2712ZI.

18. Todd Pollack et al., "Emerging COVID-19 Success Story: Vietnam's Commitment to Containment," Our World in Data, June 30, 2020, https://ourworldindata.org/covid -exemplar-vietnam-2020.

19. Emma Steen, "Tokyo Q&A: Why Is Japan Not in a Hard Lockdown over Coronavirus?" Time Out, May 12, 2020, https://www.timeout.com/tokyo/news/why -is-japan-not-in-a-hard-lockdown-over-coronavirus-051220.

20. "Japan Steps Up COVID Testing, but Some Say More Effort Needed," Al Jazeera, March 3, 2021, https://www.aljazeera.com/news/2021/3/3/japan-steps-up-covid -testing-but-some-say-more-effort-needed.

21. "Lower Prevalence of Obesity in Japan Due to Environmental Factors," Pharmaceutical Technology, January 28, 2020, https://www.pharmaceutical-technology.com/comment /low-obesity-japan/.

22. S. D. Stellman et al., "Smoking and Lung Cancer Risk in American and Japanese Men: An International Case-Control Study," *Cancer Epidemiology, Biomarkers & Prevention* 10, no. 11 (November 2001), 1193–99, https://pubmed.ncbi.nlm.nih.gov /11700268/.

23. Sawako Hibino et al., "Dynamic Change of COVID-19 Seroprevalence among Asymptomatic Population in Tokyo during the Second Wave," medRxiv, September 23, 2020, https://www.medrxiv.org/content/10.1101/2020.09.21.20198796v1.

30: Free at Last

1. "Pfizer and BioNTech Announce Vaccine Candidate against COVID-19 Achieved Success in First Interim Analysis from Phase 3 Study," Pfizer, November 9, 2020, https:// www.pfizer.com/news/press-release/press-release-detail/pfizer-and-biontech-announ ce-vaccine-candidate-against.

2. Nadia Kounang, "Pfizer Says Early Analysis Shows Its Covid-19 Vaccine Is More Than 90% Effective," CNN, November 9, 2020, https://www.cnn.com/2020/11/09/health /pfizer-covid-19-vaccine-effective/index.html.

3. Tim Loh, "Fauci Says End to Pandemic Is in Sight, Thanks to Vaccines," Bloomberg, November 12, 2020, https://www.bloomberg.com/news/articles/2020-11-12/covid -won-t-be-pandemic-for-long-thanks-to-vaccines-fauci-says.

4. Yuliya Talmazan and Erika Edwards, "'Truly Striking' : Covid-19 Vaccine Candidate 94.5 Percent Effective, Moderna Says," NBC News, November 16, 2020, https://www .nbcnews.com/health/health-news/covid-19-vaccine-candidate-94-5-percent-effective -moderna-says-n1247888.

5. "Pfizer and BioNTech Conclude Phase 3 Study of COVID-19 Vaccine Candidate, Meeting All Primary Efficacy Endpoints," Pfizer, November 18, 2020, https://www.pf izer.com/news/press-release/press-release-detail/pfizer-and-biontech-conclude-phase -3-study-covid-19-vaccine.

6. Noah Higgins-Dunn, "CDC Director Says Face Masks May Provide More Protection Than Coronavirus Vaccine," CNBC, September 16, 2020, https://www.cnbc.com/20 20/09/16/cdc-director-says-face-masks-may-provide-more-protection-than-coronavir us-vaccine-.html.

7. Philip Oltermann, "Uğur Şahin and Özlem Türeci: German 'Dream Team' behind Vaccine," *The Guardian*, November 10, 2020, https://www.theguardian.com/world /2020/nov/10/ugur-sahin-and-ozlem-tureci-german-dream-team-behind-vaccine.

8. Laurie McGinley et al., "Trump Rails against 'Medical Deep State' after Pfizer Vaccine News Comes after Election Day," *Washington Post*, November 11, 2020, https://www .washingtonpost.com/politics/2020/11/11/trump-angry-about-pfizer-vaccine/.

9. Zeke Miller, "Trump Hails Vaccine 'Miracle,' with Millions of Doses Soon," Associated Press, December 8, 2020, https://apnews.com/article/feds-pfizer-coronavirus-vaccine -doses-bb5cb23e49aa72ba9cf11b80f1c40b05.

10. Rebecca Shabad, "Pence Receives Covid Vaccine in Televised Appearance, Hails 'Medical Miracle,'" NBC News, December 18, 2020, https://www.nbcnews.com/poli tics/white-house/pence-set-receive-covid-vaccine-televised-appearance-n1251655.

11. Alex Berenson (@AlexBerenson), "Been thinking a lot...," Twitter, November 10, 2020, https://twitter.com/alexberenson/status/1326169723999051777?lang=en. Screenshot in my possession.

31: The Excerpts

1. Lisa Müller et al., "Age-Dependent Immune Response to the Biontech/Pfizer BNT162b2 COVID-19 Vaccination," medRxiv, March 5, 2021, https://www.medrxiv.org/content /10.1101/2021.03.03.21251066v1.full.

2. For example, Paul Naaber et al., "Dynamics of Antibody Response to BNT162b2 Vaccine after Six Months: A Longitudinal Prospective Study," *The Lancet*, September 5, 2021, https://www.thelancet.com/journals/lanepe/article/PIIS2666-7762(21)00185 -X/fulltext.

3. Michael L. Anderson et al., "The Effect of Influenza Vaccination for the Elderly on Hospitalization and Mortality: An Observational Study with a Regression Discontinuity Design," *Annals of Internal Medicine* 172, no. 7 (April 7, 2020): 445–52, https://pub med.ncbi.nlm.nih.gov/32120383/.

4. All figures in this section are taken from the Food and Drug Administration briefing books on the Pfizer and Moderna vaccines.

5. Ibid.

6. This was the figure at the original time of publication, in March 2021.

7. Ibid.

8. Serena Tinari, "The EMA Covid-19 Data Leak, and What It Tells Us about mRNA Instability," *British Medical Journal* 372, no. 627 (March 10, 2021), https://www.bmj .com/content/372/bmj.n627.

9. Laurens Cerulus, "EU Medicines Agency Says Hackers Manipulated Leaked Coronavirus Vaccine Data," *Politico*, January 25, 2021, https://www.politico.eu/artic le/european-medicines-agency-ema-cyberattack-coronavirus-vaccine-data/.

10. Tinari, "The EMA Covid-19 Data Link." The British authorized the Pfizer vaccine for emergency use on December 2, 2020, becoming the first country to do so. Immunizations began almost immediately. Sarah Boseley and Josh Halliday, "UK Approves Pfizer/BioNTech Covid Vaccine for Rollout Next Week," *The Guardian*, December 2, 2020, https://www.theguardian.com/society/2020/dec/02/pfizer-bionte ch-covid-vaccine-wins-licence-for-use-in-the-uk.

11. "Operation Warp Speed: Accelerated COVID-19 Vaccine Development Status and Efforts to Address Manufacturing Challenges," Government Accountability Office, February 11, 2021, https://www.gao.gov/products/gao-21-319.

12. Berkeley Lovelace Jr., "First Human Trial for Coronavirus Vaccine Begins Monday in the US," CNBC, March 16, 2020, https://www.cnbc.com/2020/03/16/first-human-tr ial-for-coronavirus-vaccine-begins-monday-in-the-us.html.

13. "German Company Begins Testing Possible Vaccine," *Times of India*, April 29, 2020, https://timesofindia.indiatimes.com/world/europe/german-company-begins-testing -possible-vaccine/articleshow/75450971.cms.

14. "Assessment Report COVID-19 Vaccine Moderna," European Medicines Agency, March 11, 2021, https://www.ema.europa.eu/en/documents/assessment-report/covid -19-vaccine-moderna-epar-public-assessment-report_en.pdf.

15. These figures all come from Pfizer's trial data, as reported in the FDA briefing book.

16. "Assessment Report COVID-19 Vaccine Moderna."

17. Uğur Şahin et al., "BNT162b2 Induces SARS-CoV-2-Neutralising Antibodies and T Cells in Humans," medRxiv, December 11, 2020, https://www.medrxiv.org/content /10.1101/2020.12.09.20245175v1.

18. "Selected Adverse Events Reported after COVID-19 Vaccination," Centers for Disease Control, https://www.cdc.gov/coronavirus/2019-ncov/vaccines/safety/adverse-events.html.

19. Matt Apuzzo et al., "Where Europe Went Wrong in Its Vaccine Rollout, and Why," *New York Times*, March 20, 2021, https://www.nytimes.com/2021/03/20/world/eu rope/europe-vaccine-rollout-astrazeneca.html.

32: Bad News

1. Molly Jong-Fast, "Who Was I Before This Pandemic—And Who Am I Now?" *Vogue*, February 13, 2021, https://www.vogue.com/article/how-the-pandemic-has-changed -me. "I mostly hid in my apartment (an enormous luxury, I know). I was scared."

2. Molly Jong-Fast, "Pandemic Fatigue Is Real—But Now Is Not the Time to Give In to It," *Vogue*, December 5, 2020, https://www.vogue.com/article/pandemic-fatigue-is-re al-but-coronavirus-vaccine-is-almost-here.

3. "Interim Considerations: Preparing for the Potential Management of Anaphylaxis after COVID-19 Vaccination," Centers for Disease Control, March 3, 2021, https://www .cdc.gov/vaccines/covid-19/clinical-considerations/managing-anaphylaxis.html#:~:tex t=CDC%20currently%20recommends%20the%20following,another%20vaccine %20or%20injectable%20therapy.

4. Bill de Blasio (@NYCMayor), "The #COVID19 vaccine is the miracle so many have waited and worked for, and will end the pandemic. Get this shot of hope and help set our city free. Out new Vaccine For All Campaign will help spread the word that the vaccine is safe, effective and free," Twitter, December 22, 2020, 11:33 a.m., https://tw itter.com/NYCMayor/status/1341421682016268290.

5. Ezekiel Emmanuel et al., "Take Whatever COVID Vaccination You Can Get. All of Them Stop Death and Hospitalization," *USA Today*, February 12, 2021, https://www.usatoday. com/story/opinion/2021/02/12/all-covid-vaccines-stop-death-severe-illness- column/6709455002/.

6. Martina Navratilova (@Martina), "Just got my first shot—Pfizer—and I am so excited and relieved and happy etc—if there are any antivaxxers out here—if you can—please get the vaccine...," Twitter, February 28, 2021, 12:46 p.m., https://twitter.com/Mar tina/status/1366082435008647169.

7. Jane C. Timm, "Fact Check: Coronavirus Vaccine Could Come This Year, Trump Says. Experts Say He Needs a 'Miracle' to Be Right," NBC News, May 15, 2020, https:// www.nbcnews.com/politics/donald-trump/fact-check-coronavirus-vaccine-could-co me-year-trump-says-experts-n1207411.

8. Caroline Kelly, "'I Will Not Take His Word for It': Kamala Harris Says She Would Not Trust Trump Alone on a Coronavirus Vaccine," CNN, September 5, 2020, https:// www.cnn.com/2020/09/05/politics/kamala-harris-not-trust-trump-vaccine-cnntv/ index.html.

9. Brian Mann, "Cuomo Says N.Y. Health Officials Will Review Any U.S.-Approved COVID-19 Vaccine," NPR, September 24, 2020, https://www.npr.org/sections/coron avirus-live-updates/2020/09/24/916565352/cuomo-says-n-y-health-officials-will-revi ew-any-u-s-approved-covid-19-vaccine.

10. Michael Specter, "Trump Is Right: Andrew Cuomo Should Accept F.D.A. Approval of a Coronavirus Vaccine," *New Yorker*, November 16, 2020, https://www.newyork er.com/news/daily-comment/trump-is-right-andrew-cuomo-should-accept-fda-appro val-of-a-coronavirus-vaccine.

11. Eric Lutz, "Trump's Rush to Release a COVID Vaccine Has Americans Worried," *Vanity Fair*, October 6, 2020, https://www.vanityfair.com/news/2020/10/trump-rush -release-covid-vaccine-americans-worried.

12. Eric Lutz, "The White House's Incompetence Is Apparently Holding Up 'Millions' of COVID Vaccines," *Vanity Fair*, December 18, 2020, https://www.vanityfair.com/ne ws/2020/12/white-house-delays-pfizer-vaccine-shipments.

13. Barbara Sibbald, "Rofecoxib (Vioxx) Voluntarily Withdrawn from Market," *Canadian Medical Association Journal* 171, no. 9 (October 24, 2006): 1027–28, https://www.nc bi.nlm.nih.gov/pmc/articles/PMC526313/.

14. Melody Petersen, "Increased Spending on Drugs Is Linked to More Advertising," *New York Times*, November 21, 2001, https://www.nytimes.com/2001/11/21/business/in creased-spending-on-drugs-is-linked-to-more-advertising.html.

15. "Study Linking Vioxx to Heart Problems Finally Published," Canadian Broadcasting Corporation, January 25, 2005, https://www.cbc.ca/news/science/study -linking-vioxx-to-heart-problems-finally-published-1.534735.

16. Harlan M. Krumholz et al., "What Have We Learnt from Vioxx?" *British Medical Journal* 334, no. 7585 (January 20, 2007): 120–23, https://www.ncbi.nlm.nih.gov/pmc /articles/PMC1779871/#ref13.

17. Lindsey Graham (@LindseyGrahamSC), "Thank God for nurses who help people in need and know how to use a needle. Thank God for those who produced these vaccines. If enough of us take it, we will get back to normal lives. Help is on the way," Twitter, December 19, 2020, 2:24 p.m., https://twitter.com/lindseygrahamsc/status/13403774 10806689792.

18. Robby Soave, "Reopen the Schools!" *Reason*, June 29, 2020, https://reason.com/20 20/06/29/reopen-schools-coronavirus-covid-19/.

19. Robby Soave (@robbysoave), "People who say 'well, the vaccine doesn't actually prevent infection' are wrong. The vaccine almost certainly prevents infection. It is akin to a cure. If you got it, you don't have to wear a mask. You will neither contract nor spread the disease," Twitter, January 18, 2020, 4:48 p.m., https://twitter.com/robbysoave/sta tus/1351285350237433856.

20. "Operation Warp Speed's Triumph," *Wall Street Journal*, March 2, 2021, https://www .wsj.com/articles/operation-warp-speeds-triumph-11614728552.

21. Ben Shapiro (@benshapiro), "Alternatively, once you are fully vaccinated, take off the mask and go live your life because the vaccines are a scientific miracle and there is no data to back a single element of the lower right side of this chart," Twitter, April 27, 2021, 5:59 p.m., https://twitter.com/benshapiro/status/1387164630234116103?lan g=en.

22. In the winter of 2021, a full year into the epidemic—and with vaccinations taking off—the public health mandarins and their media waterboys experimented with a push to encourage "double masking." Two masks would fit more tightly to the face and help block more viral particles, or so the theory went. Laurel Wamsley, "CDC Says Double-Masking Offers More Protection against the Coronavirus," NPR, February 10, 2021, https://www.npr.org/sections/coronavirus-live-updates/2021/02/10/966313710/cdc-now-recommends-double-masking-for-more-protection-against-the-coronavirus. Other outlets helpfully offered tips on the best ways to double-mask. Fortunately, this effort petered out quickly. Even the most committed Team Apocalypse reporters realized that asking people to wear two masks raised questions about how useful one might be. And two masks just seemed *silly*, a bridge too far.

23. Monica Gandhi (@MonicaGhandi9), "No time in history do we have this extraordinary detection of asymptomatic infection since latter can transmit to others. So, please be assured that YOU ARE SAFE after vaccine from what matters—disease and spreading. Two vaccinated people can be as close as 2 spoons in a drawer!" Twitter, January 9,

2021, 2:33 p.m., https://twitter.com/monicagandhi9/status/1347989801090224129?lang=en.

24. Martin Varsavsky (@martinvars), "The relevant data is not the very few who got mild Covid after full vaccination. We should explain that after millions of vaccinations there is NOT ONE fully vaccinated person, who got severe Covid, and died of Covid," Twitter, February 17, 2021, 7:01 p.m., https://twitter.com/martinvars/status/1362190510350340096.

25. Adir Yanko, "Just 4 of 660 COVID Victims Received Both Vaccine Doses—Health Ministry Data," Ynet News, February 11, 2021, https://www.ynetnews.com/health_science/article/Hkm6mJmW00.

26. Ashish K. Jha (@ashishkjha), "Am often asked about different vaccines and their efficacy. Each trial tracks, reports efficacy differently. Currently, we have preliminary results for Novovax and J&J. But what numbers matter? What should you look for? Here's one set of data to track. In a simple table," Twitter, January 31, 2021, 10:16 p.m., https://twitter.com/ashishkjha/status/1356079020878786561.

27. David Leonhardt, "Vaccine Alarmism," *New York Times*, February 19, 2021, https://www.nytimes.com/2021/02/19/briefing/ted-cruz-texas-water-iran-nuclear.html.

28. Costas Pitas, "UK Passes 100,000 COVID Deaths, with Many More to Come," Reuters, January 26, 2021, https://www.reuters.com/article/uk-health-coronavirus-britain-casualties-idUSKBN29V20D.

29. "30% of Israeli COVID-19 Deaths Were in January Alone—Health Ministry Data," *Times of Israel*, February 1, 2021, https://www.timesofisrael.com/30-of-israeli-covid-19-deaths-were-in-january-alone/.

30. Martin Vernon (@runnermandoc), "One month into the care home vaccination programme, I am deeply concerned to be seeing covid-19 infection outbreaks among first dose vaccinated resident within, and beyond 21 days of vaccination. Are any other clinicians seeing this happening?" Twitter, February 1, 2021, 3:22 p.m., https://twitter.com/runnermandoc/status/1356337026757492738.

31. Ida Rask Moustsen-Helms et al., "Vaccine Effectiveness after 1st and 2nd Dose of the BNT162b2 mRNA Covid-19 Vaccine in Long-Term Care Facility Residents and Healthcare Workers—a Danish Cohort Study," medRxiv, March 9, 2021, https://www.medrxiv.org/content/10.1101/2021.03.08.21252200v1.

32. Ciara Linnane, "U.S. Suffers Another 4,000 COVID Deaths in a Single Day as Fauci Warns about New Strains," Market Watch, January 28, 2021, https://www.marketwatch.com/story/u-s-suffers-another-4-000-covid-deaths-in-a-single-day-as-fauci-warns-about-new-strains-11611849723.

33. Tom Randall, "When Will Life Return to Normal? In 7 Years at Today's Vaccine Rates," Bloomberg, February 4, 2021, https://www.bloomberg.com/news/articles/2021-02-04/when-will-covid-pandemic-end-near-me-vaccine-coverage-calculator.

34. "About VAERS," Vaccine Adverse Event Reporting System, https://vaers.hhs.gov/about.html.

35. "I've Heard That People Have Experienced Serious Allergic Reactions to the Vaccine and Am Worried That Might Happen to Me or a Loved One. Can I Have an Allergic Reaction or Die from the Vaccine?" See Friends Again, https://www.seefriendsagain.org/allergic-reactions.

36. Beatrice Dupuy, "Data from Vaccine Reporting Site Being Misrepresented Online," Associated Press, February 4, 2021, https://apnews.com/article/fact-checking-afs:Content:9957832237.

37. "COVID-19 VaST Work Group Report—May 24, 2021," Centers for Disease Control, May 24, 2021, https://www.cdc.gov/vaccines/acip/work-groups-vast/report-2021-05-24.html.

38. Jatara McGee, "Get the Facts on the Vax: Debunking Claims about the COVID-19 Vaccines," WLWT5, September 7, 2021, https://www.wlwt.com/article/get-the-facts-on-the-vax-debunking-claims-about-the-covid-19-vaccines/37505869#.

39. Twitter removed the tweet after I complained, but I have the screenshot.

40. Michael Eisen (@mbeisen), "What utterly disgusting, murderous POSs all the prominent people in the media spreading anti-vaccine propaganda are. Alex Berenson is a murderer. Naomi Wolf is a murderer. I can't believe Twitter lets them get away with this BS," Twitter, May 20, 2021, 12:20 a.m., https://twitter.com/mbeisen/status/1395233042453524483.

41. Tom Taylor (@TomTaylorMade), "Did…did Naomi Wolf get one of her unhinged anti-vaxx theories from listening to a stranger talk about Pym particles in Avengers: Endgame?" Twitter, June 5, 2021, 8:32 a.m., https://twitter.com/TomTaylorMade/status/1401154866257403904?s=20.

42. Lev Facher, "The White House Is Set to Unveil a Wide-Reaching, Billion-Dollar Campaign Aimed at Convincing Every American to Get Vaccinated," Stat News, March 15, 2021, https://www.statnews.com/2021/03/15/white-house-unveil-a-wide-reaching-billion-dollar-campaign-convincing-every-american-to-get-vaccinated/.

43. Katie Adams, "10 Recently Launched COVID-19 Vaccine Ad Campaigns," *Becker's Hospital Review*, April 22, 2021, https://www.beckershospitalreview.com/digital-marketing/10-recently-launched-covid-19-ad-campaigns.html.

44. Morgan Hines, "'Get Back to What You Love': Google COVID-19 Vaccine Ad Garners 6.3 Million Views, Emotional Response," *USA Today*, April 5, 2021, https://www.usatoday.com/story/tech/2021/04/05/google-covid-vaccine-ad-goes-viral-get-back-what-you-love/7088232002/.

45. Walgreens, "This is Our Shot | John Legend | COVID-19 Vaccines at Walgreens," YouTube, April 16, 2021, https://www.youtube.com/watch?v=295r46gmVl0.

46. World Health Organization, "COVID-19 vaccines could save your life. Get vaccinated, as soon as it's your turn," Facebook, August 24, 2021, https://www.facebook.com/WHO/videos/1016395655764297/.

47. Mark Murphy, "Debunking Common COVID-19 Vaccines Myths and Falsehoods," Savannah Now, January 17, 2021, https://www.savannahnow.com/story/opinion/2021/01/17/physician-addresses-many-myths-and-falsehoods-covid-vaccines/6636091002

33: Truth Leaks Out

1. Han Xia et al., "Biosafety Level 4 Laboratory User Training Program, China," *Emerging Infectious Diseases* 25, no. 5 (May 2019), https://wwwnc.cdc.gov/eid/article/25/5/18-0220_article.

2. Josh Rogin, "Opinion: State Department Cables Warned of Safety Issues at Wuhan Lab Studying Bat Coronaviruses," *Washington Post*, April 14, 2020, https://www.washingtonpost.com/opinions/2020/04/14/state-department-cables-warned-safety-issues-wuhan-lab-studying-bat-coronaviruses/.

3. Jackson Ryan, "How the Coronavirus Origin Story Is Being Rewritten by a Guerrilla Twitter Group, CNET, April 15, 2021, https://www.cnet.com/features/how-the-coronavirus-origin-story-is-being-rewritten-by-a-guerrilla-twitter-group/; Peng Zhou et al., "Addendum: A Pneumonia Outbreak Associated with a New Coronavirus of

Probable Bat Origin," *Nature* 566, no. E6 (November 17, 2020), https://www.nature.com/articles/s41586-020-2951-z.

4. Jason Beaubien, "Why They're Called 'Wet Markets'—And What Health Risks They Might Pose," NPR, January 31, 2020, https://www.npr.org/sections/goatsandsoda/2020/01/31/800975655/why-theyre-called-wet-markets-and-what-health-risks-they-might-pose.

5. Rafi Letzter, "The Coronavirus Didn't Really Start at That Wuhan 'Wet Market,'" Live Science, May 28, 2020, https://www.livescience.com/covid-19-did-not-start-at-wuhan-wet-market.html.

6. Stephanie Hegarty, "The Chinese Doctor Who Tried to Warn Others about Coronavirus," BBC News, February 6, 2020, https://www.bbc.com/news/world-asia-china-51364382.

7. "China Delayed Releasing Coronavirus Info, Frustrating WHO," Associated Press, June 2, 2020, https://apnews.com/article/united-nations-health-ap-top-news-virus-outbreak-public-health-3c061794970661042b18d5aeaaed9fae.

8. Zhuang Pinghui, "Chinese Laboratory That First Shared Coronavirus Genome with World Ordered to Close for 'Rectification,' Hindering Its Covid-19 Research," *South China Morning Post*, February 28, 2020, https://www.scmp.com/news/china/society/article/3052966/chinese-laboratory-first-shared-coronavirus-genome-world-ordered.

9. Yanan Wang and Ken Moritsugu, "Human-to-Human Transmission Confirmed in China Coronavirus," Associated Press, January 19, 2020, https://apnews.com/article/pneumonia-ap-top-news-international-news-china-health-14d7dcffa205d9022fa9ea593bb2a8c5.

10. Donald G. McNeil Jr. and Zolan Kanno-Youngs, "C.D.C. and W.H.O. Offers to Help China Have Been Ignored for Weeks," *New York Times,* February 7, 2020, https://www.nytimes.com/2020/02/07/health/cdc-coronavirus-china.html.

11. Melinda Wenner Moyer, "Vaccines Are Pushing Pathogens to Evolve," Quanta Magazine, May 10, 2018, https://www.quantamagazine.org/how-vaccines-can-drive-pathogens-to-evolve-20180510/.

12. Claire Jarvis, "Which Species Transmit COVID-19 to Humans? We're Still Not Sure," *The Scientist*, March 16, 2020, https://www.the-scientist.com/news-opinion/which-species-transmit-covid-19-to-humans-were-still-not-sure-67272.

13. Bryan A. Johnson et al., "Furin Cleavage Site Is Key to SARS-CoV-2 Pathogenesis," bioRxiv, August 26, 2020, https://www.ncbi.nlm.nih.gov/pmc/articles/PMC7457603/.

14. David Cyranoski, "Profile of a Killer: The Complex Biology Powering the Coronavirus Pandemic," *Nature*, May 4, 2020, https://www.nature.com/articles/d41586-020-01315-7.

15. Carl Zimmer and James Gorman, "Fight over Covid's Origins Renews Debate on Risks of Lab Work," *New York Times*, June 20, 2021, https://www.nytimes.com/2021/06/20/science/covid-lab-leak-wuhan.html.

16. Mark Lipsitch, "Why Do Exceptionally Dangerous Gain-of-Function Experiments in Influenza?" *Methods in Molecular Biology*, 1836 (2018): 589–608, https://www.ncbi.nlm.nih.gov/pmc/articles/PMC7119956/.

17. Mark Lipsitch and Thomas V. Inglesby, "Moratorium on Research Intended to Create Novel Potential Pandemic Pathogens," *mBio* 5, no. 6 (November–December 2014), https://www.ncbi.nlm.nih.gov/pmc/articles/PMC4271556/.

18. "Experiments with the full-length and chimeric SHC014 recombinant viruses were initiated and performed before the GOF research funding pause." Vineet D. Menachery et al., "A SARS-Like Cluster of Circulating Bat Coronaviruses Shows Potential for

Human Emergence," *Natural Medicine Journal* 21, no. 12 (November 9, 2015): 1508–13, https://www.ncbi.nlm.nih.gov/pmc/articles/PMC4797993/.

19. "Gain-of-Function Deliberative Process Written Public Comments," National Institutes of Health, October 19, 2014–June 8, 2016, https://osp.od.nih.gov/wp-content/uploads /2013/06/Gain_of_Function_Deliberative_Process_Written_Public_Comments.pdf.

20. Anthony S. Fauci, Gary S. Nabel, and Francis S. Collins, "A Flu Virus Risk Worth Taking," *Washington Post*, December 30, 2011, https://www.washingtonpost.com/opi nions/a-flu-virus-risk-worth-taking/2011/12/30/gIQAM9sNRP_story.html.

21. Anthony S. Fauci, "Research on Highly Pathogenic H5N1 Influenza Virus: The Way Forward," *mBio* 3, no. 5 (September–October 2012), https://www.ncbi.nlm.nih.gov /pmc/articles/PMC3484390/.

22. Francis S. Collins, "NIH Lifts Funding Pause on Gain-of-Function Research," National Institutes of Health, December 19, 2017, https://www.nih.gov/about-nih/who-we-are /nih-director/statements/nih-lifts-funding-pause-gain-function-research.

23. Sharon Lerner et al., "NIH Documents Provide New Evidence U.S. Funded Gain-of-Function Research in Wuhan," The Intercept, September 9, 2021, https://theintercept .com/2021/09/09/covid-origins-gain-of-function-research/.

24. Y. Guan et al., "Isolation and Characterization of Viruses Related to the SARS Coronavirus from Animals in Southern China," *Science* 302, no. 5643 (October 10, 2003): 276–78, https://www.science.org/doi/abs/10.1126/science.1087139.

25. Robert Roos, "WHO Sees More Evidence of Civet Role in SARS," Center for Infectious Disease Research and Policy, January 16, 2004, https://www.cidrap.umn.edu/news-per spective/2004/01/who-sees-more-evidence-civet-role-sars.

26. Rogin, "Opinion: State Department Cables Warned of Safety Issues at Wuhan Lab."

27. Kristian G. Andersen et al., "The Proximal Origin of SARS-CoV-2," *Nature Medicine* 26 (March 17, 2020): 450–52, https://www.nature.com/articles/s41591-020-0820-9.

28. Maanvi Singh et al., "Trump Claims to Have Evidence Coronavirus Started in Chinese Lab but Offers No Details," *The Guardian*, April 30, 2020, https://www.theguardian .com/us-news/2020/apr/30/donald-trump-coronavirus-chinese-lab-claim.

29. Kathy Gilsinan, "How China Is Planning to Win Back the World," *The Atlantic*, May 2020, https://www.theatlantic.com/politics/archive/2020/05/china-disinformation-pr opaganda-united-states-xi-jinping/612085/.

30. Meg Kelly and Sarah Cahlan, "Was the New Coronavirus Accidentally Released from a Wuhan Lab? It's Doubtful," *Washington Post*, May 1, 2020, https://www.washing tonpost.com/politics/2020/05/01/was-new-coronavirus-accidentally-released-wuhan -lab-its-doubtful/.

31. Olafimihan Oshin, "Washington Post Issues Correction on 2020 Report on Tom Cotton, Lab-Leak Theory," *The Hill*, June 1, 2021, https://thehill.com/homenews /media/556418-washington-post-issues-correction-on-2020-report-on-tom-cotton-lab -leak-theory.

32. Nsikan Akpan and Victoria Jaggard, "Fauci: No Scientific Evidence the Coronavirus Was Made in a Chinese Lab," *National Geographic*, May 4, 2020, https://www .nationalgeographic.com/science/article/anthony-fauci-no-scientific-evidence-the-coro navirus-was-made-in-a-chinese-lab-cvd.

33. Nicholas G. Evans, "Where the Coronavirus Bioweapon Conspiracy Theories Really Come From," Slate, February 27, 2020, https://slate.com/technology/2020/02/corona virus-bioweapon-conspiracy-theories.html.

34. Lindsey Ellefson, "NY Times COVID Reporter Deletes Tweet Claiming 'Racist Roots' of 'Lab Leak Theory' after Backlash," The Wrap, May 27, 2021, https://www.thewrap .com/new-york-times-covid-lab-leak-apoorva-mandavilli/.

35. Guy Rosen, "An Update on Our Work to Keep People Informed and Limit Misinformation about COVID-19," Facebook, April 16, 2020, https://about.fb.com /news/2020/04/covid-19-misinfo-update/ (Update, February 8, 2021: "We are expanding the list of false claims we will remove to include additional debunked claims about the coronavirus and vaccines. This includes claims such as: COVID-19 is man-made or manufactured.")

36. Rowan Jacobsen, "Could COVID-19 Have Escaped from a Lab?" *Boston*, September 9, 2020, https://www.bostonmagazine.com/news/2020/09/09/alina-chan-broad-insti tute-coronavirus/.

37. Michaeleen Doucleff, "World Health Organization Finishes Investigation into Origins of COVID-19," NPR, February 9, 2021, https://www.npr.org/2021/02/09/9659667 86/world-health-organization-finishes-investigation-into-origins-of-covid-19.

38. Scott Gottlieb, "WHO Said What about Wuhan?" *Wall Street Journal*, February 21, 2021, https://www.wsj.com/articles/who-said-what-about-wuhan-11613933182.

39. Ibid.

40. "WHO-Convened Global Study of Origins of SARS-CoV-2: China Part," World Health Organization, March 30, 2021, https://www.who.int/publications/i/item/who -convened-global-study-of-origins-of-sars-cov-2-china-part.

41. Nicholas Wade, "Origin of Covid—Following the Clues," Medium, May 2, 2021, https://nicholaswade.medium.com/origin-of-covid-following-the-clues-6f03564c038.

42. Christina Wilkie and Rich Mendez, "Biden Orders Closer Review of Covid Origins as U.S. Intel Weighs Wuhan Lab Leak Theory," CNBC, May 26, 2021, https://www.cn bc.com/2021/05/26/biden-orders-us-intelligence-to-intensify-investigation-into-covid -19-origins.html.

43. Ellen Nakashima et al., "Biden Receives Inconclusive Intelligence Report on Covid Origins," *Washington Post*, August 4, 2021, https://www.washingtonpost.com/ politics/2021/08/24/covid-origins-biden-intelligence-review/.

44. Cristiano Lima, "Facebook No Longer Treating 'Man-Made' Covid as a Crackpot Idea," Politico, May 26, 2021, https://www.politico.com/news/2021/05/26/facebook -ban-covid-man-made-491053.

45. Julie Mazziotta, "Fauci's Emails from the Pandemic Show His Stress-Filled Days: 'Some Crazy People in This World,'" *People*, June 2, 2021, https://people.com/health/faucis -emails-from-the-pandemic-show-stress-filled-days/.

46. CNN (@CNN), "Thousands of emails from and to Dr. Fauci reveal the weight that came with his role as a rare source of frank honesty within the Trump administration's Covid-19 task force," Twitter, June 2, 2021, 7:45 a.m., https://twitter.com/cnn/status /1400055865181356052?lang=en.

47. Email correspondence between Fauci, Anthony (NIH/NIAID)[E] and Kristian G. Anderson, January 31, 2020–February 1, 2020, https://cdn.factcheck.org/ UploadedFiles/Andersen-Jan-31-email-to-Fauci.png, https://cdn.factcheck.org/ UploadedFiles/Andersen-Jan-31-email-to-Fauci.png.

48. Email correspondence of Fauci, Anthony (NIH/NIAID)[E], January–March 2020, Document Cloud, https://s3.documentcloud.org/documents/20793561/leopold-nih-foia-anthony-fauci-emails.pdf, at page 3221 (of 3234).

49. Sharon Lerner and Mara Hvistendahl, "New Details Emerge about Coronavirus Research at Wuhan Lab," The Intercept, September 6, 2021, https://theintercept.com /2021/09/06/new-details-emerge-about-coronavirus-research-at-chinese-lab/.

50. James Gorman and Carl Zimmer, "Scientist Opens Up about His Early Email to Fauci on Virus Origins," *New York Times*, June 14, 2021, https://www.nytimes.com/2021

/06/14/science/covid-lab-leak-fauci-kristian-andersen.html?action=click&module=Re
latedLinks&pgtype=Article.

34: Dodging Bullets

1. "Twitter by the Numbers: Stats, Demographics & Fun Facts," Omnicore, January 3, 2021, https://www.omnicoreagency.com/twitter-statistics/.
2. Kate Tempest, "People's Faces," *The Book of Traps and Lessons* (Republic Records, 2019).
3. Brian Fung, "Parler Has Now Been Booted by Amazon, Apple and Google," CNN, January 11, 2021, https://www.cnn.com/2021/01/09/tech/parler-suspended-apple-app -store/index.html.
4. Probably the best one they could find was an October 2020 tweet in which I wrote that the Institute for Health Metrics and Evaluation "has been wrong over and over—why would anyone credit or repeat its projection of 500,000 US Covid deaths by spring?" Sure enough, the IHME finally got one right, probably with a little help from the vaccine post-first-dose spike. In February 2021, the United States recorded its 500,000th Covid death. So be it. To make predictions is to be wrong from time to time, and on the whole my published record compares favorably to Fauci's or anyone else's.
5. "COVID-19 Advice for the Public: Getting Vaccinated," World Health Organization, June 18, 2021, archived at the WayBack Machine, http://web.archive.org/web/20210 618212957/https://www.who.int/emergencies/diseases/novel-coronavirus-2019/covid -19-vaccines/advice.
6. Nickie Louise, "WHO Says 'Children Should Not Be Vaccinated for the Moment [because] There Is Not Yet Enough Evidence on the Use of Vaccines against COVID-19,'" Tech Startups, June 21, 2021, https://techstartups.com/2021/06/21/who-says-ch ildren-should-not-be-vaccinated-for-the-moment-because-there-is-not-yet-enough-evi dence-on-the-use-of-vaccines-against-covid-19/.
7. "COVID-19 Advice for the Public: Getting Vaccinated," World Health Organization, July 14, 2021, https://www.who.int/emergencies/diseases/novel-coronavirus-2019/co vid-19-vaccines/advice.
8. McKenzie Sadeghi, "Fact Check: Claims about WHO Guidance for Vaccinating Children Are Missing Context," *USA Today*, June 25, 2021, https://www.usatoday .com/story/news/factcheck/2021/06/25/fact-check-posts-whos-stance-vaccinating-chi ldren-lack-context/7778033002/.
9. "Israel," Worldometer, https://www.worldometers.info/coronavirus/country/israel/.
10. Rossella Tercatin, "Coronavirus in Israel: Over 6,000 Dead since Beginning of Pandemic," *Jerusalem Post*, March 14, 2021, https://www.jpost.com/israel-news/coro navirus-govt-debates-expanding-number-of-returnees-destinations-661943.
11. Patrick Kingsley, "'Like a Miracle': Israel's Vaccine Success Allows Easter Crowds in Jerusalem," *New York Times*, April 3, 2021, https://www.nytimes.com/2021/04/03 /world/middleeast/easter-jerusalem-coronavirus.html.
12. Mark G. Thompson et al., "Interim Estimates of Vaccine Effectiveness of BNT162b2 and mRNA-1273 COVID-19 Vaccines in Preventing SARS-CoV-2 Infection among Health Care Personnel, First Responders, and Other Essential and Frontline Workers— Eight U.S. Locations, December 2020–March 2021," *Morbidity and Mortality Weekly Report* 70, no. 13 (April 2, 2021): 495–500, https://www.cdc.gov/mmwr/volumes/70 /wr/mm7013e3.htm.

13. Derek Thompson, "The Pandemic's Wrongest Man," *The Atlantic*, April 1, 2021, https://www.theatlantic.com/ideas/archive/2021/04/pandemics-wrongest-man/618475/.
14. "United States," Worldometer, https://www.worldometers.info/coronavirus/country/us/.
15. Noah Weiland et al., "Johnson & Johnson Vaccinations Paused after Rare Clotting Cases Emerge," *New York Times*, April 13, 2021, https://www.nytimes.com/2021/04/13/us/politics/johnson-johnson-vaccine-blood-clots-fda-cdc.html.
16. "See How Vaccinations Are Going in Your County and State," *New York Times*, https://www.nytimes.com/interactive/2020/us/covid-19-vaccine-doses.html.
17. Frank Jordans, "BioNTech Boss Strikes Upbeat Note on Europe's Vaccine Drive," Associated Press, April 28, 2021, https://apnews.com/article/europe-north-america-immunizations-coronavirus-pandemic-coronavirus-vaccine-f1eca91561f3a1be9550b79534b17741.
18. Monica Ghandi (@MonicaGhandi9), "No time in history do we have this extraordinary detection of asymptomatic infection since latter can transmit to others. So, please be assured that YOU ARE SAFE after vaccine from what matters—disease and spreading. Two vaccinated people can be as close as 2 spoons in a drawer!" Twitter, January 9, 2021, 2:33 p.m., https://twitter.com/MonicaGandhi9/status/1347989801090224129.
19. Monica Ghandi (@MonicaGhandi9), "Good to see this January 9 tweet has so much evidence behind it now in real world that vaccines block transmission since biological plausibility was ample. Here are some of the studies cited in CDC guidance that vaccines block transmission," Twitter, May 17, 2021, 10:38 a.m., https://twitter.com/MonicaGandhi9/status/1394301284556017664.
20. Alan Murray and Katherine Dunn, "The CEOs on Our World's Greatest Leaders List," *Fortune*, May 12, 2021, https://fortune.com/2021/05/12/ceo-daily-worlds-greatest-leaders/.
21. "Transcript: Coronavirus: Leadership during Crisis with Anthony S. Fauci, MD," *Washington Post*, May 20, 2021, https://www.washingtonpost.com/washington-post-live/2021/05/20/transcript-coronavirus-leadership-during-crisis-with-anthony-s-fauci-md/.
22. Jessica Bursztynsky, "Yes, It's Going to Be a Hot Vax Summer," CNBC, May 22, 2021, https://www.cnbc.com/2021/05/22/yes-its-going-to-be-a-hot-vax-summer.html.
23. Stephen Collinson, "A Vaccine Marvel Is Bringing America Back," CNN, May 25, 2021, https://www.cnn.com/2021/05/25/politics/vaccine-marvel-america-back/index.html.
24. Ian Mount et al., "Operation Overtake: How Europe Surpassed the U.S. in Its COVID Vaccination Push," *Fortune*, July 1, 2021, https://fortune.com/2021/07/01/europe-overtakes-us-covid-vaccination-push/.
25. "WHO Warns of 'Two-Track Pandemic' as Cases Decline but Vaccine Inequity Persists," UN News, June 7, 2021, https://news.un.org/en/story/2021/06/1093472.
26. Elaine K. Howley, "How to Talk to Someone Who's Hesitant to Get the COVID-19 Vaccine," *U.S. News & World Report*, May 12, 2021, https://www.usnews.com/conditions/coronavirus-and-your-health/articles/how-to-talk-to-someone-whos-hesitant-to-get-the-covid-19-vaccine.
27. "The Tuskegee Timeline," Centers for Disease Control, https://www.cdc.gov/tuskegee/timeline.htm.
28. Blake Farmer, "'It's Not a Never Thing'—White, Rural Southerners Hesitant to Get COVID Vaccine," NPR, April 15, 2021, https://www.npr.org/sections/health-shots/20

21/04/15/987412681/its-not-a-never-thing-white-rural-southerners-are-waiting-to-get-the-vaccine.

29. Adrian Horton, "John Oliver on Vaccine Hesitancy: 'We Badly Need to Convince Anyone Who Can Be Convinced,'" *The Guardian*, May 3, 2021, https://www.theguardian.com/tv-and-radio/2021/may/03/john-oliver-vaccine-hesitancy-covid.

30. Daniel Kalla, "The 'Vaccine Hesitant' Are a Threat to Society. But We Must Show Them Compassion," *Globe and Mail*, May 7, 2021, https://www.theglobeandmail.com/opinion/article-the-vaccine-hesitant-are-a-threat-to-society-but-we-must-show-them/.

31. Theresa Waldrop et al., "Fauci: Vaccinations Will Help Coronavirus Variants from Emerging," CNN, January 22, 2021, https://www.cnn.com/2021/01/21/health/us-coronavirus-thursday/index.html.

32. John P. Moore and Paul A. Offit, "SARS-CoV-2 Vaccines and the Growing Threat of Viral Variants," *Journal of the American Medical Association* 325, no. 9 (January 28, 2021): 821–22, https://jamanetwork.com/journals/jama/fullarticle/2776039.

33. Nandita Bose and Jeff Mason, "'Get a Shot, Have a Beer': Biden, Anheuser-Busch Push July Vaccination Goal," Reuters, June 2, 2021, https://www.reuters.com/business/healthcare-pharmaceuticals/biden-outline-steps-help-reach-july-4-vaccination-goal-2021-06-02/.

34. "COVID-19 Vaccine Incentives," National Governors Association, July 30, 2020, https://www.nga.org/center/publications/covid-19-vaccine-incentives/.

35. Dara Khosrowshahi, "The Road to 70 Percent: Free Vaccination Rides Begin Today," Uber, May 24, 2021, https://www.uber.com/newsroom/freevaccinerides/.

36. Allan J. Wallkey et al., "Lottery-Based Incentive in Ohio and COVID-19 Vaccination Rates," *Journal of the American Medical Association* 326, no. 8 (July 2, 2021): 766–67, https://jamanetwork.com/journals/jama/fullarticle/2781792.

37. Julia Manchester, "Biden: Coronavirus Vaccine Should Not Be Mandatory," *The Hill*, December 4, 2020, https://thehill.com/homenews/campaign/528834-biden-coronavirus-vaccine-should-not-be-mandatory.

38. "Transcript of Pelosi Weekly Press Conference Today," Nancy Pelosi Speaker of the House website, April 29, 2021, https://www.speaker.gov/newsroom/42921-2.

39. Audie Cornish et al., "You Asked, We Got Answers: The U.S. Surgeon General Takes On Your COVID-19 Questions," NPR, June 9, 2021, https://www.npr.org/2021/06/09/1004862388/you-asked-we-got-answers-the-u-s-surgeon-general-takes-on-your-covid-19-question.

40. "Table 31. Vaccination Coverage for Selected Diseases by Age 24 Months, by Race and Hispanic Origin, Poverty Level, and Location of Residence: United States, Birth Years 2010–2015," Centers for Disease Control, 2019, https://www.cdc.gov/nchs/data/hus/2019/031-508.pdf.

41. "Israel," Worldometer.

42. "Transcript: Coronavirus: Leadership during Crisis."

43. Lisa A. Jackson et al., "Evidence of Bias in Estimates of Influenza Vaccine Effectiveness in Seniors," *International Journal of Epidemiology* 35, no. 2 (April 2006): 337–44, https://pubmed.ncbi.nlm.nih.gov/16368725/.

44. "COVID-19 Vaccine Surveillance Report Week 36," Public Health England, September 9, 2021, https://assets.publishing.service.gov.uk/government/uploads/system/uploads/attachment_data/file/1016465/Vaccine_surveillance_report_-_week_36.pdf.

45. Ariel Israel et al., "Large-Scale Study of Antibody Titer Decay Following BNT162b2 mRNA Vaccine or SARS-CoV-2 Infection," medRxiv, August 22, 2021, https://www.medrxiv.org/content/10.1101/2021.08.19.21262111v1.

46. Michel C. Nussenzweig, "Natural Infection versus Vaccination: Differences in COVID Antibody Responses Emerge," The Rockefeller University, August 24, 2021, https://www.rockefeller.edu/news/30919-natural-infection-versus-vaccination-differences-in-covid-antibody-responses-emerge/.

47. Sivan Gazit et al., "Comparing SARS-CoV-2 Natural Immunity to Vaccine-Induced Immunity: Reinfections versus Breakthrough Infections," medRxiv, August 25, 2021, https://www.medrxiv.org/content/10.1101/2021.08.24.21262415v1.

48. Meredith Wadman, "Having SARS-CoV-2 Once Confers Much Greater Immunity Than a Vaccine—but Vaccination Remains Vital," *Science*, August 26, 2021, https://www.science.org/content/article/having-sars-cov-2-once-confers-much-greater-immunity-vaccine-vaccination-remains-vital.

49. Amy Spiro, "Pfizer Exec Calls Israel 'a Sort of Laboratory' for COVID Vaccines," *Times of Israel*, September 12, 2021, https://www.timesofisrael.com/pfizer-exec-calls-israel-a-sort-of-laboratory-for-covid-vaccines/.

50. "United States," Worldometer.

51. "Meet the Press—July 4, 2021," NBC News, July 4, 2021, https://www.nbcnews.com/meet-the-press/meet-press-july-4-2021-n1273065; "Surgeon General: 99.5% of Virus Deaths Are Unvaccinated People," CNN, July 18, 2021, https://www.cnn.com/videos/politics/2021/07/18/murthy-full-interview.cnn.

52. "Read: Internal CDC Document on Breakthrough Infections," *Washington Post*, July 29, 2021, https://www.washingtonpost.com/context/cdc-breakthrough-infections/94390e3a-5e45-44a5-ac40-2744e4e25f2e/?_=1, slide 4.

53. Alex Berenson, "Here We Go Again," *Unreported Truths* (Substack), July 25, 2021, https://alexberenson.substack.com/p/here-we-go-again.

54. Alex Silverman, "Many Vaccinated Americans Are Still Uncomfortable Returning to Public Activities. The U.S. Economy Needs Them," Morning Consult, May 12, 2021, https://morningconsult.com/2021/05/12/vaccinated-unvaccinated-americans-comfort-with-activities/.

55. Ibid.

56. Zeke Miller, "Biden Grappling with 'Pandemic of the Unvaccinated,'" Associated Press, July 17, 2021, https://apnews.com/article/joe-biden-health-government-and-politics-pandemics-coronavirus-pandemic-8318e3f406278f3ebf09871128cc91de.

57. Fenit Nirappil, "They're Called Mild Cases. But People with Breakthrough Covid Can Still Feel Pretty Sick," *Washington Post*, August 31, 2021, https://www.washingtonpost.com/health/2021/08/31/mild-coronavirus-breakthrough-infections/.

58. Jackie Fortier, "The Anger toward Unvaccinated People Is Personal for Some Who Got Breakthrough COVID," NPR, August 13, 2021, https://www.npr.org/2021/08/13/1027537422/the-anger-toward-unvaccinated-people-is-personal-for-some-who-got-breakthrough-c.

59. "Widow: Unvaccinated to Blame for Vaccinated Iowa Man's Death," Associated Press, September 14, 2021, https://apnews.com/article/health-coronavirus-pandemic-iowa-5afd2572d5a282c499a9a2de7ac0fe3d.

60. Berkeley Lovelace Jr., "Biden Outlines Plan to Mandate Covid Vaccines for Millions: 'Our Patience Is Wearing Thin,'" CNBC, September 9, 2021, https://www.cnbc.com/2021/09/09/biden-to-detail-new-six-pronged-plan-to-increase-us-covid-vaccination-rates-fight-virus.html.

61. Frank Bruni, "The Pizza-Paved Path to the Far Side of the Covid Pandemic," *New York Times*, September 16, 2021, https://www.nytimes.com/2021/09/16/opinion/vaccine-mandates-businesses.html?action=click&module=Well&pgtype=Homepage&section=OpEd%20Columnists.

62. Jonathan Meer, "Opinion: Don't Want the COVID-19 Vaccine? Then Pay the Full Cost If You Land in the Hospital," Market Watch, August 6, 2021, https://www.marketw atch.com/story/dont-want-the-covid-19-vaccine-then-pay-the-full-cost-if-you-land-in -the-hospital-11628206594.

63. Arthur L. Caplan and Dorit R. Reiss, "Vaccine Mandates Aren't Enough. Make Unvaccinated People Pay If They Harm Others," *Barron's*, August 3, 2021, https:// www.barrons.com/articles/coronavirus-vaccine-mask-mandate-unvaccinated-516279 39803.

64. Nancy Gibbs, "Opinion: Do the Unvaccinated Deserve Scarce ICU Beds?" *Washington Post*, September 1, 2021, https://www.washingtonpost.com/opinions/2021/09/01/do -unvaccinated-deserve-scarce-icu-beds/.

65. Lovelace Jr., "Biden Outlines Plan."

66. Melissa Quinn, "Arizona Becomes First State to Sue Biden Administration over COVID-19 Vaccine Mandates," CBS News, September 15, 2021, https://www.cbsne ws.com/news/arizona-sues-biden-administration-covid-19-vaccine-mandates/.

67. Kasen K. Riemersma et al., "Shedding of Infectious SARS-CoV-2 Despite Vaccination," medRxiv, August 24, 2021, https://www.medrxiv.org/content/10.1101/2021.07.31.21 261387v4.full.

68. Sharon LaFraniere, "U.S. to Advise Boosters for Most Americans 8 Months after Vaccination," *New York Times*, August 16, 2021, https://www.nytimes.com/2021/08 /16/us/politics/booster-shots.html.

69. Steven Nelson, "Biden, Fauci Discuss Requiring COVID Booster Shots Every 5 Months," *New York Post*, August 27, 2021, https://nypost.com/2021/08/27/biden-and -fauci-discuss-covid-19-booster-shots-every-5-months/.

70. Joanna Taylor, "Israel's Covid Chief Calls for Fourth Vaccine Dose," *The Independent*, September 6, 2021, https://www.independent.co.uk/news/world/middle-east/covid-vac cine-israel-fourth-dose-b1915076.html.

71. Sarah Owermohle, "Biden's Top-Down Booster Plan Sparks Anger at FDA," *Politico*, August 31, 2021, https://www.politico.com/news/2021/08/31/biden-booster-plan-fda -508149.

72. Philip R. Krause et al., "Considerations in Boosting COVID-19 Vaccine Immune Responses," *The Lancet*, September 13, 2021, https://www.thelancet.com/journals/lan cet/article/PIIS0140-6736(21)02046-8/fulltext.

73. Julie Steenhuysen, "Analysis: U.S. Hopes COVID Vaccine Boosters Will Decrease Not Just Deaths, but Virus Spread," Reuters, September 15, 2021, https://www.reuters.com /world/us/us-looks-covid-19-boosters-curb-virus-spread-2021-09-15/.

74. Yafei Liu et al., "The SARS-CoV-2 Delta Variant Is Poised to Acquire Complete Resistance to Wild-Type Spike Vaccines," bioRxiv, August 23, 2021, https://www. biorxiv.org/content/10.1101/2021.08.22.457114v1; Kasen K. Riemersma et al., "Shedding of Infectious SARS-CoV-2 despite Vaccination," medRxiv, August 24, 2021, https://www.medrxiv.org/content/10.1101/2021.07.31.21261387v4.

75. "Press Briefing by Press Secretary Jen Psaki and Surgeon General Dr. Vivek H. Murthy, July 15, 2021," White House, July 15, 2021, https://www.whitehouse.gov/briefing-ro om/press-briefings/2021/07/15/press-briefing-by-press-secretary-jen-psaki-and-surge on-general-dr-vivek-h-murthy-july-15-2021/. The censors generally define "misinformation" as facts that are accurate but in their eyes misleading—such as posts based on VAERS data. "Disinformation" describes statements that are factually inaccurate or actually untruthful. Because they could not refute the facts that I and others presented, they were forced to label them "misinformation."

76. John Hendel, "Congress Faces Broadband Crunch," *Politico*, July 16, 2021, https://www.politico.com/newsletters/morning-tech/2021/07/16/congress-faces-broadband-crunch-796549.

77. Ian Schwartz, "WH's Psaki: If You're Banned on One Social Media Platform, You Should Be Banned on All Others," RealClearPolitics, July 17, 2021, https://www.realclearpolitics.com/video/2021/07/17/whs_psaki_if_youre_banned_on_one_social_media_platform_you_should_be_banned_on_all_others.html.

78. C-SPAN, "President Biden: 'They're Killing People,'" YouTube, July 16, 2021, https://www.youtube.com/watch?v=gJoOtLn4goY.

79. Corona Realism (@homenkollin), "Something really odd is going on: In Europe we are seeing surges at many places where most of the population has already been vaccinated. At the same time, the 15 least vaccinated countries don't seem to face any problem. At some point, denying this problem will get painful," Twitter, July 16, 2021, 6:59 a.m., https://twitter.com/holmenkollin/status/1415989536933490688.

80. Stephen J. Thomas et al., "Six Month Safety and Efficacy of the BNT162b2 mRNA COVID-19 Vaccine," medRxiv, July 28, 2021, https://www.medrxiv.org/content/10.1101/2021.07.28.21261159v1.full.pdf.

81. Michael Ruiz, "Twitter Permanently Suspends Alex Berenson over Coronavirus Tweets," Fox Business, August 28, 2021, https://www.foxbusiness.com/media/twitter-permanently-suspends-alex-berenson-over-coronavirus-tweets.

82. Senator Elizabeth Warren, letter to Andy Jassy, Elizabeth Warren Senate website, September 7, 2021, https://www.warren.senate.gov/imo/media/doc/2021.9.7%20Letter%20to%20Amazon%20on%20COVID%20Misinformation.pdf.

35: In Conclusion: Our Own Shadows

1. Brie Stimson, "San Francisco Mayor Defiant after Caught Maskless in Nightclub despite Mandate: Don't Need 'Fun Police,'" Fox News, September 17, 2021, https://www.foxnews.com/politics/san-francisco-mayor-london-breed-maskless-nightclub-mandate-fun-police.

2. Danielle Kurtzleben, "What Is Infrastructure? It's a Gender Issue, for Starters," NPR, April 15, 2021, https://www.npr.org/2021/04/15/987229254/biden-infrastructure-push-highlights-economic-gender-gaps.

3. Francis Collins, "COVID-19 Infected Many More Americans in 2020 Than Official Tallies Show," NIH Director's Blog, September 7, 2021, https://directorsblog.nih.gov/tag/covid-19-testing/.

4. "NHE Fact Sheet: Historical NHE, 2019," Centers for Medicare and Medicaid Services, December 16, 2020, https://www.cms.gov/Research-Statistics-Data-and-Systems/Statistics-Trends-and-Reports/NationalHealthExpendData/NHE-Fact-Sheet#:~:text=Hospital%20expenditures%20grew%206.2%25%20to,than%20the%204.0%25%20in%202018. (We spent $1.2 trillion in 2019, so $1.3 trillion in 2021 is actually a conservative estimate.)

5. Leticia Miranda, "Rural Hospitals Losing Hundreds of Staff to High-Paid Traveling Nurse Jobs," NBC News, September 15, 2021, https://www.nbcnews.com/business/business-news/rural-hospitals-losing-hundreds-staff-high-paid-traveling-nurse-jobs-n1279199.

6. Jaclyn Diaz, "A N.Y. Hospital Will Stop Delivering Babies as Workers Quit over a Vaccine Mandate," NPR, September 13, 2021, https://www.npr.org/2021/09/13/1036521499/covid-workers-resign-new-york-hospital-stops-baby-delivery.

7. The stocks of Moderna and BioNTech sit near all-time highs as I write these words in lateish September. I think of myself as a cynic, but I'm a naïf in the woods compared

to the folks on Wall Street. They have decided that a "vaccine" that stops working after a few months and needs to be dosed again is the best vaccine of all, since it means endless profits for its makers—who have no legal liability for any injuries that that their vaccines might cause. See MacKenzie Sigalos, "You Can't Sue Pfizer or Moderna If You Have Severe Covid Vaccine Side Effects. The Government Likely Won't Compensate You for Damages Either," CNBC, December 17, 2020, https://www.cnbc.com/2020/12/16/covid-vaccine-side-effects-compensation-lawsuit.html.

8. "Denmark," COVID-19 Ined, https://dc-covid.site.ined.fr/en/data/denmark/.

9. Min Gao et al., "Associations between Body-Mass Index and COVID-19 Severity in 6.9 Million People in England: A Prospective, Community-Based, Cohort Study, *The Lancet* 9, no. 6 (June 1, 2021): P350–359, https://www.thelancet.com/journals/landia/article/PIIS2213-8587(21)00089-9/fulltext.

10. Philip Ewing, "Hospital Ship USNS Comfort Scheduled to Sail from New York City," NPR, April 28, 2020, https://www.npr.org/sections/coronavirus-live-updates/2020/04/28/847457974/hospital-ship-usns-comfort-scheduled-to-sail-from-new-york-city.

11. Donald G. McNeil Jr., "D.A. Henderson, Doctor Who Helped End Smallpox Scourge, Dies at 87," *New York Times*, August 21, 2016, https://www.nytimes.com/2016/08/22/us/dr-donald-a-henderson-who-helped-end-smallpox-dies-at-87.html.

12. Thomas V. Inglesby et al., "Disease Mitigation Measures in the Control of Pandemic Influenza," *Biosecurity and Bioterrorism* 4, no. 4 (2006): 366–75, https://pubmed.ncbi.nlm.nih.gov/17238820/.

13. Mark Landler and Stephen Castle, "Britons, Unfazed by High Covid Rates, Weigh Their 'Price of Freedom,'" *New York Times*, August 28, 2021, https://www.nytimes.com/2021/08/28/world/europe/coronavirus-britain-uk.html.

14. Damien Cave, "Australia Is Betting on Remote Quarantine. Here's What I Learned on the Inside," *New York Times*, August 20, 2021, https://www.nytimes.com/2021/08/20/world/australia/howard-springs-quarantine.html.

15. Abram Van Engen, "How America Became 'a City upon a Hill,'" *Humanities* 41, no. 1 (winter 2020), https://www.neh.gov/article/how-america-became-city-upon-hill.

Index